A SHORT
PAEDIATRICS

UNIVERSITY MEDICAL TEXTS

General Editors
SELWYN TAYLOR
DM, MCh, FRCS, Hon FRCS(Ed), Hon FCS(SA)
Dean Emeritus, Royal Postgraduate Medical School,
Consulting Surgeon, Hammersmith Hospital

HOWARD ROGERS
MA, MB, BChir, PhD, MRCP
Reader in Clinical Pharmacology, Guy's Hospital Medical School
(UMS Guy's and St Thomas's Hospitals)

A selection of titles in the University Medical Texts series is given below.
A complete list is available from the publisher.

A Short Textbook of Medicine
J. C. HOUSTON MD, FRCP
C. L. JOINER MD, FRCP
J. R. TROUNCE MD, FRCP

A Short Textbook of Surgery
SELWYN TAYLOR DM, MCh (Oxon), FRCS
LEONARD COTTON MCh (Oxon), FRCS

A Short Textbook of Psychiatry
LINFORD REES BSc, MD, FRCP, DPM

A Short Textbook of Medical Microbiology
D. C. TURK DM, MRCP, FRCPath
I. A. PORTER MD, FRCPath
B. I. DUERDEN BSc (Med. Sci.), MD, MRCPath
T. M. S. REID BMed. Biol, MB, ChB, MRCPath

A Short Textbook of Preventive Medicine for the Tropics
A. O. LUCAS BSc, MD, DPH, DTM&H, FRCP, SMHyg, FMCPH
H. M. GILLES MD, FRCP, FFCM, FMCPH, DTM&H

A SHORT TEXTBOOK OF
PAEDIATRICS

Second Edition

PINCUS CATZEL
MB, BCh, FRCP, DCH
Principal Paediatrician, Johannesburg Hospital, South Africa

IAN ROBERTS
MB, BS, MRCP
Consultant Paediatrician, Royal Hospital, Chesterfield

HODDER AND STOUGHTON
LONDON SYDNEY AUCKLAND TORONTO

Cover illustration: showing an electronmicrograph of a longitudinal section through three vertebrate cardiac muscle cells. Courtesy of Y. Uehara, G. R. Campbell and G. Burnstock, Department of Anatomy, University College, London.

British Library Cataloguing in Publication Data

Catzel, Pincus
 A short textbook of paediatrics. —2nd ed.
 1. Pediatrics
 I. Title   II. Roberts, Ian
 618.92   RJ45

ISBN 0 340 33921 7

First edition 1976
Third impression 1981
Second edition 1984
Second impression 1987

Typeset 10/11 pt Times Roman (Monophoto) by Macmillan India Ltd., Bangalore

Printed in Great Britain for Hodder and Stoughton Educational, a division of Hodder and Stoughton Ltd., Mill Road, Dunton Green, Sevenoaks, Kent by Richard Clay Ltd., Bungay, Suffolk

EDITOR'S FOREWORD

When this book was first published seven years ago it was pointed out that the title of 'paediatrics', rather than 'child health', had been chosen quite deliberately. That this was the right decision is supported by the book's subsequent performance.

Now a new edition reflecting the changed attitudes and practices of the 1980s has been called for and in producing it Doctor Catzel has been joined by Doctor Ian Roberts. These two paediatricians, one working in South Africa, the other in England, have collaborated to produce an excellent amalgam of child care spanning the whole globe. The book has been brought up to date throughout and this has necessitated much rewriting of the text; Professor Lucy Wagstaff has provided a chapter on paediatric community care.

It must indeed be rare for a new edition of a book to be shorter than its predecessor, but for once this is the case. This new edition has been reduced by 10 %, entirely due to compression and rewriting. The text has been reset in the new style of the series and this has produced a very attractive introduction to the subject. Another interesting change in presentation is the guide to further reading in Appendix II. This replaces the lists at the end of individual chapters—lists which, with updating, were beginning to get rather out of hand.

This new edition will prove a worthy successor to Doctor Catzel's original volume.

Selwyn Taylor

AUTHORS' PREFACE

'The essence of knowledge is, having acquired it, to apply it'
Confucius

A Short Textbook of Paediatrics is a guide to the diagnosis and treatment of diseases of childhood as seen in both temperate and tropical countries. In view of the present day emphasis on community paediatrics, we asked Professor Lucy Wagstaff to write a chapter on the subject in order to balance the presentation. It is hoped that this will overcome some of the criticisms of the first edition.

Extensive updating and revision has improved the book considerably. We hope that this second edition will meet not only the needs of students of clinical paediatrics but also those practitioners and postgraduate students who require an overall review of the subject.

Pincus Catzel
Ian Roberts

Note: Whenever adult doses of drugs are given in this book the paediatric dose should be estimated by means of the *percentage method*. See page 392.

ACKNOWLEDGEMENTS

We would like to thank J. D. L. Hansen, Professor of Paediatrics and Head of the Department of Paediatrics at the University of Witwatersrand and the Johannesburg Hospital, members of his department and the other university departments for help and advice in preparing this manuscript. Our thanks also go to the following for their courteous help in revising individual areas of the book:

Renée Bernstein (genetics), Colin Block (bacterial infections), John B. Barlow (mitral valve prolapse), Jennifer Cartwright (growth and development), John Chappell (surgical disorders), T. F. B. Collins (tuberculosis), R. Dansky (diseases of the cardiovascular system), J. H. S. Gear (rickettsial and viral diseases), Renée Heitner (blood and intestinal tract), Joy Isdale (abdominal masses in childhood), Trefor Jenkins (genetics), W. J. Kalk (endocrine disorders), S. E. Levin (cardiovascular system), June Lloyd (inherited metabolic diseases), Lorna McDougall (blood and its disorders), John Pettifor (all aspects of Vitamin D), John Pretorius (ENT problems), A. R. Rabson (advice on allergy and immunology), Harry Reef (central nervous system), I. Reef (complete revision of chapters on allergy and the respiratory system), J. E. Sahakian (hyperlipoproteinaemias), Peter D. Thomson (diseases of the genito-urinary tract and fluid and electrolyte balance), Hessel Utian (cardiovascular system and central nervous system), Lucy Wagstaff (community paediatrics) and Richard West (inherited metabolic diseases).

We would also like to thank our respective secretaries, Marion Berry and Margaret White, for their impeccable typing and the staff of Hodder and Stoughton Educational for seeing the book through to production.

Pincus Catzel
Ian Roberts

CONTENTS

CHAPTER 1

HUMAN GENETICS

The child is the end-product of interplay between his genetic constitution and his environment. No inheritance, however promising, can reach fruition unless tenderly nurtured and cared for. However, a child born with an altered genetic constitution, as in Down's syndrome and cystic fibrosis, will also need special protection and care if he is to survive and fulfil his potential.

It is therefore necessary for the practitioner to become familiar with the language of human genetics so that he can support the abnormal child and his family. Genetic counselling for parents demands a great deal of knowledge, patience and human understanding and should be undertaken only by those practitioners with a special interest in the subject.

CLASSIFICATION OF CONGENITAL ABNORMALITY

1 *Genetic*
   (a) Single gene abnormalities which follow laws of Mendelian inheritance (7 %).
   (b) Multifactorial abnormalities, e.g. congenital dislocation of the hips, neural tube defects and congenital hypertrophic pyloric stenosis (15–20 %).
   (c) Chromosomal abnormalities e.g. Down's syndrome (25 %).
2 *Non-genetic*
   Prenatal teratogens e.g. rubella, phenytoin (15–20 %).
3 *Uncertain aetiology.*

Congenital abnormalities may be detected at birth (e.g. hare-lip) or shortly thereafter (e.g. congenital deafness, cataracts, congenital hypertrophic pyloric stenosis and renal tract anomalies). In some of these a definite chromosomal abnormality can be detected (up to 25 %). Other congenital anomalies are not inherited but may be caused by damage to the embryo in the first trimester of pregnancy by a virus such as rubella or cytomegalovirus, a parasite such as *Toxoplasma gondii* or drugs such as phenytoin or cytotoxic agents. None of these conditions can be reversed by treatment though some can be prevented; rubella, for instance, can be prevented by vaccination of all fertile females who have not previously contracted the disease. Greater care in the use of drugs during early pregnancy may prevent other abnormalities.

Chromosomes carry the hereditary material known as genes. These are arranged linearly along the chromosome, each occupying a specific locus. Each gene is made up of deoxyribonucleic acid (DNA) whose nucleotide bases guanine, cytosine, adenine and thymine are arranged in sequences known as the 'triplet code'. This sequence forms a template from which RNA transfers the 'message' on the chromosome in the nucleus to the ribosome in the cell's cytoplasm, and interprets it in the form of an amino acid sequence. The amino acids are built up to form enzymes and other proteins.

The Watson-Crick model pictures the DNA in the form of a double helix. When the cell divides the helix unwinds and reduplicates itself (replication) to form two new cells with two complete sets of paired chromosomes. After sexual division (meiosis) each sex cell contains only one half of the chromosome material. An autosome is any chromosome other than a sex chromosome. In somatic cells there are twenty-two pairs of autosomes plus one pair of sex chromosomes, whereas the sex cells (gametes) contain twenty-two single autosomes plus one sex chromosome, either X or Y.

Genes exist in pairs known as alleles. If the host bears two identical genes for a particular trait such as brown eyes or the Rhesus (Rh) factor, he is known as homozygous. If each gene is different (blue eyes and brown eyes or Rh positive and negative) the host is heterozygous for that trait. The genotype is the allelic composition of the host's cells. The phenotype is the expression of the genotype, as in eye colour, Rh status, finger length or hair character.

A single gene is thought to determine the synthesis of a single polypeptide chain. Mutation results in the substitution of one amino acid residue in this chain. Thus, for example, the only difference between sickle-cell haemoglobin and normal haemoglobin is that one peptide of the former contains valine instead of glutamic acid.

INHERITANCE

Mendelian inheritance may be one of three types:

1 Autosomal dominant trait

For example achondroplasia, arachnodactyly, Sturge-Weber syndrome, Thomsen's disease and hereditary spherocytosis. An affected heterozygous individual mating with a normal individual may produce a normal or an affected child in a 1 : 1 ratio (Fig. 1.1(A)). Normal children will have all normal offspring. Occasionally a generation may be skipped due to variability in expression and penetrance, so that an apparently normal person has an affected child.

Autosomal co-dominant traits exist when two genes dominate over a recessive gene, for example blood group antigens A and B dominate over blood group O.

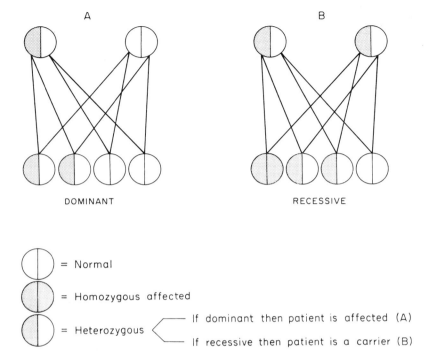

Fig. 1.1 Autosomal inheritance. In dominant inheritance heterozygotes manifest the trait. In recessive inheritance only the homozygote manifests the trait. The heterozygote is a carrier and can transmit the trait to its offspring

2 Autosomal recessive trait

For example Hurler's syndrome, Tay Sachs' disease, sickle-cell anaemia, thalassaemia major, retinitis pigmentosa, cystic fibrosis of the pancreas, galactosaemia, phenylketonuria and most other inborn errors of metabolism. The disease is only recognisable when the gene is present in the homozygous state.

In Fig. 1.1(B) the parents are both heterozygous and are apparently normal. They are, however, carriers of the trait and their offspring include one homozygote who manifests the disease, two heterozygotes who are outwardly normal but carry the disease (carrier state) and one entirely normal individual. The carrier state can often be detected; in Tay Sachs' disease, for instance, the enzyme hexosaminidase is 50% reduced in quantity in carriers.

It can be seen from the above that the recessive homozygous state is uncommon. To produce it two carriers must mate, thus the incidence of first cousin marriages is very high in such cases. In the normal population the incidence of cousin marriages is less than 0.4 %. Amongst parents who have produced affected offspring for a recessive gene, it may be as high as 35 %.

3 X-linked traits

These may be recessive or dominant. Recessive X-linked traits are transmitted by carrier females to 50 % of their sons who will be affected and 50 % of their daughters who will be carriers, as in haemophilia, Duchenne's muscular dystrophy, G-6-PD deficiency and hypophosphataemic vitamin D resistant rickets (Fig. 1.2). Dominant X-linked traits are transmitted in the same manner but are expressed phenotypically in the carrier female and are usually lethal in affected males (e.g. incontinentia pigmenti).

Many congenital diseases such as diabetes mellitus are multifactorial—they depend on more than one gene and environmental factors for their expression and are thus not as easy to define as the above diagrams suggest.

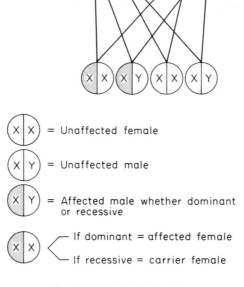

Fig. 1.2 X-linked inheritance

THE HUMAN KARYOTYPE

The human karyotype is the arrangement of the 46 human chromosomes into specific groups. This is demonstrated by photographing them during metaphase, making enlarged prints, cutting out each chromosome and then pairing them. These are placed in seven groups A to G (the Denver Classification) as in Fig. 1.3(a). Each chromosome is numbered by its specific banding pattern (Paris Conference, 1971) as in Fig. 1.3(b).

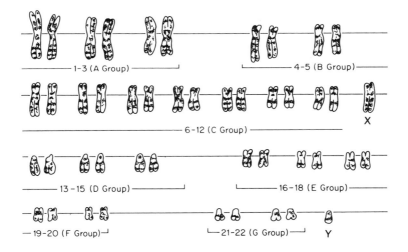

Fig. 1.3(a) Normal male karyotype (courtesy of Dr Renée Bernstein)

The total number of chromosomes in each somatic cell is 46 (the diploid number) made up of 22 pairs of chromosomes called autosomes and a pair of sex chromosomes designated XX in the female and XY in the male. The term 'haploid' refers to the number of chromosomes in the germinal (sex) cells (ova or sperm). In man this is 23, which is half the diploid number.

NUCLEAR SEX CHROMATIN

Barr bodies (X-chromatin) 1 μm in diameter are found in the nuclei of females. Cells containing the distinctive mass are called X-chromatin positive cells, whereas those without are termed X-chromatin negative. Barr bodies occur in 15–45 % of interphase nuclei of squamous cells from buccal mucosa of females. A similar body, called a 'drumstick' is found as appendages on 1–3 % polymorphonuclear leucocytes in females.

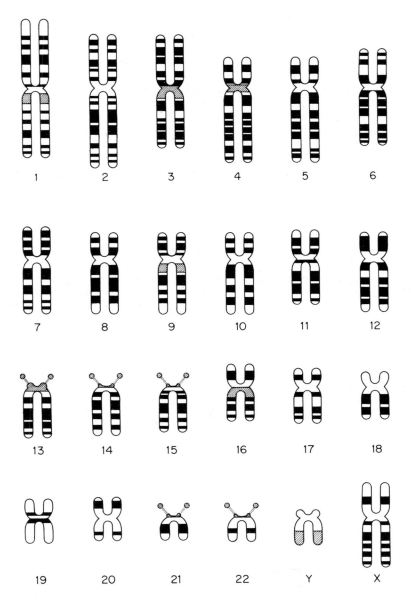

Fig. 1.3(b) Diagrammatic representation of chromosome bands (Paris Conference, 1971)

Barr bodies and drumsticks represent the inactive X chromosomes in normal females. They are never seen in normal (XY) males or in Turner's syndrome (XO). In Klinefelter's syndrome (XXY) they are found because one of the two X-chromosomes is inactivated.

CHROMOSOMAL ABNORMALITIES

It is estimated that at least 1 in 200 live-born infants has a chromosomal abnormality sufficient to cause serious physical or mental defects. All these abnormalities can be detected antenatally but it is practically impossible to eliminate these genetic diseases because one cannot predict all the pregnancies which should be screened. One is limited therefore to screening 'high risk' families.

Alterations to the chromosome may be in number or in structure.

1 Changes in number (aneuploidy)

In Down's syndrome there is an additional homologue on chromosome 21 hence the name trisomy-21. It is due to non-disjunction—that is, the failure of the homologous chromosome 21 to go to the opposite pole during meiosis (Fig. 1.4). Increasing age is a factor in non-disjunction. Trisomy-18 and trisomy-13 also have been documented but are very rare because they are usually lethal.

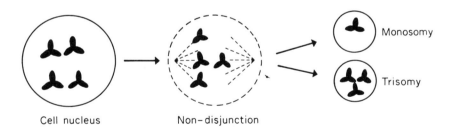

Fig. 1.4 Non-disjunction leading to trisomy and monosomy

Loss of a chromosome (monosomy) occurs in Turner's syndrome, where an X chromosome is absent, while Klinefelter's syndrome exhibits an extra X due to non-disjunction of the X chromosome. Mosaicism is an anomaly of chromosome division occurring after fertilisation resulting in cells containing different numbers of chromosomes.

At least 50% of first trimester spontaneous abortions have a chromosomal abnormality incompatible with life.

2 Structural changes

Translocation (the commonest structural change) is the exchange of genetic material between any two chromosomes. Usually the chromosome number of 46 is maintained but in the type of translocation known as 'centric fusion' the chromosome number may be reduced. Down's syndrome in young mothers is commonly due to translocation. The commoner form of this disorder, which is associated with elderly parents, is due to trisomy-21 (see Fig. 1.4). Partial deletion of chromosome 5 occurs in 'cat-cry' syndrome. Ring forms occur when both ends of a chromosome are lost.

Many alterations in structure or number are incompatible with life, and are detected in aborted fetuses. However, it should be recognised that 1 in 1000 people has a chromosomal rearrangement which does not produce obvious clinical effects because there is no loss or gain of genetic material. They are known as balanced translocation carriers. They are, however, at high risk to produce abnormal gametes and hence abnormal offspring. In fact they are usually detected only after they have produced an abnormal infant, such as a baby with Down's syndrome. For subsequent children, such parents can be offered prenatal diagnosis and selective abortion in countries where this is permitted.

PRENATAL DIAGNOSIS

By the 16th–17th week of pregnancy it is possible to obtain 10–20 ml amniotic fluid by means of transabdominal puncture of the uterine cavity. The fluid is examined for biochemical abnormalities while the cells, which are fetal in origin, are cultured and examined for chromosomal and, where indicated, biochemical abnormalities. The risk to both mother and fetus seems negligible in skilled hands. All women over 40 years of age and perhaps even younger, and all women who have already had a child with these disorders, should be offered amniocentesis with a view to therapeutic abortion, if they so wish.

Fetal sex can be determined antenatally by chromosome studies. This may be important in certain X-linked recessive traits where only the male is affected by the disease, e.g. haemophilia and Duchenne's muscular dystrophy.

The following are some of the disorders which have yielded to antenatal diagnosis:

1 Chromosomal disorders

The most notable is Down's syndrome which, it is stated, results from 1 in 70 pregnancies in women over the age of 40 and 1 in 40 over the age of 45.

2 Metabolic diseases

(a) Tay Sachs' disease (amaurotic family idiocy)
(b) Mucopolysaccharidoses
(c) Gaucher's disease
(d) Glycogen storage disease and galactosaemia
(e) Maple syrup urine disease, and many others.

3 Neural tube defects

Anencephaly, meningomyelocele and other congenital neural tube defects, associated with a leak of cerebrospinal fluid into the amniotic fluid, can be diagnosed in the second trimester of pregnancy in a large percent of cases by the increased presence in this fluid of alphafetoprotein—a fetal-specific alpha-1-globulin, which normally disappears after birth. Exomphalos and congenital nephrosis may also raise the alphafetoprotein level.

DERMATOGLYPHICS

Dermatoglyphics is the study of handprints. As every reader of detective stories knows, no two sets of fingerprints are identical. The formation of dermal ridges is determined by many genes and those that are of interest to the clinician are the ridge patterns on the fingers and flexion patterns of the palms. Characteristic ridge patterns have been found in trisomy-21 and certain X-linked disorders. Single palmar creases are found in 70% of children with Down's syndrome, but may be present in 5% of normal individuals. The Sydney line is sometimes found in retarded children but is a non-specific finding as is a single palmar crease (Fig. 1.5). It is

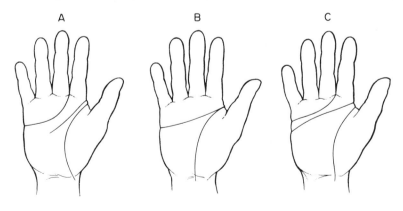

NORMAL PALMAR CREASE   SINGLE PALMAR CREASE   SYDNEY LINE

Fig. 1.5 Dermatoglyphic hand patterns

important therefore to include inspection of the palms of the hands as part of the paediatric examination.

GENETIC COUNSELLING

Genetic counselling may be requested by couples who have produced an abnormal child or fear that they may produce one because of the presence of such an abnormality in the family history or population group. Sometimes the counsellor may be approached by a middle-aged couple who still want children or by parents who are afflicted by repeated abortions. He may be asked to judge the wisdom of a first cousin marriage. The risks involved in having a genetically abnormal child must be carefully weighed for the parents. The factors to be considered include:

1 The severity of the abnormality.
2 The risk of it recurring, e.g. is it a 50:50 chance or a small risk of less than 1 in 10?
3 Can it be treated? For example some congenital heart disorders require major surgery; phenylketonuria can be effectively treated by a suitable diet but the diet may be difficult to maintain.
4 Socio-economic status, education and religious persuasion.
5 The age of the parents and whether or not they already have a normal child.
6 The laws of the country relating to abortion.

The practitioner should discuss the facts in language which the parents can understand; the decision must be theirs alone.

Recently the term selective abortion has come into vogue, referring to termination of pregnancy after studies, including amniocentesis, indicate congenital abnormality. If the disease is carried by the male only, then only the male will be aborted, the female being allowed to carry to term.

If the risks of having an affected baby are too high the parents should consider the possibility of sterilisation or contraception to prevent further offspring. In some circumstances artificial insemination may be appropriate while in others the parents should consider adopting or fostering a baby.

CHAPTER 2

THE HISTORY AND EXAMINATION
OF THE CHILD

THE HISTORY

The history of a child is usually obtained from the mother. Sometimes the patient is accompanied by the father or other relative or guardian and the history becomes that much less reliable. The child can often supply important information if he is approached properly. The questioner should be relaxed and talk to the child 'eye to eye' and use normal conversational English, not high-pitched 'baby-talk'. The child likes to be treated in an adult way although *he* knows that *you* know that he is still a child. A friendly smile and conversation can achieve a great deal.

The history chart should contain the following information—full name of child, sex, date and place of birth, parents' name and initials, address and telephone number, occupation, race and religion. The latter is important because Jewish and Moslem patients are not permitted to eat pork products. Some insulins and brands of ACTH are made from this animal but are acceptable by injection. Jehovah's Witnesses are not permitted to have blood transfusions, a prohibition which can cause many problems.

In hospital practice the name and address of the referring practitioner should be noted so that reports may be sent to him promptly. The patient may be seen at several departments or clinics and treatment may be duplicated if the patient's own general practitioner is not kept informed.

The main complaint

The first question to ask is 'What is your complaint?' The answer should be recorded exactly as stated, not translated into medical jargon; for example 'he wets his bed every night', not 'nocturnal enuresis'.

The opening gambit is followed by the history of the present complaint. How and when did it begin? How did it develop? Is it getting worse? The mother should not be hurried and should be given every opportunity to talk freely.

Each complaint should be explored systematically. Aggravating or relieving factors should be considered. The examiner has to assess the child *via* the mother and he must therefore consider her reliability. Direct questions should be avoided initially, but later they may be essential. For example, if the mother says that her child has a headache the examiner is entitled to ask for its location, type, intensity, spread and frequency.

Perinatal health

Maternal illnesses acquired before or after conception may have affected the child. Toxaemia, diabetes mellitus, blood group incompatability between the parents and exposure to X-rays should be reviewed. Infections such as rubella, cytomegalovirus, or the use of drugs in early pregnancy may be significant. The child's birth-weight and gestation should be recorded. Was birth normal or not? Did the baby breathe and cry immediately? Did he stay in hospital longer than usual? Any deviation from normal such as pallor, cyanosis, jaundice, abnormal cry, convulsions, injuries or excessive mucus should be noted. The use of sedatives, analgesics or anaesthetics during labour is important in relation to the need for resuscitation of the baby. If necessary, the record of confinement should be examined.

Postnatal development, feeding and excretion

The subsequent physical, mental, emotional and social development will be recorded according to the needs of the case. If the child is brought in for ringworm or other minor ailment, his milestones would be only cursorily reviewed to check that he is normal. However, factors such as overcrowding, which are important in the spread of ringworm, would be emphasised. On the other hand, if the complaint is that of poor performance at school, then of course the child's milestones of development must be assessed with infinite patience.

While considering the child's development the history of his feeding should be included. Was he breast or bottle fed? When and how was he weaned? Some details of the present diet should be included to determine if it is reasonably well balanced and whether the mother's story matches the child's appearance.

It is logical to follow an interest in the patient's appetite with an interest in his excretory activities. When was he toilet trained and is he dry by day and night? Is he liable to attacks of abdominal pain, and does he vomit easily? Is there burning or frequency of micturition? Is the urine dark or light or cloudy? What are the stools like?

Previous illnesses and immunisations

These should be recorded in order of appearance with their complications. In particular, diseases which give lasting immunity such as measles, mumps, roseola infantum, German measles and chickenpox should be noted and questions asked about inoculations against the usual diseases (diphtheria, pertussis, tetanus, BCG, poliomyelitis, measles, mumps and rubella) and recent drug administration. Is there a history of drug sensitivity?

Operations and accidents

The nature, severity and complications should be recorded.

The family history

Many ailments run in families or are inherited. A family tree is useful in such cases and may give evidence of consanguinity. The health of the parents, grandparents and siblings should be recorded when relevant. Their relationship to each other, particularly those who live in the same abode, may be of deep psychological significance. In the case of infectious disease, the health of contacts must be inquired into. The occurrence of tuberculosis, allergic disorders, rheumatic fever, cardiovascular and renal diseases, congenital anomalies, epilepsy, mental retardation and neoplastic diseases are all important.

Social history

This includes the family income, housing, school and play facilities. The occupation of the parents may be important, as well as the history of travel abroad, for instance to a tropical area.

Habits

Eating habits, sleep, exercise, bowel and bladder habits should be recorded and abnormal habits such as bed-wetting, encopresis, nightmares and night-terrors, masturbation, breath-holding, pica, tics and temper tantrums should be elicited carefully.

Systematic review

To ensure that nothing important has been left out, it is worth while reviewing each system in turn. Starting with the ear, nose and throat (including teething and tonsils), proceeding to the cardiovascular and respiratory systems, the gastro-intestinal and genito-urinary tracts, endocrine organs and central nervous system. The main points to be elucidated will be found in the appropriate chapters.

With increasing practice the ability to take histories, and even more importantly to interpret them, improves. Questioning becomes more selective and a sixth sense develops. Intuition is as important to a physician as intensive logical thinking.

THE PHYSICAL EXAMINATION

The examination of the patient begins when he enters the consulting room by observing general appearance, movements and relationship with his parent, without upsetting the child by staring at him. This observation should be continued during the taking of the history for it will often reveal if the patient is acutely ill, interested in his surroundings, apprehensive, hyperactive or apathetic.

It is worth while having a few well-selected toys hidden away to be produced at appropriate moments, to keep the patient interested and amused. These toys should be colourful, simple, sturdy and interesting enough to hold the child's attention for long periods. A baby can be deposited in a playpen or held by the mother on her lap. Older children should be kept busy with puzzles or crayon and paper. It may be a good opportunity to get them to 'Draw-a-Man' (p. 60).

The child may be examined initially sitting or lying on his mother's lap, or on the couch. Clothing should be removed bit by bit in a shy child but the examination is not complete until the whole body from the hair of the head to the tips of the toes has been inspected and examined. Most children will let their mothers remove all their clothes in one go, provided they can keep their underpants on. The sequence of examination depends on the child. If he is quiet one should listen to the heart, palpate the abdomen and examine the central nervous system. Uncomfortable procedures such as examination of the ear, nose and throat or the rectum should be left to last, with constant reassurances that it will only be 'a little uncomfortable'. If one says that the examination won't be sore at all and in fact it is, the patient's confidence may be lost. During crying vocal fremitus can often be felt and inspiratory breath sounds are better heard than when the child is quiet.

Essentials of the examination

The height and weight in centimetres and kilogrammes, the head circumference, the temperature, pulse, respiratory rate and blood pressure should be taken in all cases. These measurements are checked at each visit and compared with standard charts.

The normal rectal temperature is up to 37.5°C, which is 0.5°C higher than oral and 1.0°C higher than axillary. The latter is the safest and least traumatic.

General appearance

The examiner should first assess the nutrition and hydration, and observe whether or not the patient is acutely ill. If he can walk, is his posture, gait and co-ordination normal? In the case of a baby are his milestones (sitting, smiling, babbling) normal? An infant follows a light by 4 weeks, holds his head firmly by 10 weeks, sits alone by 6 months and can walk by 12–15 months. More detailed milestones will be discussed on page 57.

Any obvious abnormality such as mongoloid face, chest deformity or skin disorder are noted. The extremities should be examined for deformity, clubbing or cyanosis of the fingers, and the phalanges should be counted! Measurements are important in paediatrics. Each student should know the width of his own fingers so that he can use them as a standard for measuring the sizes of enlarged livers, spleens, tumours and even the distance of the apical impulse of the heart from the mid-line.

Skin

1 Colour (cyanosis, pallor, jaundice).
2 Pigmentation, local or generalised (café-au-lait, blue spots, albinism).
3 Tissue turgor (inelasticity suggests dehydration, wrinkling suggests recent weight loss, striae suggest sudden weight gain); pitting oedema requires firmer pressure to elicit than in the adult.
4 Rashes (exanthemata, urticaria, specific skin diseases).

The scalp should be carefully examined for alterations in hair texture and colour, as well as for local lesions and the presence of nits.

Lymph nodes

Systematic examination of *all* lymph nodes is essential. The axillary and epitrochlear nodes, and the inguinal and popliteal nodes, should not be missed. In Hodgkin's disease one sometimes finds lymph nodes in unexpected places.

This is a good opportunity to search for *subcutaneous nodules* over bony prominences, especially along the occiput and around the elbows when rheumatic fever or rheumatoid arthritis is suspected.

Head and neck

The size, shape and circumference of the skull should be noted. Any abnormality such as premature closure of the fontanelles, frontal bossing, craniotabes, alterations in hair texture or presence of a bruit should be recorded and followed up; for example, if craniotabes is detected one should search for other signs of rickets, syphilis, osteogenesis imperfecta or prematurity. Transillumination of the head in a dark room should be done if a cerebral anomaly such as hydrocephalus or subdural effusion is suspected. Increased tension of the fontanelle may suggest meningitis but could be caused by benign intracranial hypertension secondary to drug therapy. A depressed fontanelle should suggest dehydration.

The face

The face is examined for obvious abnormalities such as asymmetry, slanting of the eyes (mongoloid or ante-mongoloid), hypertelorism (increased space between the eyes), epicanthic folds, depressed or abnormal nasal bridge, sinus tenderness, nasolabial fold asymmetry, facial nerve irritability (Chvostek's sign) and any tics or habit spasms. Is the face alive with intelligence or dull, as occurs with an 'adenoid face'?

(handwritten margin note, right side): craniotabes — ↓ mineralization of skull — softness of bone

(handwritten note, bottom left): tetany

Bitot spots - foamy gray Δ spots of keratinized epithelium on conjunctiva due to Vit A deficien...

The eyes

The eyes especially should be examined for nystagmus, squint, blocked tear duct, infection, Bitot's spots on the conjunctiva, Brushfield's spots or a Kayser-Fleischer ring around the iris. To get the baby to open his eyes he should be held above one's head in the prone position (Doll's eye reflex). The reaction of the pupils to light and accommodation, the presence of a dislocated or opaque lens or of corneal opacities are noted. A careful fundoscopic examination should be done where indicated. With care this can be performed on a sleeping baby if one uses a dim light in a darkened room. One per cent cyclopentolate hydrochloride eye drops may be necessary to dilate the pupil. The disc is normally pale in babies.

The nose

The most important things about the nose are its patency, the presence of a discharge, activity of the ala nasae and size and colour of the turbinates. A bad smell coming from the nose is nearly always due to a foreign body.

The mouth

An unusual shape or presence of hare-lip or naevi should be noted. Lesions at the corner of the mouth, ulcers on the buccal mucous membrane, tongue or pharynx are important. The gums and teeth should be carefully examined as well as the opening of Stensen's duct at the level of the second upper molar. Epstein's pearls, Bohn's nodules and enanthems (especially Koplik's spots) should be noted. The hard and soft palate, the fauces and tonsils should be viewed with a proper light, and the presence of a post-nasal drip recorded.

The child should be asked to put out his tongue and the surface examined carefully. In a baby the movement of the tongue can be observed by dropping water onto it. If the tip of the tongue passes over the alveolar margin, the baby is not tongue-tied. Sometimes when a baby or child yells it is possible to view the pharynx without the aid of a spatula. The mother may hold the child's head, arms and legs against her to prevent their movement (Fig. 2.1).

The ears

Abnormal ears may be associated with other anomalies, so their size, shape and position should be noted. The young child may be held by the mother as shown in Fig. 2.2. To examine the ear drum in a baby the ear is pulled backwards and downwards to straighten out the canal; in older children the ear is pulled backwards, then upwards to view the drum. The anatomical markings and light reflex should be noted (Fig. 20.1). If discharge is present a swab should be taken for culture and the ear cleaned so that the presence of a perforation can be observed. Excessive wax may be removed by inserting a softening agent and syringing or by

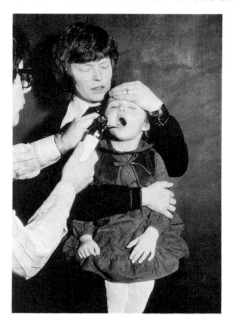

Fig. 2.1 Examining the mouth

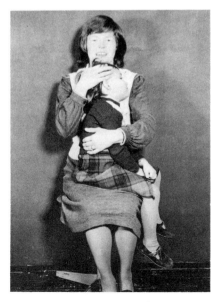

Fig. 2.2 Examining the ear

gently poking out with a Jobson-Horne probe. The hearing should be tested (does he respond to a whispered command?) and the mastoid bone should always be percussed for tenderness.

The neck

By four months of age the head should sit firmly on the neck. If the head is floppy one should consider the possibility of cerebral palsy or general hypotonia. The chin should be able to touch each shoulder easily. If not, the sternomastoid should be examined for a tumour to account for the torticollis. Swelling of the cervical lymph nodes and thyroid, abnormal sinuses or fistulas and cystic masses should be carefully evaluated. Is the trachea central, if not has it been pulled or pushed? Webbing of the neck or other congenital anomalies need to be noted. The venous and arterial pulsation should be assessed. Neck stiffness should be excluded.

The chest

The size, shape and symmetry of the chest are noted with special reference to abnormalities such as rib or suprasternal retraction, Harrison's sulcus, ricketty rosary, pigeon breast or depressed sternum. One should also examine the shoulder girdle.

The respiratory system

This system should be examined for rate, rhythm and type of breathing, shortness of breath, prolongation of expiration, reduced chest expansion or fixity of the chest. In babies respiration is mainly abdominal. Vocal fremitus, dullness or resonance on percussion should be assessed. Very light percussion yields more information than heavy. Alteration in breath sound on auscultation should be recorded and evaluated. The presence of adventitious sounds such as rhonchi and crepitations indicates the presence of mucus or inflammatory products in the respiratory tract. It should be remembered that in children breath sounds are coarser than in adults and may have a jerky 'cog-wheel' character. Often bronchial-like breathing or some prolongation of expiration may be heard normally. Listening to the breathing with the bell of a stethoscope 2 cm from the open mouth will determine whether or not these sounds are normal. This exaggerates the expiratory sound. Listening over the trachea mimics amphoric breathing. In testing for vocal fremitus, the word 'ninety-nine' brings out nasal sounds, the word 'coca-cola' the guttural throat sounds and 'pepsi-cola' the sybilants.

The cardiovascular system

The cardiovascular system should be examined as a whole, starting with the pulses, blood pressure and neck veins. One should look for oedema of the eyes, sacrum and feet and for the presence of dyspnoea, and note

rachitic rosary – succession of beadlike prominences along costal margin in rickets

the size and shape of the heart and any unusual bulging or pulsation. The heart sounds, murmurs and adventitious sounds should be carefully evaluated. While listening to the heart or feeling the pulse the child is asked to take a deep breath so that sinus arrhythmia can be evaluated. Each heart sound in the mitral, tricuspid, aortic and pulmonary areas should be examined systematically. Any murmurs should be carefully timed and characterised, and their transmission noted.

The abdomen

The abdomen should be relaxed and this can be achieved in babies by giving them a bottle from which to drink. Distension, movement with respiration, visible peristalsis and abnormal venous flow are noted. Hernias at the umbilicus, inguinal and femoral region are searched for. Local tenderness or rebound tenderness may be important signs of peritoneal inflammation. The liver, spleen, kidneys and tumours should be searched for. In babies and young children the tip of the spleen is palpated far more laterally than in older children. Enlargement of the liver should be determined in the mid-line as well as in the right nipple line. Hyper-resonance and shifting dullness should be assessed and one should listen for alteration in bowel sounds.

The genitalia

The genitalia should be carefully examined. In the male the foreskin is examined by gently pulling, not pushing (see Fig. 16.1). In fat boys the penis may be buried in fat and look smaller than it actually is. The urethral opening should be located in both sexes. The testes should be carefully palpated with *warm* hands in the male; the introitus inspected in the female. Any discharge should be cultured.

Rectal examination

This should be done with a gloved index finger, well lubricated with petroleum jelly. The ball of the finger is pressed flat against the anal opening until it 'gives' and the finger slips into the rectum. With care the index finger will slip into the rectum of quite small babies. If it is forced in, however, it may tear the mucous membrane, therefore it is wiser to use the little finger first.

The anus should be carefully inspected for fissures, especially in constipated babies. On inserting the finger the anal tone can be assessed. The cervix is usually palpable in girls. Local tenderness is cautiously felt for.

The examining glove should be examined on withdrawal of the finger for faeces, blood and mucus.

The spine

The posture and presence of spinal curves, dimples, sinuses or cysts, hairy naevi and other abnormalities should be noted. Stiffness of the neck or back must be assessed. Older children can be asked to kiss their knees, an impossible procedure if the neck or back is rigid.

The limbs

These should be checked for abnormalities of length, size or shape. The fingers and toes should be deliberately counted. Bow-legs and knock-knees are commonly found, though are not often pathological. The range of movement of all joints should be assessed. The nails should be examined and the pattern on the palms of the hands and feet noted.

The nervous system

A full neurological examination should be done when indicated. This involves assessment of cerebral function, examination of the cranial nerves, deep and superficial reflexes, motor power, involuntary movements, and so on. The normal milestones of development should be assessed in all children. In the newborn the primitive reflexes should be tested for.

Summary

A complete and detailed history and examination is the *sine qua non* of the consultant paediatrician. The general practitioner does not usually have the time for this and therefore learns to be selective in taking the history and examination. When based on a good knowledge of paediatrics this will usually be satisfactory and the practitioner misses little of importance. But if a patient comes back a second or third time, a more thorough investigation is warranted. It cannot be over-emphasised that most errors of diagnosis are made by not *listening* properly and by not *examining* properly.

Paediatric pitfalls

1 No examination is complete until the patient has been inspected from head to toes, without his clothes.

2 No examination is complete without blood pressure, temperature, height, weight and head circumference.

3 Rectal examination should never be omitted in a child with abdominal pain.

4 The ears should always be examined in a child that coughs. Dried wax on the drum can cause reflex vagal irritation.

5 In the newborn baby the thighs should be abducted fully (to exclude hip disease) and the femoral pulses felt (to exclude coarctation).

6 The examination of the urine should never ever be omitted. Dysuria and frequency of micturition may be due to urethritis and threadworms and not necessarily to urinary infection.

7 The tonsils should never be assessed when they are acutely inflamed. Tonsils (as well as other lymph tissues) are normally large in children—they atrophy after the age of 10.

8 If a child seems retarded, make sure that he is not deaf or blind.

9 Beware of the baby with a floppy neck—he may have cerebral palsy.

10 The commonest cause of vomiting in small children is acute tonsillitis.

CHAPTER 3

ANTENATAL PAEDIATRICS AND CARE OF THE NEWBORN CHILD

The perinatal mortality rate is the number of stillbirths and the number of neonatal deaths in the first week of life per 1000 births. This rate has steadily declined and has now reached single figures in Sweden. The rate has been used as a crude measure of socio-economic progress, and a measure of the standard of obstetric and neonatal care. It is not surprising that much higher rates are to be found in under-developed countries.

The causes of most stillbirths are unknown. It can happen when there has been intra-uterine growth failure, revealed or concealed fetal anoxia, or when there has been a maternal disease such as diabetes mellitus.

Women who are very young, old or single and unsupported, of high parity, primiparous, or of low social class are more likely to lose their baby. They are also more liable to have low birth-weight babies (less than 2.5 kg), either pre-term or light-for-dates. About 5 % of babies are born early and the associated complications of prematurity account for the largest group in which neonatal death may be preventable. Deaths in full-term babies occur because of congenital abnormalities, infections, birth asphyxia, birth trauma, and diseases such as severe haemolytic disease.

In order to improve the quality and quantity of surviving infants attention has been focused on the health of the mother and her fetus, as well as on the care of the live baby.

FETAL SURVEILLANCE

Diagnostic amniocentesis may be offered to women in whom the risk of having an abnormal baby is high, provided they are prepared to follow an adverse result with a therapeutic abortion. The procedure carries a 1 in 200 risk of spontaneous abortion but at least a third of these fetuses are abnormal. Chromosomal disorders may be detected by culturing the amniotic fetal cells and examining their chromosomes. This is most often done in women over 40 who have a 1 in 70 chance of bearing a baby with Down's syndrome. Less commonly, the cultured cells may be analysed biochemically and it is now possible to diagnose metabolic disorders such as X-linked Hunter's syndrome and recessive disorders like Tay Sachs' disease prenatally. Between 16 and 18 weeks

exomphalos — hernia of abdominal viscera into the umbilical cord

gestation a raised maternal serum alphafetoprotein may be an indication for amniocentesis. Raised amniotic fluid levels are found with early neural tube defects, exomphalos and Turner's syndrome. Occasionally it is necessary to look for external fetal abnormalities directly through a fetoscope. Using this instrument fetal blood may be sampled for the antenatal diagnosis of inheritable haemoglobinopathies.

Spectroscopic examination of amniotic fluid gives a measure of bilirubin concentration which can be related to gestational age. This technique can be modified to assess the severity of haemolytic disease of affected babies at a given gestation, and so help the obstetrician decide if an intra-uterine transfusion or induction of labour is indicated.

The likelihood of an infant developing hyaline membrane disease can be predicted by measuring the phospholipids, lecithin and sphingomyelin which pass into amniotic fluid from the fetal lung. There is an increase in lecithin production between 34 and 36 weeks gestation which exceeds the rise in sphingomyelin. When the lecithin-sphingomyelin ratio is more than 2 the chances of an infant developing hyaline membrane disease is about 1 in 50, but more than half get it when the ratio is less than 2.

Fetal growth can be assessed by measuring the biparietal diameter of the skull using an ultrasonic A-scan. Serial measurements between 20 to 30 weeks gestation are used to assess gestation and later in pregnancy measurements of fetal head growth rates help to identify those babies with severe fetal growth retardation. The mothers of such babies excrete diminished amounts of oestriol in their urine. This hormonal end-product is derived from the fetal adrenal gland and the placenta and should increase throughout pregnancy. Low levels at a given gestation indicate poor placental function and the need for intervention.

In order to detect and prevent prolonged fetal anoxia in labour the obstetrician actively looks for evidence of fetal distress. The fetal heart rate can be monitored by using ultrasound, which records the echoes from fetal blood vessels; alternatively a phonocardiogram resting on the maternal abdominal wall will record the heart rate. Changes in intra-uterine pressure may be recorded via the abdominal wall also, or directly through a probe inserted into the amniotic cavity by way of the cervix. When the fetal heart rate falls outside the normal range, 120–160 beats per minute, or alters significantly or for prolonged periods following uterine contraction, fetal distress is present and delivery may have to be hastened.

Fetal anoxia, secondary to fetal distress, may be heralded by changes in the fetal ECG or EEG which can be recorded from electrodes applied to the presenting fetal scalp.

FACTORS DISTURBING FETAL DEVELOPMENT

Pregnancy is most likely to be successful if the mother and her placenta are functioning normally. If the mother has a serious illness like cyanotic congenital heart disease, renal failure, hypertension or toxaemia of pregnancy, her baby may fail to grow well and become light for gestational age. Infants of diabetic mothers may be large-for-dates and have an increased morbidity and mortality. The mother with myasthenia gravis, idiopathic thrombocytopenic purpura or thyrotoxicosis may have a baby who is affected by these diseases because the agents responsible for them have passed across the placenta.

All drugs taken by women of child-bearing years should be regarded as potentially teratogenic. The fetus is at greatest risk during the ten week period of organogenesis following conception, but of course the actual date of conception is invariably not known until the first period is missed. Heavy smokers have small babies while alcoholics may have small babies with smaller heads, mental disorders and general somatic abnormalities. Androgens and progesterones cause virilisation of girls and the anticonvulsants phenytoin and tridione cause mental disorders. The dangers of antineoplastic drugs and antithyroid drugs are obvious. Antibiotics should be prescribed to young women with caution. Co-trimoxazole is a folic acid antagonist. Streptomycin causes deafness. Rifampicin may cause neural tube defects and tetracycline taken in the last trimester discolours the fetal teeth.

Most drugs taken about the time of birth pass across to the baby and may affect it during the early neonatal period. Opiates and diazepam used in labour suppress the baby's respiration. The infant of a drug-addicted mother is likely to develop withdrawal symptoms within a week of separation from his source of supply. A few drugs, such as heparin and insulin do not pass to the baby. Some maternal infections are also teratogenic but congenital rubella can be prevented by immunising the mother against it before conception. Congenital syphilis can be prevented if the maternal infection is recognised and treated during pregnancy.

The dangers of fetal damage from diagnostic or therapeutic radiation can be minimised if one always bears in mind that a woman may be pregnant before submitting her to investigation or treatment by this means.

CARE OF THE NEWBORN BABY ON ARRIVAL

The delivery room should be kept warm and fully equipped to deal with any neonatal emergency, for problem babies tend to arrive in the middle of the night!

When the baby is small or pre-term or when there has been fetal distress and an abnormal method of delivery, an asphyxiated baby can be anticipated, and a doctor or nurse trained in resuscitating the newborn should be on hand to take over his care. Resuscitation equipment should be checked beforehand and warmed with an overhead radiant heater. When the baby's head is delivered the nose, mouth and pharynx should be gently sucked clear with a soft catheter. After the cord has been divided one must ensure that it is securely clamped about 2 cm from the umbilicus. If the clamp slips there may be a dramatic bleed. Vitamin K_1 0.5 mg to 1 mg i.m. should be given to prevent haemorrhagic disease of the newborn.

The Apgar score

While the baby is being dried with a warm towel on the resuscitation trolley he can be assessed by counting the Apgar Score (Table 3.1) initially one minute after his delivery.

Table 3.1 The Apgar Score

Sign	Points scored		
	0	*1*	*2*
1 Appearance (colour)	Pale or blue	Body pink, extremities blue	Pink
2 Pulse	Absent	Less than 100	More than 100
3 Grimace (when catheter enters nostril)	None	Grimaces	Sneezes or cries
4 Activity and tone	Limp	Some flexion of extremities	Active motion
5 Respiration	Absent	Slow, irregular	Good cry

If he scores seven or more no intervention is necessary. Six or less is an indication for resuscitation and this should proceed at once if he scores less than three or is less than 32 weeks gestation. One should ensure that he is not asphyxiated as a result of opiates given to the mother, as 0.01 mg/kg i.v. of naloxone hydrochloride will reverse it.

Resuscitation

The baby often begins to breathe as the airways are cleared under direct vision. Violent handling wastes time and is to be condemned. If the baby is not breathing within two minutes he should be intubated with the largest possible endotracheal tube. He is then ventilated at a

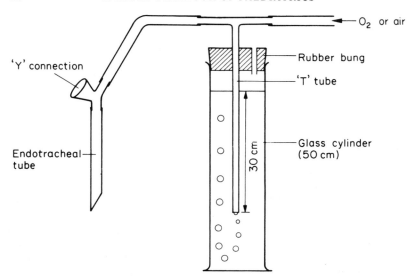

Fig. 3.1 Water manometer

rate of 30 puffs per minute using oxygen or air. The gas flow rate should be 2 litres per minute. The apparatus used is shown in Fig. 3.1.

The gas passes down the endotracheal tube when the 'Y' connection is momentarily occluded with the finger, long enough to achieve small but visible movement of the chest wall. To prevent over-distension of the lungs the circuit is attached to a 'T' tube sunk in a column of water. When a pressure of 30 cmH_2O (4.0 kPa) is reached the excess gas bubbles off and the baby's lungs are protected. Generally, the pressure can be reduced from 30 to 20 cmH_2O (4.0–2.7 kPa) after a few puffs.

If the baby becomes pink and the heart rate rises, spontaneous respirations can be anticipated. Failure to pink-up and a slowing heart rate suggest the need for further action. The position of the endotracheal tube must then be checked. If the Apgar Score remains dramatically low the baby should be given dextrose (1 g/kg) and sodium bicarbonate (3 mmol/kg) through a peripheral vein to correct hypoglycaemia and acidosis.

If cardiac arrest occurs external cardiac massage should be attempted by placing the hand under the baby's back and pressing the sternum one to two centimetres with the thumb. There should be two to three compressions between each ventilation. One should not let the baby die before needling the chest for a pneumothorax. Some severely asphyxiated babies require prolonged assistance with a mechanical ventilator. Their progress can be monitored by estimating their blood sugar and blood gases. Blood letting is facilitated by catheterising an umbilical artery.

Following delivery there should be a rapid but thorough examination of the baby. Healthy babies can then be handed to their mothers. Sick babies however, will need transfer to the Special Care Nursery. The mother must be kept informed about her baby's condition.

EXAMINATION OF THE NORMAL NEWBORN

The baby should be looked at as a whole to exclude major congenital abnormality and to ensure that he is of normal proportions. A full-term baby kicks and cries vigorously soon after birth. The skin is covered with thick cheesy *vernix caseosa* which may be removed by bathing but will spontaneously dry and fall off as powder. Peripheral cyanosis is the rule and should cause no concern if the mucus membranes are pink. The skin is red and the contours rounded. Quivering movements of the chin and lips are common.

Some moulding of the skull is to be expected, the parietal bones usually over-riding the frontal and occipital ones. Oedema of the presenting parts, due to pressure of the pelvic brim, is common. On the skull the oedematous part is called the *caput succedaneum* (or 'caput'). It disappears in three to four days and should not be confused with a *cephalhaematoma* which lasts for many weeks (p. 41).

The eyes must be inspected. A congenital cataract may be present, one eye may be bigger than the other or there might be a congenital glaucoma. The ear is more or less the same length as the nose. If there is breathing difficulty a soft nasal catheter is passed to exclude obstruction due to choanal atresia.

On the hard palate two small white nodules (Epstein's pearls) may be seen. They consist of epithelial cells and disappear spontaneously. *Naevi* on the eyelids and nape of the neck will also disappear and are called stork marks.

The newborn baby breathes 40 to 60 times per minute. Normal respiration is mainly diaphragmatic and the pattern and depth of breathing provides valuable information. Auscultation of breath sounds tend to be harsh but air exchange is normal. Bronchial breathing is commonly heard over the upper sternum and between the scapulae due to the proximity of the trachea. For a few hours after birth fine crepitations may sometimes be heard in the lungs of normal babies due to unabsorbed lung fluid.

The normal heart rate is 120 beats per minute, varying from 80 to 160 per minute. Sinus arrhythmia is usually very marked. Sounds over the pulmonary area are usually louder than the aortic sounds; P_2 may even have a booming quality. Murmurs may be heard which vary from day to day and may disappear permanently. They do not often have any pathological significance.

The normal abdomen distends easily with gas. The liver edge is commonly palpable to 1 cm below the costal margin and the tip of the spleen can be felt in about 10 % of newborns. The kidneys, too, are easily palpable and may be felt in 50 % of newborns if the abdomen is deeply palpated bimanually. The bladder is intra-abdominal and easily emptied on pressure.

The extremities may be folded easily into the fetal position. The deformities caused by this correct themselves within the first week or two of life. They must be carefully distinguished from more serious fixed deformities such as club foot.

The central nervous system of the normal baby is characterised by reflex activities such as sucking, swallowing and breathing. If the cheek is gently touched the head will turn *towards* the hand as though seeking his mother's breast (*rooting reflex*). Any sudden movement or loud noise elicits the *Moro (startle) reflex*. There is a general extension of the trunk, abduction of the arms and fingers, often with a quivering motion, followed by adduction and return to normal posture. The legs also abduct and adduct but less actively than the arms. The *grasp reflex* is elicited by inserting a finger into the palm of the hand. The grasp is so strong that the baby can sometimes be lifted up. Numerous other reflexes can be elicited, such as the *tonic neck reflex*, the *stepping reflex* and *postural righting reflexes*. Disturbances may indicate brain damage. The deep reflexes are usually present but the plantar response can be very misleading as both flexor and extensor responses are easily obtainable. It depends how hard one scratches the sole of the foot and on other factors. In the normal newborn it should be possible to abduct fully the flexed hips, thus excluding some cases of congenital dislocation of the hips. The presence of strong femoral pulses which can be felt at the same time excludes coarctation of the aorta. The anus should be inspected in all cases; taking the rectal temperature will determine its patency. The external genitalia and inguinal regions should be carefully assessed. The features of low birth-weight babies are described in Chapter 4.

THE BABY OF LOW BIRTH-WEIGHT

The baby born before 37 completed weeks, from the first day of the last menstrual period, is called pre-term, from 37 to 41 weeks term, and after 42 weeks post-term. The birth-weight at any particular gestation is variable and should be plotted on a percentile chart (Fig. 4.1). Babies whose weights are above the 90th percentile and called 'large-for-dates' and those below the 10th percentile 'light-for-dates'. It follows then that 10% of all babies are light-for-dates. A baby who weighs less than 2.5 kg at birth is called 'low birth-weight'. In developed countries about two-thirds of these are pre-term and the remainder light-for-dates. The latter may behave differently from pre-term babies and are considered separately.

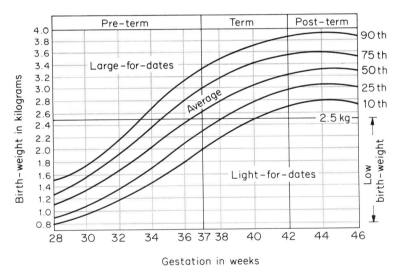

Fig. 4.1 A percentile chart showing the classification of babies by birth-weight and gestation (multiple sources)

LIGHT-FOR-DATES BABIES

The majority of light-for-dates babies are perfectly healthy and just happen to be light. The tendency to produce light-for-dates babies may be familial, though it happens more often in the very young primipara and with multiple pregnancy. For the latter, special percentile charts are available. Light-for-dates babies are found if there has been intra-uterine growth retardation, a major congenital abnormality or a congenital infection, and these conditions should be thought of when examining the baby for the first time.

Obstetricians try to select out light-for-dates babies for close antenatal surveillance because of the risks of underlying fetal abnormality and intra-uterine death. There is also a greater risk of *birth asphyxia* and *aspiration of meconium* into the lungs with the first breath. If there is any meconium to be seen on the skin the airway should be inspected immediately with a laryngoscope and any meconium present carefully sucked out. A further problem to be anticipated is *hypoglycaemia* which generally occurs in the first forty-eight hours. This complication is largely prevented by feeding the baby within two hours of birth and by monitoring the blood sugar every four hours and intervening when it falls. If the baby looks red the haemoglobin and packed cell volume should be measured to exclude *polycythaemia*. Blood viscosity increases sharply when the packed cell volume is over 70%, and spontaneous thrombosis should be prevented by removing a portion of the baby's blood and replacing it with plasma. Spontaneous *pulmonary haemorrhage* occasionally occurs and is heralded by blood welling out of the airway. Treatment is with intermittent positive pressure ventilation (IPPV) but the condition is usually fatal.

THE PRE-TERM BABY

Pre-term delivery may result from maternal obstetric problems, such as cervical incompetence and ante-partum haemorrhage, or from induction of labour performed for conditions such as rhesus iso-immunisation. In most cases the cause of pre-term delivery is unknown and cannot be prevented. It is clear from Fig. 4.1 that the earlier a baby is born the lighter he will be, although a large baby at 34 weeks can weigh the same as a small baby at 40 weeks gestation. Asiatic babies tend to be smaller than Caucasians.

APPEARANCE OF THE PRE-TERM BABY

The earlier a baby is born the more obviously he appears different from his term counterpart (Fig. 4.2). He is small and looks red, for his haemoglobin is high and the skin is thin and shiny. The skin tends to hang in folds due to lack of subcutaneous fat. He is covered in a fine downy hair called *lanugo*. There are few creases on the sole of the foot which may be oedematous. The bones of the vault are soft, the fontanelle is large and

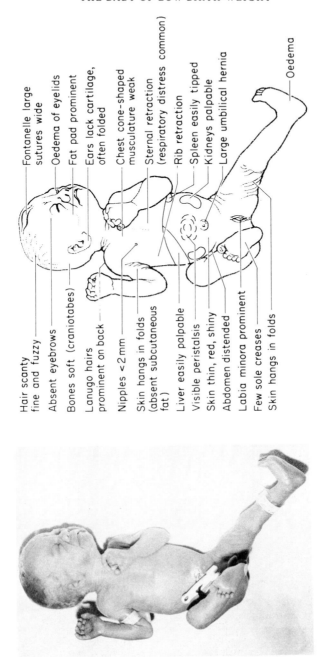

Hair scanty
fine and fuzzy

Absent eyebrows

Bones soft (craniotabes)

Lanugo hairs
prominent on back

Nipples <2 mm

Skin hangs in folds
(absent subcutaneous
fat)

Liver easily palpable

Visible peristalsis

Skin thin, red, shiny

Abdomen distended

Labia minora prominent

Few sole creases

Skin hangs in folds

Fontanelle large
sutures wide

Oedema of eyelids

Fat pad prominent

Ears lack cartilage,
often folded

Chest cone-shaped
musculature weak

Sternal retraction
(respiratory distress common)

Rib retraction

Spleen easily tipped

Kidneys palpable

Large umbilical hernia

Oedema

Fig. 4.2 Appearance and characteristics of the pre-term baby

the sutures wide. The ear is poorly cartilaginised and simply formed. Breast tissue is absent and the nipples are small. The liver, spleen and kidneys are easily palpable. Peristaltic waves may be seen through the abdominal wall and there may be an umbilical hernia. Girls have prominent labia minor and in boys the testes are undescended or high in the inguinal canal. The supine pre-term baby assumes a frog-like position. He is hypotonic and there is paucity of spontaneous limb movement. The rooting and sucking reflexes may be weak and if he is less than 35 weeks gestation he may need to be tube fed. When a pre-term baby is recognised his gestation should be carefully assessed before plotting his head, length and weight percentiles.

ESTIMATION OF GESTATIONAL AGE

Most estimates are based on the baby's morphological appearance and neurological state and should be accurate to within two weeks of the true gestational age. An assessment is unreliable if the baby is ill, and the examination is best performed some hours after delivery on a wakeful baby.

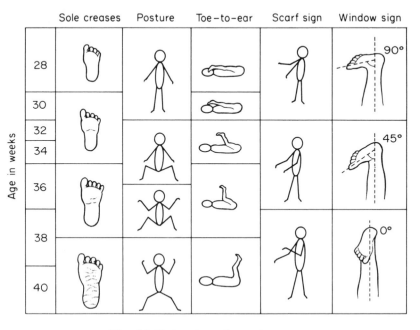

Fig. 4.3 Estimation of gestational age

The best estimate of gestational age is made by measuring the morphological appearance in combination with the neurological state and details of an accurate method have been described by V. Dubowitz (Journal of Paediatrics, 77, 1, 1970). Some signs are listed below and should be used in conjunction with Fig. 4.3.

1 Clinical

Crown-sole length in cm × 0.8 = gestational age in weeks.

(a) *Sole of foot*—if only an anterior transverse crease is found, baby is less than 36 weeks; if the sole is covered in creases he is 40 weeks or more.

(b) *Scalp hair*—fine and fuzzy before 38 weeks, becomes increasingly coarser and silkier thereafter.

(c) *Ear lobes*—no cartilage before 36 weeks, some between 36–38 weeks and ear quite stiff and firm by full term.

(d) *Breast nodules*—not palpable before 36 weeks, 2–4 mm by 38 weeks and 6–7 mm at term.

(e) *Testes* in lower inguinal canal by 36 weeks, in scrotum by 39 weeks.

2 Reflexes

(a) *Sucking and swallowing* are weak and poorly synchronised before 32 weeks, but quite strong and synchronised after 34 weeks.

(b) *Rooting reflex* is slow before 32 weeks but becomes brisk and active by 34 weeks.

(c) *Moro reflex* is weak before 32 weeks, complete thereafter.

(d) *Crossed extension reflex* produces only slight flexion before 32 weeks, full flexion by 34 weeks, flexion followed by extension by 38 weeks and the full reflex by term, i.e. flexion-extension-adduction with fanning of toes.

3 Tone

(a) *Posture*—before 32 weeks baby is completely hypotonic, lying flat on back, arms and legs extended. Gradually flexion at the hips and knees occurs so that by 34 weeks baby lies in a frog-like position. By 36 weeks the elbows also tend to flex. The baby becomes increasingly hypertonic and by 40 weeks there is relatively little movement of the limbs.

(b) *Toe-to-ear manoeuvre*—before 34 weeks, if the baby's extended legs are flexed at the hips his toes will reach to near his ears. Gradually his hips become less supple so that at 40 weeks his thigh can only be flexed to 90° off the table, if the leg and thigh are in a straight line.

(c) *'Scarf sign'*—before 32 weeks, with baby flat on his back, either arm can be moved across the baby so that the elbows reach beyond the edge of the body on the opposite side. By 38 weeks the elbow reaches only to the mid-line and at 40 weeks it can only be placed just short of the mid-line.

(d) *The 'window sign'*—before 32 weeks the hand can be flexed to about 90° on the forearm, by 36 weeks it can be flexed to about 45° and at term full flexion is possible. The same applies to dorsiflexion of the foot at the ankle.

NURSING THE LOW BIRTH-WEIGHT BABY

Except in hot countries, babies weighing less than 1.8 kg should be nursed initially in an incubator. The advantages of an incubator are that the baby can be observed easily at eye level in an environment where the temperature, humidity and oxygen concentration can be controlled. Minimal handling is a rule. Unnecessary interference with the baby can cause hypothermia, apnoea and cross-infection.

Food

Breast or expressed breast milk is better than modified cows milk. Most babies less than 35 weeks gestation are unable to suck so should be fed using a feeding tube. This may be nasogastric, orogastric or nasojejunal. If there are long-term nutritional problems parenteral feeding can be used. The first feed should be given within two hours to prevent hypoglycaemia. Frequency of feeds will depend on the baby's birth-weight as shown in Table 4.1.

The amount of milk fed to the baby depends on his age and weight. Babies differ and the figures suggested in Table 4.2 are offered as a basic guide.

Relatively large quantities of feed are given to low birth-weight babies to ensure that the rapidly growing brain receives adequate nutrients. The baby's first feed can be milk provided there is no suspicion of oesophageal atresia which causes excessive oral secretions. The baby's nutritional progress is measured by weighing on alternate days. He should not lose

Table 4.1 Frequency of milk feeds

Birth weight	Frequency
Less than 2.3 kg	3-hourly
Less than 1.8 kg	2-hourly
Less than 1.5 kg	Hourly
Less than 1.2 kg	Nasogastric or nasojejunal drip feed

Table 4.2 Quantity of milk feed per day

Day of life	Low birth-weight baby ml/kg	Normal baby ml/kg
1	60	45
2	90	60
3	120	75
4	150	90
5	Increase as tolerated	120
6	and according	150 usually
7	to weight	sufficient
8	↓	
9		
10	180, increasing as necessary to 250	

more than 10 % of his birth-weight and he should regain his birth-weight within ten to fourteen days. Some very small babies who are slow to gain weight may have a metabolic acidosis but they thrive once this is corrected with sodium bicarbonate. Vitamin supplements may be started in the neonatal period and continued throughout the first year. Iron supplements may be given until weaning to prevent a late iron deficiency anaemia.

Temperature control

Light babies lack subcutaneous white fat and brown fat and if they are also pre-term they have an immature thermoregulatory centre so may not be able to shiver or sweat. The environmental temperature in which the baby is nursed will depend on his age, weight and gestation and is known as the thermoneutral environment. In temperate climates babies weighing over 2 kg can usually be dressed safely in a room temperature of 27°C but lighter infants may need the protection of an incubator and should be attached to a continuous reading thermometer.

Jaundice

All pre-term babies become jaundiced because their liver enzyme systems are immature and unconjugated bilirubin is not efficiently conjugated until four to five days have passed. Jaundice may be aggravated by polycythaemia, bruising, infection and haemolysis. As hyperbilirubinaemia can lead to kernicterus (p. 48) the colour of the baby should be noted frequently and the bilirubin estimated if the jaundice appears early or is deepening quickly.

Respiration

Pre-term babies are likely to develop hyaline membrane disease (see below). In this disease signs of respiratory distress are always present within four hours. The baby should be nursed either prone or supine in an incubator. The chest and abdomen should be exposed to observe the respiratory effort. Babies of less than 34 weeks gestation are liable to recurrent apnoeic attacks and should be nursed on an apnoea alarm which is a device for measuring the time interval between breaths. The alarm is set to ring when the interval is prolonged.

Hypoglycaemia

This is most likely to occur in a sick pre-term baby, light-for-dates baby or a baby with rhesus iso-immunisation. It may be anticipated before symptoms occur by regular estimation of blood sugar (see p. 44).

Infection

Neonates, particularly those of low birth-weight, have an immature immunological system and are likely to acquire infections. Breast feeding will offer some protection but such small babies should be nursed in a clean environment where the equipment is regularly sterilised and where the ventilation system is clean. Slavish attention to hand washing before and after touching the baby is the most important factor in preventing infection.

SPECIAL PROBLEMS OF THE PRE-TERM BABY

Hyaline membrane disease

This is the commonest cause of the respiratory distress syndrome (Chapter 5). Rare in term babies, it increases in frequency the shorter the gestation period. The baby is unable to maintain open alveoli due to deficiency of surfactant so that the lung tends to collapse at the end of each breath. This leads to the cardinal signs of expiratory grunting, cyanosis, rib recession and tachypnoea. Signs of the disease begin within four hours of birth and a chest X-ray will show the collapsed alveoli as a ground glass shadow with air bronchograms. Surfactant deficiency is, in some measure, reduced by giving the fetus (via the mother) dexamethasone forty-eight hours before delivery, and also by resuscitating early at birth to prevent breakdown of surfactant which occurs with hypoxia. The principle of management is to tide the baby over his first week when he should be able to produce enough surfactant on his own. He should be nursed in an incubator and be tube-fed. Hypoxia is prevented by nursing in humidified oxygen, the concentration of which is measured. The baby's arterial oxygen tension should be kept between 6–12 kPa (44–90 mmHg). This is facilitated by using a transcutaneous skin oxygen monitor or a continuous reading monitor inserted into an umbilical artery. Alternatively, four hourly samples from an umbilical arterial catheter can be taken for analysis. The arterial pH and CO_2 should be measured intermittently so that the tendency towards acidosis can be corrected with bicarbonate or by adjusting the baby's ventilation. When the ambient oxygen concentration reaches 60% and the arterial tension falls to 6 kPa (44 mmHg) oxygenation can be improved by applying continuous distending pressure of up to 10 cmH$_2$O (0.9 kPa) to the airway by using either nasal prongs, a facial mask or a head box, or by applying pressure directly down an endotracheal tube. If the baby deteriorates in spite of these measures intermittent positive pressure ventilation (IPPV) can be used, but the complications of ventilator therapy are serious.

Jaundice

See Chapter 5.

Oxygen toxicity

behind the lens

Oxygen therapy can cause retrolental fibroplasia, a condition in which the peripheral retinal vessels become first stretched then tortuous and dilated. Retinal haemorrhage occurs. New vessels grow into the vitreous and retinal detachment can occur with progressive fibrosis which leads to loss of vision. Minor changes may be extremely difficult to detect and may not appear until some months after exposure to oxygen. Unfortunately, retrolental fibroplasia can occur at any oxygen concentration or gestation but is most likely to appear in the very pre-term baby treated with high oxygen concentrations for prolonged periods. It is therefore mandatory that the arterial oxygen tension is regularly measured to prevent hyperoxaemia.

Anaemia

The neonatal haemoglobin level falls steadily for the first three months of life until the bone marrow produces enough red cells to replace those lost. The haemoglobin level of the pre-term baby falls faster, partly because there is a quicker doubling of his size and partly due to a dilutional effect. The anaemia is exacerbated by sepsis, bruising and, in sick babies, by frequent blood sampling (professorial anaemia). The haemoglobin and packed cell volume should be checked regularly and top-up transfusion given when the PCV falls below 40%, or the haemoglobin less than 7 g/dl.

Intraventricular haemorrhage (IVH)

This occurs in up to 35 % of babies born before 34 weeks gestation and can be detected by ultrasound scan in the first few days of life. Predisposing factors include the respiratory distress syndrome, acidosis and hypercapnia. The majority of bleeds are small and do not cause any detectable handicap but large bleeds cause cerebral palsy, hydrocephalus or death. Methods of reducing the incidence and severity of IVH are under investigation.

Necrotising enterocolitis

This is an uncommon but increasingly recognised disorder found in babies who have suffered from hypoxia. It may follow interference to the blood supply to the gut after umbilical vessel catheterisation and exchange transfusion. It may result from invasion of the gut by anaerobic organisms after ischaemia. The baby develops abdominal distension, vomiting and bloody diarrhoea. Abdominal X-ray shows intramural air and sometimes air in the portal tract, or the peritoneum after perforation. Treatment is by feeding the baby parenterally and giving penicillin, gentamicin and metronidazole. Surgical treatment may be necessary for perforation or stricture.

PROGNOSIS OF LOW BIRTH-WEIGHT BABIES

The decline in perinatal mortality which has occurred with improved obstetric and neonatal care has been accompanied by a reduction in the number of handicapped children. The majority of babies who are born pre-term can expect to survive as normal individuals and there can be little doubt that investment in their welfare is highly cost-effective. Between 10–30 % of babies weighing less than 1 kg at birth who survive have a major handicap. Light-for-dates babies do not fare as well as babies who have grown appropriately for their gestation.

CHAPTER 5

DISORDERS OF THE NEONATE

CONGENITAL ANOMALIES THAT THREATEN THE LIFE OF THE NEONATE

Choanal atresia

Choanal atresia is a congenital malformation in which the posterior nares are obstructed by a mucosal or bony plate. In bilateral cases the infant cannot breathe through the nose and shows signs of asphyxia with cyanosis and rib retraction. The cyanosis is aggravated by attempts at feeding. The diagnosis is confirmed by finding that it is impossible to pass a nasal catheter. The baby should be nursed prone with an oropharyngeal airway in place and be given oxygen therapy if hypoxia persists. Surgical treatment should be organised urgently as delay in opening the choana may be fatal.

Micrognathia

Micrognathia means a small lower jaw. It may result in a posterior displacement of the tongue with obstruction of the posterior pharynx. When associated with a cleft or a high-arched palate it is called a Pierre Robin syndrome. It may cause respiratory embarrassment unless the tongue is prevented from falling back. Nursing in the prone position or suturing the tongue to the mandible may be life-saving in severe cases.

Intestinal obstruction (See Chapter 15)

The cardinal features of bowel blockage in the neonate are vomiting and abdominal distension. Bile appears in the vomitus if the obstruction is distal to the ampulla of Vater. Sometimes small amounts of light-coloured meconium may be passed. The obstruction may be complete or incomplete. It may be due to atresia or stenosis of the bowel or there may be errors of rotation associated with volvulus. Babies with rectal atresia may not vomit for two to three days but the absence of meconium and progressive abdominal distension should be noticed early. In all cases of suspected intestinal obstruction a nasogastric tube should be passed to allow for free drainage of gastric contents and to prevent aspiration. A straight X-ray of the abdomen of the baby hanging by the arms should be taken. An experienced radiologist can sometimes locate the site of the obstruction on these plates alone. Fluid levels are common to all forms of obstruction but are occasionally seen in normal babies. Laparotomy may be the only way to make a definite diagnosis but the baby must be carefully prepared for operation. In the newborn baby intestinal obstruction may be mimicked by umbilical infection, which produces a picture similar to paralytic ileus. Inspection of the infected umbilicus reveals the diagnosis. Another pitfall is the presence of a hardened meconium plug which can cause obstruction. This can usually be removed by careful colonic lavage. Rarely, Hirschprung's disease (p. 245) may present as intestinal obstruction.

Omphalocele (Exomphalos)

Omphalocele is a defect of the umbilical ring through which the bowel and other abdominal organs may protrude. It may be associated with chromosomal abnormalities, which should be excluded. The defect may vary from a few centimetres in diameter to extensive involvement of the abdominal wall. The protruding organs are covered by a thin layer of peritoneum which is easily infected. The abdominal cavity itself is very small so surgical repair may be very difficult or impossible, unless the remaining abdominal wall can be stretched sufficiently to permit replacement of the abdominal contents. Alternatively, the defect may be covered with a synthetic material such as Silastic, which can be rolled up so that the bowel is gradually pushed back into the abdominal cavity over a period of several weeks.

Diaphragmatic hernia

Progressive dyspnoea, cyanosis, and respiratory difficulty may be caused by loops of bowel entering the chest. Most cases occur on the left side through the foramen of Bochdalek because the size of the liver on the right covers quite large defects. It is possible, however, for a large part of the liver to enter the chest and cause trouble. The diagnosis is usually made radiologically. One must be careful not to confuse loops of bowel with 'cysts' in the lung. Treatment consists of *early* surgery because the condition of the baby may change dramatically as a result of swallowing air or taking a feed. A nasogastric tube should be passed in all cases prior to surgery. As with omphalocele, it may be very difficult to return the loops of bowel into the relatively small, unexpanded abdominal cavity, unless it is stretched.

Congenital heart disease (see Chapter 11)

The majority of asymptomatic acyanotic neonates who develop heart murmurs in the first few days of life have single valvular lesions or coarctation of the aorta. Those who develop murmurs towards the end of the first week prove to have left-to-right shunts such as persistent ductus arteriosus. Life-threatening and more complex lesions are likely if heart failure or cyanosis are present. Heart murmurs *may* be absent.

Most acyanotic abnormalities can be diagnosed clinically with the aid of a chest X-ray and an electrocardiogram. Babies with heart failure or cyanosis should be referred urgently to a paediatric cardiac unit for further investigation and treatment, as they can deteriorate rapidly. Echocardiography, contrast radiography and cardiac catheterisation are usually necessary to establish an accurate anatomical diagnosis. The baby is best able to withstand these investigations if he is kept warm, fed and in acid-base balance. Heart failure should be treated with digoxin and diuretics whilst awaiting definitive surgical correction.

Neural tube defects (see p. 151)

Congenital defects are often multiple so that if one defect is found the baby should be carefully examined for others. They may be associated with chromosomal abnormalities which should also be looked for in order that accurate genetic advice can be given to the parents.

BIRTH INJURIES

Haemorrhage

Haemorrhage may occur under the periosteum of one or more of the cranial bones, causing a swelling which is limited by the attachment of the periosteum to bone (*cephalhaematoma*). Blood loss may be sufficient to cause anaemia and require a blood transfusion. Reabsorption of the blood can aggravate jaundice and it is important to check serum bilirubin levels in order to prevent kernicterus. The swelling usually clears in 6–8 weeks though a hard bony ridge may persist for months.

Intracranial haemorrhages may occur as a result of a difficult birth. Symptoms depend on the size and site of the bleeding. A tear in the middle meningeal artery will cause an *extradural haemorrhage*, while involvement of other vessels may lead to *subdural, subarachnoid, intracerebral* or *intraventricular bleeding.*

Symptoms may be minimal or the patient may present with anorexia, vomiting, failure to thrive, cerebral (high-pitched) cry, irritability, stupor or convulsions. Signs of anaemia or shock may be present and sometimes neurological signs including cranial nerve palsy may be detected. Slow or rapid enlargement of the head and bulging of the fontanelle should be looked for.

Diagnosis may be confirmed by lumbar puncture, subdural taps, sonar or by means of computerised axial tomography (CAT scan). Treatment depends on the underlying site of the haemorrhage. Oxygen should be given for hypoxia and vitamin K_1 for hypoprothrom-binaemia. Subdural effusions should be tapped. Hyperbilirubinaemia must be treated to prevent kernicterus. In cases of cerebral oedema the use of phenobarbitone, mannitol and dexamethasone should be considered.

Erb's paralysis

Erb's paralysis is a flaccid paralysis of the deltoid, supra and infra-spinatus, the biceps and supinator muscles due to stretching or damage to the fifth and sixth cervical roots of the brachial plexus during delivery. This is usually associated with breech delivery when the shoulder is pulled down. The arm hangs to the side with the forearm pronated and the hand 'in a position ready to receive a tip' (porter's tip). In the severest cases the root of the phrenic nerve may be torn, leading to paralysis of the diaphragm on the affected side. The Moro reflex is, of course, absent on the affected side.

Most cases of Erb's paralysis get better spontaneously within weeks but paralysis can be permanent. Mothers should be taught to give the baby passive physiotherapy.

Klumpke's paralysis

Klumpke's paralysis is rare and involves the eighth cervical and first thoracic roots of the brachial plexus, with or without damage to the cervical sympathetic plexus.

Facial nerve paralysis

Facial nerve paralysis may be secondary to compression of the seventh nerve by the bony pelvis or forceps during delivery. It is usually temporary, but when the facial nerve is paralysed from an upper motor neurone lesion the paralysis is permanent.

INFECTIONS OF THE NEWBORN

Congenital infections

The fetus may be invaded by almost any microbe which infects his mother. Infections which most commonly cause permanent damage are cytomegalovirus (CMV), toxoplasmosis, syphilis and rubella. They may cause general signs of fetal growth retardation, hepatosplenomegaly and purpura as well as specific signs such as chorioretinitis and microcephaly in toxoplasmosis, and congenital heart disease with deafness and blindness in rubella. Diagnosis is by serological investigation.

If a mother is a carrier of hepatitis B surface antigen her baby should be given anti-HBsIg immediately, as he is liable to become infected.

Acquired infections

The baby may be affected by an ascending vaginal infection before delivery, especially after prolonged rupture of the membranes. Neonates most at risk are those born after instrumental delivery or who are of low birth-weight and artificially fed. Signs of infection are often non-specific and insidious but the baby may deteriorate rapidly. There may be exaggerated jaundice, changes in body temperature, hypotonia, excess loss of weight or failure to gain weight, vomiting, diarrhoea or splenomegaly. Infections often seen are pneumonia, urinary tract infection and meningitis, frequently associated with a septicaemia.

Group B beta-haemolytic streptococcal infection is becoming increasingly common. Two-thirds of cases present in the first two days of life (early infection) and one-third after ten days (late infection). Early infection can present with fever, unexpected apnoeic attacks or with respiratory distress which may have the radiological features of hyaline membrane disease. Streptococcal meningitis occurs in 30 % of cases. The prognosis is poor and 70 % die within thirty-six hours. *Late onset infection* with group B streptococci can cause meningitis, asymptomatic bacteraemia, otitis media, ethmoiditis, conjunctivitis, cellulitis, breast abscess, empyema, septic arthritis, impetigo or osteomyelitis. Late infection probably results from cross infection in the nursery.

Most organisms responsible for neonatal bacteraemia can cause meningitis including *E. Coli, Streptococcus agalactiae* and *Listeria monocytogenes*. Although *Listeria* is rare it can produce a distinguishable clinical picture. The mother may have a 'flu-like illness and the amniotic fluid may be tinged green. The baby has respiratory depression, a skin rash and ulceration of the pharynx.

Whenever infection is suspected full investigation is mandatory and should include appropriate external swabs for culture, blood culture, suprapubic examination of urine and a lumbar puncture. A full blood count should be performed because the earliest signs of infection may be suspected with changes in the neutrophil count or the appearance of immature cells forms. Chest X-ray may demonstrate pneumonia. Treatment should begin early without awaiting results of culture. Antibiotics should be given systemically and should cover a broad spectrum, such as penicillin and gentamicin, or cefotaxime.

Haemorrhage in the newborn

A large feto-maternal bleed or bleeding from the umbilical stump may present as a pale, shocked baby with acidotic breathing. Blood transfusion is urgent and in an emergency blood group O Rh negative blood should be given, 20 ml per kg via the umbilical vein.

Blood loss may occur at other sites too, such as the gastro-intestinal tract, renal tract or into the skin or brain. Gastro-intestinal bleeding may result from a surgical condition such as volvulus. Swallowed maternal blood can cause confusion, but can be distinguished from neonatal blood by measuring its adult haemoglobin content.

Thrombocytopenia may present with purpura and is treated with platelet transfusion. Thrombocytopenia may be transitory and secondary to maternal disease or iso-immunisation, or it may be associated with a congenital infection. It may also be part of a more generalised disorder such as disseminated intravascular coagulation (DIC). Babies with DIC are usually ill with severe infection, and coagulation studies show low fibrinogen, low prothrombin and low partial thromboplastin time. Treatment is that of the underlying disease. Exchange transfusion with fresh donor blood and anticoagulants may be required. Platelet transfusions are necessary for severe thrombocytopenia.

Vitamin K deficiency nearly always occurs in breast-fed babies (see p. 80). Bleeding usually occurs in the first few days of life but may be delayed for several weeks. The prothrombin time is prolonged and the disorder is corrected by giving 1 mg of vitamin K_1 intravenously. Some centres administer vitamin K to every newborn baby prophylactically by intramuscular injection.

The inherited coagulation disorders rarely cause bleeding in the newborn period. They are diagnosed by factor assay in plasma. Fresh, frozen plasma and cryoprecipitate can be given after specimens have been taken for investigation.

Vaginal bleeding is usually a harmless symptom due to oestrogen withdrawal.

METABOLIC DISORDERS IN THE NEONATE

Neonatal hypoglycaemia

Hypoglycaemia occurs when the blood sugar falls below 1.6 mmol/l (30 mg/dl) in the term baby or 1.1 mmol/l (20 mg/dl) in the pre-term baby. It is common in infants of diabetic mothers and in light-for-dates babies. The baby may be asymptomatic, or develop symptoms of pallor, jitteriness, hypotonia, apnoea or convulsions. Symptomatic hypoglycaemia may result in permanent brain damage. Babies at risk should have regular blood sugar estimations using Dextrostix. The incidence of hypoglycaemia can be reduced by *early* feeding of all newborns with milk and by giving extra glucose by mouth if the blood sugar falls. Symptomatic hypoglycaemia is treated with 1 g/kg of intravenous glucose into a peripheral vein. Oral glucose has also been successfully used. Recurrent hypoglycaemia should be treated with an intravenous glucose infusion and the dose tailed off slowly. Rapid withdrawal of glucose can lead to rebound hypoglycaemia. In severe cases the use of glucagon should be considered. The dose is 0.1–0.2 mg subcutaneously.

Neonatal hypocalcaemia

Signs of hypocalcaemia are anorexia, apathy, jitteriness or frank, short, generalised convulsions. The serum calcium will be less than 1.8 mmol/l. *Early onset* hypocalcaemia occurs within a few days of life and is found in pre-term babies, ill babies and in those fed intravenously. In the *classical late onset* type of hypocalcaemia symptoms occur between five to ten days of life in babies fed on unmodified cow's milk. This condition probably results from hyperphosphataemia due to the high phosphate content of the milk. When this happens modified cows milk or breast milk should be substituted for the cows milk. Hypocalcaemia may be treated by giving up to 10 ml/kg/day of 10 % calcium gluconate orally or alfacalcidol 0.05 μg/kg/day. Intravenous calcium as a bolus is hazardous and should rarely be necessary.

Neonatal hyperbilirubinaemia

Neonatal jaundice may be due to haemolytic disease, deficiency of certain enzymes in the liver, obstruction of the bile passages or infection. An increase in indirect acting bilirubin in the serum is particularly dangerous because it leads to kernicterus. In full-term babies the indirect serum bilirubin should never be allowed to rise above 360 μmols/l of blood, while in small pre-term infants the figure is lower, varying from 160 to 270 μmols/l. When the serum bilirubin reaches these critical levels an exchange transfusion is advised.

Haemolytic disease of the newborn

Haemolytic disease of the newborn is caused by incompatible red blood cells from the baby crossing the placenta and stimulating antibody formation in the mother. It may occur after abortion, external version or a normal delivery. The antibodies are harmless to the mother but may return to the baby's circulation and cause variable degrees of haemolysis. The most serious disease is caused by *Rhesus incompatibility* between a Rhesus negative mother and a Rhesus positive fetus. Any Rhesus factor can produce antibodies (c, d, e, C, D, E) but D is the most important one. The first maternal sensitisation takes about three days to develop therefore her first baby is rarely affected. In a subsequent pregnancy her Rh IgG antibody will haemolyse susceptible red cells in the fetus. When the baby is affected three grades of severity are recognised:

1 *Hydrops fetalis*, in which profound anaemia leads to cardiac failure, gross hepatosplenomegaly and generalised oedema, ascites and pleural effusion.
2 *Icterus gravis neonatorum*—the commonest form—in which haemolysis leads to rapidly deepening jaundice which starts within twelve hours of birth.

3 *Congenital haemolytic anaemia*, which is associated with a *slowly* progressive anaemia and mild jaundice.

Diagnosis and treatment

Rhesus incompatibility can be anticipated by screening all pregnant women who are Rhesus negative for Rh IgG antibody. In affected women rising titres can usually be demonstrated as pregnancy advances. If the fetus is affected serial amniocentesis should be performed to measure the optical density of bile pigment in the fluid using a spectrophotometer. This measurement can be used to estimate how badly the fetus is affected. In severely affected cases the fetus will become hydropic. In this situation fresh donor cells can be injected across the uterus into the fetal peritoneal cavity where the cells are absorbed intact into the baby's circulation. This procedure improves the fetal anaemia and helps tide the baby over until birth is induced. Immediate exchange transfusion can then be done. Less severely affected babies will develop *icterus gravis neonatorum* and these babies should be delivered at about 36 weeks gestation. At birth the diagnosis should be confirmed by cord blood group, haemoglobin, bilirubin and a Coomb's test which will be positive. A cord blood bilirubin of more than 70 μmols/l or a haemoglobin of less than 14 g/dl is an indication for urgent exchange transfusion. The mildest cases of rhesus incompatibility develop *congenital haemolytic anaemia*. In all cases of suspected haemolytic disease the serum bilirubin should be measured at frequent intervals and an exchange transfusion performed if the bilirubin approaches dangerous levels (360 μmols/l in a term baby). In some cases several exchange transfusions are necessary.

Prevention of Rhesus sensitisation

Damaging Rhesus sensitisation can be prevented by giving susceptible mothers anti-rhesus IgG antibody (anti-D antibody) after abortion or delivery so that any circulating Rhesus antigen can be mopped up.

Haemolytic disease is also caused by *ABO incompatibility*. In this condition the mother is blood group O and the baby is either A or B. Feto-maternal transfusion can sensitise the mother to produce IgM and often IgG antibody against A or B. The IgG antibody develops rapidly and passes back to the baby and causes haemolysis within a few hours. Affected babies cannot easily be predicted but fortunately they are not severely ill at birth. A Coomb's test is usually negative. The baby may have a large spleen and develop early jaundice. Exchange transfusion may be necessary to prevent kernicterus. Mothers may also become sensitive to other fetal blood antigens, such as Kell, Kidd and Duffy, but cases are rare. Excess neonatal erythrocyte haemolysis may also be due to congenital abnormalities in the red cells, as in *glucose-6-phosphate dehydrogenase (G-6-PD) deficiency* and *hereditary spherocytosis*.

Physiological jaundice

In the newborn there is a relative deficiency of *glucuronyl-transferase*, the enzyme which glucuronidates bilirubin in the liver, and so indirect bilirubin collects in the plasma. The more premature the baby the greater the deficiency (jaundice of prematurity) and some degree of jaundice is invariable in the pre-term baby. It may be aggravated by the normal breakdown of fetal haemoglobin which increases the bilirubin load to the liver. Jaundice appears clinically on the third or fourth day, reaches its peak on the sixth day and then fades. The infant may be sleepy and reluctant to feed. A few babies may require treatment.

Other causes of neonatal jaundice

Congenital or acquired infections may present as prolonged or excessive jaundice and should lead to a full infection screen. Certain *drugs* such as sulphonamides and vitamin K analogues may displace bilirubin from protein binding sites and lead to hyperbilirubinaemia. Occasionally babies who are fed with breast milk develop jaundice which clears when the breast feeding is discontinued but returns when it is re-introduced. It is thought that the milk contains liver enzyme inhibitors. Breast feeding can safely be continued provided the bilirubin does not approach dangerous levels. Jaundice may also be caused by gastro-intestinal *bleeding*, cephalhaematoma and extensive bruising, due to reabsorption of bile pigments. Babies who are jaundiced and acidotic should be investigated to exclude an *inborn error of metabolism* such as galactosaemia. A diagnosis can only be made after metabolic investigation.

Management

Neonatal jaundice is very common and the majority of babies have physiological jaundice. Jaundice occurring in the first two days of life or worsening after a few days, or a serum bilirubin over 300 μmols/l in a term baby are indications for further investigation. The serum bilirubin should be measured in all but mild cases. Any underlying disease should be treated. In hyperbilirubinaemia the neonate should be adequately fed and hydrated.

Moderately severe jaundice can be treated with *phototherapy*. In this treatment blue light (wave length 400–500 nm) is shone onto jaundiced skin and converts unconjugated bilirubin into other soluble, and therefore harmless, products and the baby's total unconjugated bilirubin falls. The baby's body temperature should be monitored during phototherapy and his fluid intake increased by 25 % to compensate for increased insensible water loss. His eyes should be covered to protect them from the light.

If the baby's bilirubin approaches dangerous levels in spite of phototherapy an *exchange transfusion* should be performed to prevent kernicterus. The technique should be learned in a properly equipped neonatal unit. In this procedure a large catheter is placed into the inferior vena cava via the umbilical vein. The baby's affected blood is exchanged with compatible donor blood so that circulating bilirubin is removed and any anaemia corrected.

Prolonged neonatal jaundice

Significant jaundice persisting beyond three weeks may be a presenting sign of *hypothyroidism* and this eminently treatable disorder should be excluded by estimating thyroxine and thyroid stimulating hormone. In *neonatal hepatitis* babies become increasingly yellow by two to three weeks but manage to conjugate most of the bilirubin so are not liable to get kernicterus. If there is an obstructive element in the hepatitis the skin colour may become greenish and the stools pale. The liver may be enlarged and the baby may fail to thrive. The hepatitis may be due to a congenital infection or alpha-1-antitrypsin deficiency but often no cause is found. Though most babies recover spontaneously some progress to hepatic cirrhosis.

The clinical features of neonatal hepatitis may be indistinguishable from obstructive jaundice secondary to *congenital atresia of the bile ducts*. Differentiation between these disorders usually has to be made before six weeks of life when the infants should be submitted to laparotomy, open liver biopsy and operative cholangiogram. The vast majority have intrahepatic atresia and can be offered hepatic porto-jejunostomy. This operation is claimed to improve bile flow if done within 60 days of life. Otherwise treatment is medical with fat soluble vitamin supplements and a medium chain triglyceride milk, the fat from which may be absorbed directly into the lymphatic system. Survival may be prolonged for a few years. A few babies will be found to have *extra hepatic biliary atresia* and this may be corrected surgically.

Kernicterus

Kernicterus is a disorder in which the basal ganglia are damaged by an accumulation of unconjugated bilirubin (see p. 45). The commonest cause is haemolytic disease. Pre-term babies and ill babies are more susceptible than full-term babies. The warning signs are drowsiness, refusal to suck and hypotonia; spasticity, opisthotonos or fever may occur. Convulsions, coma or death may supervene or apparent recovery take place. Evidence of extra pyramidal involvement in the form of athetosis may develop before the first birthday. Deafness is common. Kernicterus may be prevented by timely exchange transfusion for unconjugated hyperbilirubinaemia.

The respiratory distress syndrome (RDS)

Features of this syndrome are tachypnoea, rib recession and cyanosis. Causes are:- hyaline membrane disease (see p. 36), wet lung syndrome, pneumothorax, aspiration syndrome, pneumonia and diaphragmatic hernia.

The clinical history and physical signs may give clues about the aetiology. In *hyaline membrane disease* an expiratory grunt is present and signs are always found by four hours of age. In *wet lung syndrome* affected babies have a transient tachypnoea for a day or so until their excess fetal lung fluid is reabsorbed. Most clinically significant *pneumothoraces* follow assisted ventilation. The onset is within the first few days of life but may be insidious or acute. The classical physical signs of pneumothorax may be difficult to elicit. A rapid diagnosis may be made by transilluminating the chest. *Aspiration syndrome* is usually due to meconium or milk and may follow asphyxia or an apnoeic attack. *Pneumonia* may follow prolonged rupture of the membranes; infecting organisms include pneumococci, *Haemophilus influenzae* and group B beta-haemolytic streptococci. In *diaphragmatic hernia* severe respiratory distress may be present from birth, sometimes bowel sounds are heard in the chest and the abdomen is scaphoid. Rarer causes of respiratory distress syndrome include lobar emphysema, congenital lung cysts and pulmonary oedema.

In all cases of respiratory distress syndrome it is essential to perform a chest X-ray to help differentiate the different causes. Sometimes two causes may be present in one baby.

Treatment

The general principles of nursing care and oxygen therapy are identical to those described under hyaline membrane disease (p. 36). Pneumothoraces, if large, will need drainage, a diaphragmatic hernia needs surgical repair, congenital pneumonia is treated by systemic antibiotics. Aspiration syndrome is generally treated in the same way as hyaline membrane disease but may be complicated by pneumothorax and infection.

THE INFANT OF A DIABETIC MOTHER

Diabetes mellitus (or gestational diabetes) in the mother may be associated with sterility or a high rate of fetal loss due to abortion or stillbirth. The outlook for these babies is greatly improved if the mother is 'well controlled' throughout her pregnancy. The infant of a poorly controlled diabetic is large-for-date, appears bloated and plethoric. There is an increased incidence of hyaline membrane disease, polycythaemia and congenital malformations. Diabetes mellitus may occur in later life.

The infant of a diabetic mother's obesity results from excess sugar received from the mother *in utero*. The baby's islets of Langerhans exhibit an increase in number and a hypertrophic response to this high sugar. When, however, the sugar supply is suddenly cut off at birth hypoglycaemia occurs. Hypoglycaemia can be prevented by feeding the baby early.

NEONATAL COLD INJURY

Babies most likely to suffer cold injury are born at home in winter but exposure to cold is not unknown in hospital practice, particularly if the baby has been resuscitated. As a routine the baby's temperature should be recorded using a low reading thermometer (down to $25°C$). A normal body temperature at birth will not protect the baby from hypothermia if he is not adequately swaddled and placed in a suitably warm environment. In established hypothermia the baby becomes lethargic and refuses to feed. Though the skin feels cold he may appear deceptively pink in the face, hands and feet, which become oedematous.

Treatment
The baby should be rewarmed slowly using clothes, an incubator and, if necessary, a radiant heat source. Hypoglycaemia should be prevented by dextrose infusion and associated electrolyte and pH disturbances should be corrected.

CYANOSIS IN THE NEWBORN

Peripheral cyanosis is common and is due to coldness of the extremities. It disappears on warming. *Central cyanosis* may best be detected by examining the tongue or trunk in bright sunlight. It may be due to any of the causes of respiratory distress and if this is the case can often be abolished by giving the baby 100 % oxygen to breathe for a few minutes. When the cyanosis is due to congenital heart disease it deepens when the baby cries. Respiratory signs are often absent but there is usually a tachycardia.

   Cyanotic attacks are by definition of short duration. They may follow transient airways obstruction and may be the presenting feature of pulmonary aspiration. They may also occur if there is oesophageal atresia or choanal atresia. A cyanotic episode may be a sign of an *apnoeic attack*. The baby first stops breathing then goes blue and he remains hypoxic until the attack is aborted. In these cases the cause should be elucidated. It may occur spontaneously but may be secondary to overheating or infection or may be a manifestation of a fit. Lastly, methaemoglobinaemia, whether congenital or acquired, produces cyanosis without dyspnoea or distress and may be due to nitrites in water, aniline dyes or the drug phenytoin.

FITS IN THE NEWBORN

Convulsions may be difficult to recognise in the newborn. There may be a cyanotic attack, stiffness, flaccidity, eye rolling, blinking or abnormal posturing. Such signs occurring in the neonatal period should be fully investigated. The date of onset of the fit may be a strong indication as to its cause (see Table 5.1).

Table 5.1 Causes of neonatal convulsions related to age at onset

Date of onset	Causes
First few days	Cerebral birth injury (e.g. anoxia), hypoglycaemia
Middle of first week	Septicaemia (meningitis), kernicterus
End of first week	Low calcium, magnesium or inborn errors of metabolism
Any time	Congenital infection

Treatment is of the underlying cause. Over-stimulation should be avoided. Phenobarbitone 6–8 mg/kg/day in two divided doses is a safe and effective anticonvulsant.

THE FETAL PHENYTOIN SYNDROME

About 10% of children born to mothers on long-term phenytoin therapy for epilepsy develop a characteristic syndrome. Growth may be retarded, the fontanelle is wide, scalp hair is profuse and hypertelorism may be present. The nasal bridge is broad and flat; abnormal, low set ears may be present and the neck may be short and webbed. Hypoplasia of the distal phalanges with altered palmar creases may be noted. Congenital dislocation of the hips may be present. It is associated with increased frequency of neuroblastoma due to disturbance of the neural crest *in utero*.

The fetal alcohol syndrome

Chronic alcoholism, especially weekend 'binges', may cause a characteristic picture similar to the fetal phenytoin syndrome. Microcephaly, short palpebral fissures, maxillary hypoplasia and congenital heart lesions are often present. Mental disorder is common whereas in the fetal phenytoin syndrome it is rare. Epicanthic folds may be present in both.

hypertelorism~ abnormally widely spaced eyes

CHAPTER 6

GROWTH AND DEVELOPMENT

Growth is the increase in size which occurs in infancy and childhood, the *rate* of growth varying from organ to organ; for example the brain grows most rapidly in the first year of life, slowing down progressively with age. The head circumference in the newborn averages 35 cm, at 9 months is 45 cm and at 15 years is only 55 cm. Thus the increase in head circumference from birth to 9 months is the same as from 9 months to 15 years!

The term *development* includes physical growth, as well as maturation of function, emotional and social behaviour. Each of these functions is compared with the normal development of other children of the same age. These norms are referred to as the normal *milestones of development*. They are the end result of the constant play between heredity and environment. Thus congenital deafness may lead to mutism, while lack of environmental stimulation in a child with normal hearing may retard speech development.

PHYSICAL GROWTH

For practical purposes physical growth is estimated by regular measurement of weight and length. In babies the maximum skull circumference should also be measured regularly. In special circumstances other measurements such as skin fold thickness, span, upper and lower segment ratios and chest circumference may be required.

Children do not grow at a constant rate. Growth is most rapid (for weight and length) in early infancy and at puberty. In order to determine if a child is of 'normal' size his measurements should be plotted onto a *percentile chart* appropriate for age and sex. Figures 6.1 and 6.2 show percentile charts for weight and height respectively, for boys aged 2–18 years. If a child's measurement lies on the 50th percentile he is of 'average size'. The 5th and 95th percentile lines are approximately ± 2 standard deviations. If a child's weight falls on the 5th percentile then, at that age, 95% of children are heavier, but only 5% lighter. A normally proportioned child will have similar weight and height percentiles. Parental size should be taken into account.

The *rate of growth* can be assessed by plotting several measurements of different ages. After infancy the normal child grows on or parallel to a percentile line. If he deviates grossly from the average or there is a change in rate of growth, further examination and investigation is necessary, for example obesity or failure to thrive (see pp. 71–73).

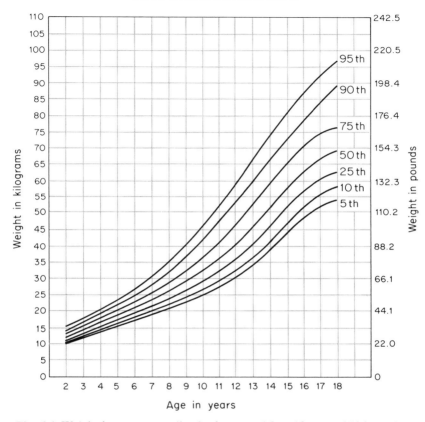

Fig. 6.1 Weight by age percentiles for boys aged 2 to 18 years. (Girls tend to weigh slightly less than boys until 8 years of age, see Table 6.1)

Quick rules for rough estimation of weight and height

Weight in kg = (Age in years + 3) × 2.3
Weight in lb = (Age in years + 3) × 5
Height in cm = 50 cm at birth, 75 cm at 1 year, 100 cm at 4 years,
125 cm at 8 years and 150 cm at 12 years.

or A child is 100 cm at 4 years of age
and gains 5 cm per annum.
See also Table 6.1.

Head circumference

As mentioned already, regular measurement of the maximum skull circumference is particularly important in infancy when growth is most

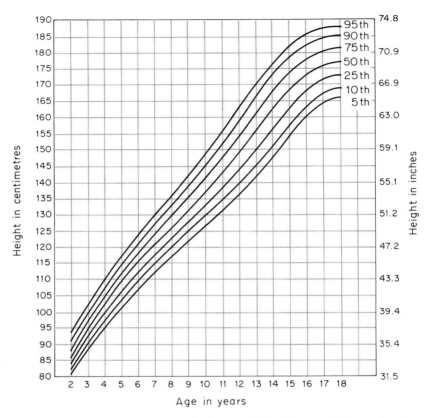

Fig. 6.2 Height by age percentiles for boys aged 2 to 18 years. (Girls tend to be slightly shorter than boys under 9 years of age, see Table 6.1)

rapid. The skull circumference percentile should be compared to the child's weight and length percentile as well as the parents' head circumference percentile. High or low percentiles may indicate micro- or macrocephaly. Changes in *rate* of growth may show that the child is *developing* micro- or macrocephaly.

Figure 6.3 shows the head circumference percentiles for boys up to 3 years of age. Girls heads are slightly smaller, their 95th percentile approximates to the boys' 75th percentile (see also Table 6.2).

Eruption of the teeth

Primary teeth
The primary teeth begin calcifying in the fifth and sixth fetal months. The lower central incisors cut at about 6 months, the rest of the incisors

Table 6.1 Height and weight tables (the ranges given in brackets are between the 5th and 95th percentiles, approximated)

Age	Weight in kg				Height in cm			
	Boys		Girls		Boys		Girls	
Full term	(2.6–4.3)	3.5	(2.4–4.0)		(47–55)	50	(46–54)	
2 months	(4.0–6.6)	4.5	(3.5–6.0)		(55–64)	58	(52–62)	
4 months	(5.0–8.4)	6.5	(4.8–7.4)		(59–67)	62	(56–66)	
8 months	(7–10)	8.5	(6.6–10)		(67–76)	69	(65–74)	
1 year	(8.5–12)	10	(7.8–11.2)		(72–81)	75	(70–79)	
1½ years	(9.5–13.5)	11	(9–12.8)		(77–88)	80	(76–86)	
2 years	(10.5–14.6)	12	(9.8–14.1)		(82–94)	85	(82–92)	
3 years	(12–17)	15	(11–16)		(91–103)	95	(90–102)	
4 years	(14–20)	16	(13–20)		(95–110)	100	(95–108)	
5 years	(15–23)	18	(15–22)		(102–117)	110	(101–116)	
6 years	(17–27)	20	(16–25)		(108–124)	115	(106–123)	
7 years	(18–30)	23	(17–30)		(113–130)	120	(112–130)	
8 years	(20–35)	25	(20–35)		(118–136)	125	(117–136)	
9 years	(22–40)	28	(22–40)		(126–143)	130	(122–143)	
10 years	(25–45)	30	(24–47)		(127–148)	140	(127–150)	
11 years	(27–52)	36	(27–54)		(132–155)	145	(134–156)	
12 years	(30–58)	39	(30–61)		(137–163)	150	(140–163)	
15 years	(44–80)	50	(41–78)		(155–182)	165	(150–173)	

following between 7 and 11 months. The first molars cut at about a year and the second molars at about 2 years. The canines cut at 18 months. There are twenty teeth by 2 years.

Permanent teeth
Eruption of permanent teeth occurs in the following order:

First molars at 6 years
Incisors (central and lateral) at 7–8 years
Cuspids (canines) and premolars at 9–13 years
Second molars at 12 years
Third molars at 18 years or later

There are thirty-two permanent teeth of which twenty-eight cut before puberty. Some permanent teeth begin calcifying shortly before birth, others at 3 years. The third molars may not start calcifying until after 7–10 years.

Bone growth and maturation

Bone age may be predicted with a good degree of accuracy from X-rays of the long bones, but this requires a great deal of experience. It requires a

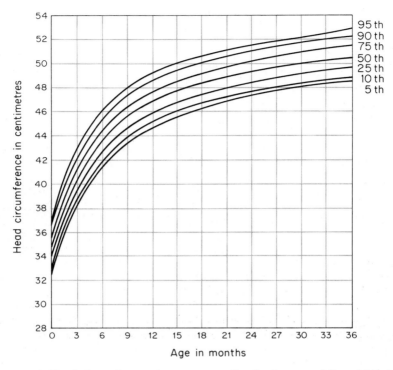

Fig. 6.3 Head circumference by age percentiles for boys aged from birth to 36 months

Table 6.2 Approxiate skull circumference

Age	Skull circumference (cm)
Pre-term	30
Full-term	35
3 months	40
9 months	45
3 years	50
15 years	55
Adult	60

knowledge of the normal ossification centres at different ages, and the various times at which the epiphyses fuse with the zone of provisional calcification. Thus the proximal epiphysis of the tibia is usually present at birth whereas that of the fibula does not appear until about 4 years of age.

Fusion of these epiphyses takes place between 15 and 18 years in boys and 13 and 16 years in girls.

Detailed analysis of skeletal maturation may be required in endocrine diseases, various types of dwarfism and chromosomal abnormalities. It is best left in the hands of a skilled radiologist.

MILESTONES OF DEVELOPMENT

Every practitioner with an interest in children can make a 'Do-it-Yourself Testing Kit' for estimating a baby's maturation. It consists of six wooden cubes, each side being about 2.5 cm in length, a rattle and a bell to attract the baby's attention, a couple of marbles, two or three small, non-rolling objects to test ability to grasp with finger and thumb, a plastic cup to drop small objects into, a golf ball, a tennis ball, an 'ABC' picture book, drawing paper (A4 size or larger), pencil and crayons. These are kept on a tray or in a box. For greater sophistication the reader is referred to R. S. Illingworth's *The Development of the Infant and Young Child— Normal and Abnormal* (Churchill Livingstone, 1980).

For proper assessment the baby or child must be at ease, the mother relaxed and the atmosphere comfortable. The tests are started well below the infant's ability and gradually increased in complexity. If time is limited the tests may be spread over several visits (Table 6.3).

By comparing what the child does with what the mother says he does at home, one can obtain a fairly good idea of the child's achievement. In patients who are difficult to assess, uncooperative or show borderline results, referral to a suitable child assessment clinic for proper testing is advised (see below).

Personal–social tests

A baby smiles spontaneously between 3–5 months, resists a toy being pulled away from him between 6–10 months, plays 'peek-a-boo' from 7–10 months, 'pat-a-cake' 10–13 months and plays ball with the examiner before 15 months. He drinks from a cup messily from 9 months, without spilling before 16 months, uses a spoon skilfully by 2 years, and washes and dries his hands before 3 years. He removes some clothes before 2 years, buttons up by $4\frac{1}{2}$ years. Most children can tie laces by 3 years and dress without supervision by 5 years.

In the preceding tests up to 90% of normal babies achieve the correct responses in the time shown. Many in fact can do them much sooner. Thus when we say that a baby walks well by 14 months, this means that 90% of normal babies do so, 10% take a little longer and must be carefully sifted from abnormal babies who takes very much longer, say 18 months or more. The fact that a few babies walk well before 11 or 12

Table 6.3 Milestones of development

Test	Response
A Gross motor	(90 per cent of babies achieve these responses in time shown.)
1 Lay baby prone; note attempt to lift head and upper part of body	Lifts head 30° by 4 weeks Lifts head 45° by 10 weeks Lifts head 90° by 14 weeks Pushes chest up with arms 12–18 weeks. By 6 months most babies rise almost to 'hands-and-knees' position. May roll over to supine. By 9 months attempts to crawl forwards (but may go into reverse). Crawls 'bottoms-up' by 1 year
2 Lay baby supine and observe	By 3 months may regard own hand; by 6 months may put his foot in his mouth. By 9 months may spontaneously lift head and sit up
(a) Move bright object slowly across baby's line of sight, 30 cm above head, to and fro	Eye follows to mid-line (90°) by 7 weeks; past mid-line by 10 weeks; follows full 180° from 2 to 4 months
(b) Hold object still	Looks at it with interest from 10 weeks on. Reaches for object before 5 months
(c) Grasp hands and pull to sitting position	Head lags behind until about 6 weeks. Thereafter neck increasingly strong. As one starts pulling on hands, neck is seen to 'stiffen' so that head and body pull up together by 5 months
(d) Observe in sitting position	Sits with support, head steady by 3–4 months; sits without support from 6–8 months but leans forward to keep balance and may fall sideways until 9 or 10 months
(e) Pull to standing position	Newborn makes 'stepping movements' until 3–6 weeks of age (reflex action); bears increasing amount of weight on leg from 3–8 months, stands holding on with full weight on legs from 8–10 months, and stands momentarily from 10–12 months. Walks holding onto furniture any time from $7\frac{1}{2}$ to $12\frac{1}{2}$ months. Stands alone well and walks alone well by 15 months
3 'Walk backwards'	Does this by 18–22 months
4 Place patient on steps	Can climb up stairs by 23 months
5 Place ball on floor	Walks into large ball when trying to kick at it by 24 months
6 'Throw ball overhand'	Does this by 2–$2\frac{1}{2}$ years
7 'Pedal tricycle'	Does this by 3 years

Table 6.3 (*Contd.*)

Test	Response
8 'Balance on one foot'	Can balance on 1 foot for 1 second by $3\frac{1}{4}$ years, for 5 seconds by $4\frac{1}{2}$ years and for 10 seconds between 5–6 years
9 Bounce tennis ball	Few catch it before $3\frac{1}{2}$ years, most can catch it by 6 years
B Finer movements	
1 Let patient sit on low chair at table and place a few cubes on it.	Takes 2 cubes by $7\frac{1}{2}$ months, bangs them together before 1 year. Makes tower of 2 cubes before 20 months, 6 cubes by 2 years and 10 cubes by $3\frac{1}{2}$ years. Imitates bridge by 4 years
2 Touch rattle to baby's finger tips	Grasps it before $4\frac{1}{2}$ months, transfers it to other hand when offered 2nd object before 8 months.
3 Place marble or small object on table	Looks at it before 6 months, pokes at objects at 9 months, makes pincer at 12 months (finger-thumb grasp)
(a) Put cup nearby	Puts marble in cup by 1 year, turns it out by 15 months
4 Give patient pencil and paper. Have cards with vertical line, circle, '+' sign and square ready to pass to him	Scribbles until 2 years, copies vertical line by 3 years, circle by 3 years, '+' sign by $4\frac{1}{2}$ years and square before 6 years.
C Language tests	
1 Ring bell	Responds to sound before 1 month
2 Tickle in play	Laughs by 3 months, squeals by 4 months
3 Call baby by his name	Turns to voice by 8 months
4 Say 'Mama'	Repeats 'Mama' before 13 months
5 Name one part of body	Points to one named part by 23 months
6 Point at picture in ABC book	Names 1 or 2 pictures by $1\frac{1}{2}$ years. If given book at 18 months, turns pages 2 or 3 at a time; turns pages singly by $2\frac{1}{2}$ years
7 Point to colours	Recognises 3 colours by 5 years
8 Ask for name	Gives 1st and 2nd name by 4 years

months is evidence of early maturation and not necessarily of a high intelligence. Beware of the mother who reads Spock!

Failure to perform these tests properly may be due to a number of factors. The patient may be tired, ill or unhappy at the time of testing. He may be in a 'negative phase' and refuse to perform. He may be deaf or partially deaf, short-sighted or mentally disordered. He may suffer from inability to concentrate, such as occurs in 'minimal brain dysfunction'. In all cases of doubt, specialised help should be sought. Babies do not 'grow out' of their disabilities—they must be treated skilfully.

The draw-a-man test

For children aged 4–12 years a useful supplementary test is the Goodenough 'Draw-A-Man Test'. The child is given pencil and paper and asked casually to 'draw a man'. The instruction must not be qualified in any way, and the mother must not interfere by adding her bit. A point is given for each detail present.

Head present
Outline more than a circle
Eyes present
    Brow and lashes shown
    Pupil shown
    Correct proportion
    Glance directed to front in pro-
        file view
Ears present
    Correct position and proportion
Nose present
    Nostrils indicated
Mouth present
    Teeth indicated
Hair shown
    Detail present
Chin and forehead shown
    Projection of chin present
Profile with not more than one
    error

Clothing present
Two articles of clothing, none transparent. Four or more articles indicated. Costume complete without incongruity. Firm lines with no overlap at points of junction. Features symmetrical and correct position

Trunk present
Length > breadth.

Shoulders indicated.
More than crude circle.
Neck present
    Neck continuous with head and
        trunk

Arms present
Arms attached to trunk at
    correct point.
Hand shown separately from fore-
    arm and fingers.
Fingers shown
    Correct number
    Shown in two dimensions
    Opposition of thumb shown
    Elbow and shoulder joints
    Arms in proportion

Legs present
Attached to trunk
Knee or hip joint shown
Legs in proportion
Feet in proportion
Heel shown

Both arms and legs in two dimensions. Outline of arms and legs without narrowing at junction with trunk

Example
A child drew the man shown in Fig. 6.4. Points are given for: 1 Head; 2 Eyes; 3 Nose; 4 Mouth; 5 Trunk; 6 Trunk length greater than

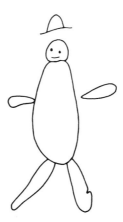

Fig. 6.4 The 'draw-a-man' test

breadth; 7 Arms; 8 Legs; 9 Legs attached to trunk; 10 Both arms and legs in two dimensions; 11 Firm lines.

Score = 11 points.

Each patient starts with 36 months credit. He is given 3 months for each point ($11 \times 3 = 33$ months). Thus he gets $36 + 33$ months = 69 months.

This boy's actual age was 66 months.

His IQ is $\dfrac{\text{Mental Age}}{\text{Chronological Age}} \times 100$

$$= \frac{69}{66} \times 100 = 104.$$

A variation of this test is to ask the patient to 'Draw a tree'. It is strange that enuretic children usually do not draw a tree standing firmly in the soil, but leaning over.

Growing up

'The first Birthday is, of course, a great occasion. . . . But biologically speaking the one-year-old baby is in the midstream of developmental changes which do not come to their fulfilment until about the age of 15 months.'

Arnold Gesell

By fifteen months babies are utterly charming but utterly exhausting to their parents. They crawl, they can walk on a broad base, they love throwing things on the floor, they mess with their food, can say 'Mama' and 'Dada', poke their fingers into holes (like electrical outlets), are learning to handle their bodies, their hands and their minds with increasing skill. And they do the most exasperating things with a happy irresistible gurgle.

By two years they can string two or three words together, can obey simple orders like 'take it to Mummy' and love opening drawers and cupboards. It is an *exploring* age. By two and a half they become very *negative* but this may be because it is easier to say 'no' than 'yes'. It is also an age of obsessions—stories must be repeated *exactly*. The three-year-old is quite skilled and many are toilet trained, but the nicest of all ages is usually four. The child is active, lively and imaginative. He often hero-worships his father, assuring everyone that he is the 'strongest man in the world' and, in fact, exaggerates about everything. He climbs, jumps, counts to 4, repeats nursery rhymes and is in general very lovable. Alas this does not last long and the happy extrovert becomes a nagging introvert at five years. The alternation between extroversion and introversion is very marked in some children, but may be passed unnoticed in emotionally deprived or retarded children who tend to be emotionally 'flat'.

Each age through childhood has its own special characteristics and the interested reader should consult more detailed works.

Discipline has been defined as an educative means by which the parent teaches the child how to become a self-respecting, likeable and socially responsible adult. It is unfortunate that the pioneer work of Gesell should have been so misinterpreted as to lead to the assumption that discipline was not necessary. Any misdemeanour by a child was looked on benignly as 'only a phase of development' through which the child had to pass. Thus if a child messed food on the walls, one had to swallow one's anger (perhaps getting an ulcer in the process) in the belief that the phase would pass. Fortunately there is a swing now in the opposite direction, and it is realised that discipline is not only good for the growing child, but even better as a safety valve for the parent! However, one does not want to replace the naughty undisciplined child with a disciplined but battered one.

CHILD ASSESSMENT CLINICS

Children with chronic mental or physical handicaps and children with abnormal patterns of development invariably require the services of a whole range of different professional workers. These children and their families may be confronted with diverse medical, social, emotional and educational problems which the child assessment clinic is designed to meet. The ways in which child assessment clinics operate vary from area to area depending on local circumstances.

The staff of the child assessment clinic may include a paediatrician, community health doctor, nurses, orthoptist, audiologist, speech therapist, occupational therapist, physiotherapist as well as the social worker, clinical and educational psychologist. The orthopaedic surgeon, ophthalmologist, ENT surgeon, child psychiatrist and family doctor are also closely involved in the work of the clinic.

Whenever a child is referred to such a clinic he is seen by the appropriate members of staff. This usually takes several days, but sometimes a prolonged period of observation is necessary. At the conclusion of the initial assessment the findings are discussed by the assessment team at a conference. In this way children with multiple or complex problems can be fully screened by a multidisciplinary team and a cohesive plan of management worked out.

The parents should be told the findings of the assessment team and the recommendations discussed with them. Where appropriate genetic advice can be given and prognosis discussed. Some parents like a written report to refer back to later on. Arrangements can then be made for the child to receive treatment (e.g. physiotherapy). The clinic can arrange contacts with peripatetic teachers and social workers, for example, and arrange for reviews at the clinic.

CHAPTER 7

INFANT FEEDING AND DISORDERS OF NUTRITION

BREAST FEEDING

Breast feeding is the best way to nourish a human infant. The main advantages of breast milk are its 'naturalness', its digestibility, its sterility and the fact that it requires no special preparation. It is the natural sequel to transplacental nutrition, babies thrive on it and have softer stools. Colic, gastroenteritis and respiratory syncytial virus infection are uncommon in breast-fed babies. The value of the intimate bond forged between mother and baby during breast feeding cannot be over-estimated.

However, in modern times breast feeding does demand some sacrifice. The mother requires privacy, she cannot delegate the job to someone else and may expect sleepless nights until the baby settles into a routine. She also risks engorged breasts, cracked nipples and mastitis. She cannot go out to work while breast feeding unless special arrangements are made for the baby, and social engagements have to be limited for the same reason.

Contra-indications to breast feeding

If the baby is pre-term he may be too weak to suck. Micrognathia and cleft palate are mechanical obstacles. Rarely, phenylketonuria, galactosaemia, maple syrup urine disease and other metabolic disorders require special dietary management.

Debilitating disease in the mother such as tuberculosis, heart disease, thyrotoxicosis, diabetes mellitus, cancer or acute infections make breast feeding hazardous for the mother, while mastitis or breast abscess is painful and requires rest. If one breast is infected it may be possible for the mother to feed her baby with the other. However, it may be necessary to empty the breasts partially to prevent congestion—this can be done manually so that baby is not brought into contact with the infected breast.

Breast milk

The earliest secretion from the breast is *colostrum*—a yellow, sticky, oily substance. A drop or two may dry on the nipple as early as the fourth month of pregnancy and forms a brown scaly deposit on the nipple. This should be wiped off with warm soapy water and the nipple treated with lanolin cream. Spirits should *never* be dabbed onto the nipples to harden them as this predisposes to cracking and infection. The nipples should be kept soft.

Colostrum 'comes in' 48 hours after delivery. It contains twice as much protein (mostly casein) as breast milk, about two-thirds the quantity of lactose and fat, more vitamin A, C and E but less of the other vitamins. It is mildly laxative and, like breast milk, it contains immunoglobulin A, lactoferrin, lysozyme and antiviral substances which all offer the baby some protection against infection.

After four or five days, colostrum changes over to breast milk, a white fluid with a bluish tinge. Normal breast milk never has the full-bodied rich white appearance of cows' milk and often leads to the complaint by mothers that it is 'too watery' or is not nourishing enough for the baby. The differences between the two should be explained. It should be emphasised that cows' milk is designed for calves and breast milk for human babies.

Human milk has half to a third the quantity of calcium and phosphorus, but most of it is in soluble form. Breast milk is distinctly sweeter, contains less than a third of the electrolytes and has much less protein caseinogen than cows' milk. It is therefore much more digestible and less likely to cause oedema (Table 7.1).

Table 7.1 Composition of milk per 100 ml

Milk type	Protein g	Fat g	Carbohydrate g	Sodium mg	Calcium mg	Energy kcal
Breast	1.2	3.8	7.0	15	30	66
Cow's	3.4	3.8	4.8	60	120	66

Note: 66 kcal = approx. 280 kJ

A number of drugs are excreted into breast milk in quantities sufficient to be significant. These include phenytoin (Epanutin), iodides (notably in certain cough mixtures), antithyroid preparations, anticoagulants of the coumarin type, ergot, reserpine, certain laxatives, antineoplastic drugs, cortisone and sex hormones. Adverse reactions in the baby have been reported with sulphonamides, tetracycline, chloramphenicol and iso-niazid. Most other drugs are secreted in small quantities, particularly if they are highly bound to protein. Although the majority of women on drugs may safely breast feed it is wise to observe the baby for possible adverse effects.

The best stimulus to milk formation is breast feeding. The baby is put to the breast every three hours initially and five to ten minutes at each breast is usually more than adequate to empty them. Often, in anticipation of feeding, the mother feels the breast fill with a pleasurable sensation. This is called the 'draught' or 'let-down reflex'.

When a baby feeds at the breast three actions are noted. First, the jaw 'bites' on the areola which compresses the milk sacs. Secondly, the nipple is drawn into the mouth and elongated. Thirdly, the tongue massages the elongated nipple against the hard palate ensuring a continuous flow of milk into the back of the throat. The majority of the milk is taken within the first 2–3 minutes, but the baby should be allowed up to 10 minutes on each breast. Prolonged feeding may lead to tender nipples which crack easily.

Manual expression of breast milk

Manual expression may be necessary to stimulate milk production, to collect milk for a pre-term baby, or to treat breast engorgement (Fig. 7.1).

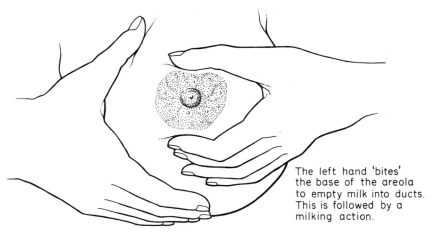

The left hand 'bites' the base of the areola to empty milk into ducts. This is followed by a milking action.

The right hand presses the breast against the chest wall to steady it.

Fig. 7.1 Manual expression of breast milk

The mother grasps the breast between finger and thumb of both hands and with the lower hand gently presses it against the chest wall. It is massaged with the other hand towards the nipple. The rim of the areola is then grasped between the tips of the finger and thumb to compress the milk sinuses (like the bite of baby's gums). This is then pressed against the chest wall and, if properly done, milk should flow. A smooth milking action is soon acquired.

Breast engorgement

Early breast engorgement is mainly vascular but obstruction due to thickened colostrum may be a factor. It is more common amongst primipara. It can be prevented by antenatal expression of colostrum which prevents the ducts from becoming clogged up. If the patient is seen for the first time with swollen, engorged, painful breasts, the engorgement should be relieved by manual expression to establish a free flow of milk. Treatment should be aimed at providing adequate support for the breasts and giving analgesics. The application of hot and cold moist towels to the breast with firm but gentle pressure to relieve pain may be necessary to 'break up the knots'. Maternal fluids can be reduced or a diuretic given. Occasionally it is necessary to inhibit prolactin production by prescribing bromocriptine.

Some problems with breast feeding

Retracted nipple should be diagnosed early in pregnancy, certainly before the sixth month. It may be treated by fitting a Waller Shield over the nipple and keeping it in place by day with a well-fitting bra. It gradually forces the nipple out. Some shields, such as the 'Mexican hat' can be fitted over the nipple at feeding time if the retraction persists.

Painful and cracked nipples can be prevented by washing the breasts properly after feeding. They are treated with an antiseptic such as 0.2 % chlorhexidine. *Breast abscesses* should be drained surgically.

Excess milk may choke the baby. It is treated by having the mother express the first 15–30 ml before each feed.

The mother may complain that her baby has diarrhoea. In actual fact it may be quite normal for breast fed babies to pass a stool after every feed (gastrocolic reflex). Some babies have *infrequent* stools but this does not matter if the stool is soft and easily passed.

Test feeding

In order to determine whether or not a baby is getting enough milk to drink he should be weighed both before and after a feed, the difference in weight being the quantity of feed taken in. Obviously the baby must be weighed with exactly the same clothing, and if he passes urine or stools during the feed, he should be weighed together with these. The procedure should be repeated with each feed over a 24-hour period, as the quantity taken in by the baby varies with each feed. Thus the baby may drink much more in the morning than in the evening. The average infant requires 150–180 ml of milk per kg of body-weight per 24 hours.

Test feeding should not be done too readily as it makes the mother anxious and shows that her attendants are worried.

Underfeeding

A hungry baby is a dissatisfied baby. He is restless and tends to wake at frequent intervals. His weight gain becomes stationary for a while and he then begins to lose weight. The stools tend to become constipated and may be small and tinged with green (*hunger stools*). He gulps his feeds, swallows air and may regurgitate part of his feed, thus aggravating the situation. The restlessness may be interpreted as 'colic' and the baby may be given anticolic medicines in error. Diagnosis may be confirmed by test weighing for 24 hours.

Treatment of underfeeding

One can attempt to increase the flow of breast milk by increasing the mother's fluid intake, by reassurance (especially if it is a first baby) and by stripping the breast after each feed, i.e. after baby has finished sucking to manually express the remaining milk—an empty breast is the best stimulus to milk formation. A relaxed, calm and contented mother also helps, but this is becoming increasingly difficult to achieve in modern society.

The alternative is to supplement the feed with modified cows' milk. Whether one gives a few ounces of milk *after* each breast feed, or whether one replaces alternate breast feeds with a bottle, is a matter of preference, and should be decided in consultation with the mother. It should be emphasised that hunger cannot be cured by prolonging breast feeding beyond 10 minutes per breast, as by this time the breast is usually quite empty.

Overfeeding

Overfeeding may be due to an over-abundance of breast milk and it can be cured by getting the mother to express the first ounce of feed or by increasing the intervals between feeds. Most cases, however, are due to supplementing milk feeds with solids at too early an age. As a result there may be an excess gain in weight initially. Some babies simply get fat, but other develop intestinal distress which is interpreted incorrectly as hunger. One commonly hears of a baby being fed almost continuously day and night 'because he is always hungry'! Many babies protest by vomiting and the weight gain becomes stationary. It is a serious fault to treat the vomiting with anti-emetics when the answer is to rationalise the feed. Many parents equate fatness with good health, so advice about reducing the caloric intake should be given tactfully but firmly. One should emphasise that overweight babies are more susceptible to respiratory infections.

ARTIFICIAL FEEDING

The basis for most artificial feeding is cows' milk. It should always be modified to make it suitable for human babies as follows:

1 It may be diluted with water, usually to two-thirds strength.
2 4% or 5% sugar is added to make up the calories lost by dilution. The end product should have 20 Calories per ounce (1 Cal = 1 kcal; 1 kcal = 4.2 kJ; 1 fl oz = 30 ml).
3 It should be sterilised by boiling. This also precipitates the casein, which can be removed, and makes the milk more digestible.

Example
Make up a feed for a 4 kg baby. A 4 kg infant requires 150 ml/kg/24 hours.

$$\text{Total fluid required} = 4 \times 150 \text{ ml/day}$$
$$= 600 \text{ ml/day}$$

Of this amount two-thirds or 400 ml is cows' milk and 200 ml is water.

The total can be divided by the number of feeds the baby has per day. At first the baby likes to be fed 3–4-hourly throughout the day and night, but by six weeks he is usually satisfied with just five feeds a day, so the family is able to get more sleep.

$$\frac{600}{5} = 120 \text{ ml (4 oz) per feed.}$$

The formula written down for the mother would be:

Cow's milk	400 ml
Water	200 ml
Sugar	30 g (6 level teaspoons)

NB 5% sugar is 5 g/100 ml ∴ 600 ml should contain 6 × 5 = 30 g. Give 120 ml (4 fl oz) of mixture every 4 hours.

Powdered milk

Manufacturers modify cows milk in a variety of ways in order to make it more like human milk (Humanised milk). It is fortified with vitamins A, C, D and iron. The powder is stable, its composition is relatively constant and it is suitable for infant feeding. Each brand has its own particular feature, but none of the milks made for normal babies has a clear advantage over the others. The retail prices vary considerably.

The milk is made up by adding one level scoop of powder per 1 fl oz (30 ml) of cooled boiled water and mixing. It is not necessary to add vitamins, iron or sugar. Clearly, mothers who wish to bottle feed have to be taught how to clean the bottles and teats and how to make up the feeds. Such knowledge is not easily acquired by reading the back of the milk packet or tin.

Special formulae

Special milks are most often prescribed for lactose intolerance or cows' milk allergy. They are usually both lactose-free and cows' milk protein-free. Certain rare diseases require other formulations. These are listed in alphabetical order in the British National Formulary.

Warning
Mothers should be instructed never to mix their scoops, (in other words, the scoop from one tin should never be used for measuring the product of another manufacturer). Mothers should also ensure that they measure *level* scoops, avoid compressing the powder and not add any additional scoops of powder otherwise their baby may receive a dangerously high solute load.

WEANING

Weaning is the process by which infants become accustomed to taking foods other than milk and should usually begin between 4 to 6 months of age. It is not unusual in some parts of Africa and India to see a two or three year old walk up to his mother, or even grandmother, pull out her teat and have a quick suck. Early weaning may lead to obesity.

In our opinion a baby's first food after milk should not be a starchy one. Apple sauce, mashed banana or a finely sieved coloured vegetable such as peas or green beans make good starters. These may be given when the baby weighs 5–6 kg. A teaspoonful is given *before* the midday bottle. If it is well-taken the amount is slowly increased until baby can consume 2 or 3 tablespoonsful. Initially only one of the above foods is given, as babies are not easily bored by food and do not require variety to keep them happy. New feeds should be added *one at a time* and given for at least a week so that, should allergies occur, they are quickly detected and eliminated.

When baby takes his 'lunch' well, he may be given a baby-cereal for breakfast. Within a short time he will settle down to three meals a day, each being followed by a bottle containing 5 or 6 fl oz (150–180 ml) of milk. Between the main meals he may have a bottle or cup of water or fruit juice. Babies should *not* drink more than 24 fl oz (720 ml) of milk per 24 hours, otherwise they will become too easily satisfied with their liquid diet and become finicky about solids. Too often one hears the complaint, 'he wont't eat a thing', only to find that the patient drinks 2–3 pints of milk per 24 hours! It is impossible to eat if one's stomach is filled with clotted milk.

Vitamin and mineral supplements

In the United Kingdom supplements of vitamins A, C and D are recommended for babies through their first 5 years of life unless there is *no doubt* that the child is receiving an adequate intake. Deficiency states are unlikely to occur in term breast-fed infants, or infants fed on 'humanised' milk provided they are weaned by 6–8 months. All low birth-weight babies should have supplements of vitamins A, C, D and iron as their requirements are relatively greater and their stores much less. Iron should be given from 1 to 6 months of age. Very low birth-weight babies also need supplements of vitamin E and folic acid.

PROBLEMS IN NUTRITION

Obesity

Obese children have an excessive amount of subcutaneous fat which makes them heavy in proportion to their height. Such children usually have a weight above the 97th percentile for their age. The commonest cause is overeating. There may be a genetic predisposition in some patients, but this may be due to a family tendency to overeat. It is not known why some people eat excessive calories and still remain thin. They must utilise their energy intake very inefficiently.

Rarely obesity may be a feature of a more generalised morphological abnormality as in the Prader-Willi syndrome, and the Lawrence-Moon-Biedl syndrome when there is also mental disorder. Very rarely is it a presenting sign of an endocrine problem such as Cushing's disease, hypothyroidism or a hypothalamic lesion.

The fat child has a double chin, excess deposits of fat around the breast, abdomen and hips. In fat boys the penis looks deceptively small because it is buried in fat. The skin fold thicknesses are increased and may be plotted on to standard charts. The proximal extremities are large whereas the hands and feet seem relatively small. *Emotional problems* commonly underly overeating but whether this is cause or effect must be assessed in each patient individually.

Treatment

Dietary counselling and *expert* handling of the child's emotional problems are essential to success. It is usually necessary to alter the child's eating habits permanently. A large number of children relapse and then become reluctant to attend the doctor for follow-up. Drug therapy should not be used for primary obesity in children.

Failure to thrive

A child is deemed to be failing to thrive when there is significant slowing in his rate of growth. Weight is usually affected before height. It is not possible to demonstrate a slowing in the rate of growth on a percentile chart when the child first presents if no previous measurements are available. However, the child may be failing to thrive if there is a large discrepancy between his weight and height percentiles or if his weight is below the third percentile. Whenever short stature is the predominant feature dwarfism should be suspected.

In infancy failure to thrive is often due to a feeding problem. The feed may be inadequate in quantity or quality. The technique may be wrong and this can only be detected by actually watching a feed in progress. Some babies are extremely finicky. They have small appetites because they are basically small people and no amount of feeding will fatten them up. The problem may be complicated by a blocked nose, cleft palate or abnormally small jaw. Organic disease should always be excluded, such as chronic infections, especially of the urinary tract. Tuberculosis, syphilis and bilharzia are still commonly found in some countries and should not be forgotten. Congenital disorders of the heart, bowel, urinary tract, cerebral palsy or metabolic diseases such as galactosaemia, infantile renal acidosis or hypothyroidism should be excluded. If failure to thrive occurs after the introduction of gluten into the diet coeliac disease may be the cause. In fibrocystic disease there are usually obvious respiratory symptoms.

Emotional deprivation is an important cause of failure to thrive. The diagnosis can only be made if a full social history is taken and a social enquiry is made into the family. Obviously this should be done before the child is submitted to unpleasant investigations. Characteristically such infants put on weight quickly after coming into hospital. Despite intensive investigation there remains a small number of patients in whom no cause for the failure to thrive can be detected. Some of these grow up to be small adults, others suddenly make a spurt at puberty and grow up to be perfectly normal. Where no obvious cause can be found the situation should be explained carefully to the parents.

Infantile colic

The baby with intestinal colic complains of his discomfort by crying, going red in the face and by drawing his legs up towards his abdomen. The disorder is chronic and should be distinguished from acute surgical conditions like intussusception and also from infantile spasms.

Pain may occur during or after a feed and may be due to the baby feeding too quickly. The rate at which milk is delivered to the breast-fed baby can be reduced if the mother expresses about 30 ml from her breast before starting the feed. Infantile colic may be due to excess wind and this too can be lessened by slowing the rate at which the baby feeds. 'Windy' babies are also helped by lying them prone after a feed so that excess air in the stomach rises to the fundus and escapes painlessly up the oesophagus.

Evening colic is a self-limiting disorder, of unknown cause, which disappears by the time the baby is three months old. It is sometimes called 'three month colic'. The colic begins after the 6 pm feed and is not relieved by feeding or 'winding'. The baby's tired parents find their child difficult to settle and have to comfort him until he finally falls asleep in the late evening. Dicyclomine 5–10 mg before the evening feed often relieves symptoms.

DEFICIENCY STATES

Vitamin Deficiencies

1 Vitamin A

Vitamin A deficiency is characterised by failure to gain weight, night blindness and xerophthalmia. The conjunctivae are dry, wrinkle easily and Bitot's spots, which have a foamy appearance, may be found near the cornea. Keratomalacia (softening of the cornea) with destruction of the anterior chamber of the eye may occur. The skin may be dry, scaly and show prominent follicles. Diagnosis is confirmed by finding low vitamin A levels in the serum and by impairment of dark adaptation.

Treatment

Ten times the normal daily requirement for vitamin A should be given for 10 days. Thus 15 000 to 45 000 i.u. is required daily. In severe cases the first dose should be given intramuscularly. In malabsorption syndrome, in which the fat-soluble vitamin is not readily absorbed, water-soluble forms of the vitamin are available. Overdosage should be avoided as it causes increased intracranial pressure, desquamation of the palms and soles, subcutaneous masses, jaundice and exfoliation of hair.

2 Vitamin D

Deficiency of vitamin D causes rickets. Rickets is a group of disorders characterised by failure of mineralisation of growth cartilage (osteoid) usually associated with a skeletal deformity, hypophosphataemia and generalised hypotonia. Osteomalacia is failure of mineralisation of endosteal bone surface and occurs after the epiphysis has fused. In man vitamin D is derived from the diet and from the skin through the action of ultra-violet light. It is hydroxylated by the liver and then converted into its active form (1,25-dihydroxycholecalciferol ($1,25-(OH)_2D_3$)) by the kidney.

This hormone acts on the gastro-intestinal tract where it stimulates the absorption of calcium and phosphorus, and on bone where synergistic action with parathyroid hormone causes increased bone resorption. Both these actions help to maintain a normal serum calcium concentration.

Causes of rickets

1 Vitamin D deficiency due to:
   (a) Inadequate sunlight
   (b) Inadequate vitamin D in diet
   (c) Malabsorption syndromes.
2 Increased vitamin D metabolism due to liver enzyme induction by anticonvulsants, e.g. phenytoin, phenobarbitone.
3 Failure to produce 1,25-dihydroxycholecalciferol due to:
   (a) Vitamin dependency rickets
   (b) Renal failure.
4 Increased phosphate loss due to:
   (a) Hypophosphatemic vitamin D resistant rickets
   (b) Fanconi's syndrome.
5 Lack of alkaline phosphatase due to hypophosphatasia (rare).

Vitamin D deficient rickets

This form of rickets is seen in countries where there is limited sunlight or a high degree of atmospheric pollution. With the advent of vitamin D supplementation of milk and margarine and other foods vitamin D deficiency is less commonly seen in developed countries although it is still a problem in the Asian population in Britain. In developing countries the custom of covering infants to protect them from sunlight or the custom of purdah prevents an adequate exposure to ultra-violet light and thus increases the risk of developing rickets or osteomalacia. Neonatal rickets can occur in babies of very low birth-weight especially those who have received prolonged intravenous feeding.

Clinical features
Infantile rickets usually occurs between six months and two years of age, though in pre-term babies it may occur as early as two to three months. Pallor of the skin, due to lack of sunshine, and sweating of the forehead may be early signs. The head has a squarish appearance due to frontal bossing while wide sutures suggest a 'hot-cross bun'. The anterior fontanelle may not close until long after 18 months. Craniotabes is common. The primary dentition may show enamel defects and caries; the permanent teeth, which normally start cutting after six years of age, may show horizontal lines of discolouration and hypoplasia due to rickets in babyhood.

Ricketty rosary is swelling of the costo-chondral junctions. The epiphyses of the long bones are thickened and this is best detected at the wrist. The weight-bearing bones (arms in crawling infants, legs when they walk) become bowed. In the legs one finds knock-knees with lateral and forward bowing of the lower third of the leg.

Generalised hypotonia with lax ligaments is usual, resulting in a 'floppy' baby. Traction by the diaphragm causes depression and flaring of the lower ribs (Harrison's sulcus). This pushes the liver and spleen downwards so that they are palpable.

Radiology

Rickets is characterised by the overproduction of osteoid which fails to calcify. It is often diagnosed primarily by the radiologist when an X-ray of the chest happens to show broadening and cupping of the rib ends or of the inferior angle of the scapula. The best site for diagnosing rickets is the wrist. (See Fig. 7.2).

The distal ends of the long bones appear widened and cupped ('champagne glass appearance'). The space between the epiphysis and diaphysis is increased because the thick rachitic metaphysis is uncalcified and therefore radio-translucent. There is general decalcification of the skeleton leading to pathological fractures which heal with callus formation. The appearance of periostitis is due, not to inflammation, but to the presence of uncalcified osteoid under the periosteum.

With healing, a zone of preparatory calcification appears, proximal to the epiphyseal cartilage. Calcification of the osteoid proceeds from the diaphysis towards this line.

Clinical pathology

The plasma inorganic phosphate falls below 1.1 mmol/l (normal 1.4–2.1 mmol/l). The serum calcium is usually within normal limits (2.2–2.7 mmol/l) but this is attained at the expense of bone calcium. In some cases, however, the serum calcium falls to 1.8 mmol/l or less and tetany results. This may also occur during early *healing* when large quantities of calcium are suddenly withdrawn from the plasma to be deposited in bone.

The serum alkaline phosphatase level may be regarded as an indication of activity in rickets. In normal infants it is under 25 King Armstrong units. In severe rickets it may rise to over 100 KA units. With healing it slowly returns to normal.

Treatment

Rickets is often associated with other evidence of malnutrition, therefore a well-balanced diet, including iron and other vitamin supplements should be prescibed when indicated. Vitamin D 2500–5000 i.u. daily should produce healing in 4–6 weeks. If not, the possibility of other causes of rickets should be considered. Additional calcium may be given but is not usually essential, unless tetany co-exists.

Overdosage with vitamin D causes hypercalcaemia. This complication may lead to extensive deposition of calcium in the tissues. The serum calcium should be monitored during treatment. If it becomes high treatment should be stopped. Very high levels of serum calcium may quickly be reduced by giving prednisolone 20–30 mg/day. Calcitonin may be of use. Maintenance of an adequate urinary output is essential.

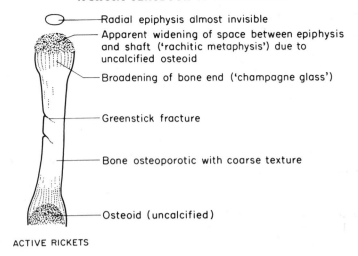

Radial epiphysis almost invisible

Apparent widening of space between epiphysis and shaft ('rachitic metaphysis') due to uncalcified osteoid

Broadening of bone end ('champagne glass')

Greenstick fracture

Bone osteoporotic with coarse texture

Osteoid (uncalcified)

ACTIVE RICKETS

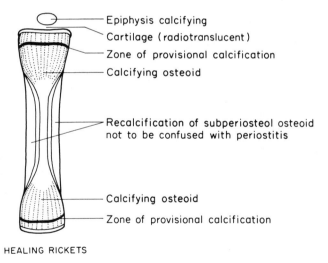

Epiphysis calcifying

Cartilage (radiotranslucent)

Zone of provisional calcification

Calcifying osteoid

Recalcification of subperiosteol osteoid not to be confused with periostitis

Calcifying osteoid

Zone of provisional calcification

HEALING RICKETS

Fig. 7.2 Infantile rickets

Rickets due to renal failure

Renal rickets is a failure of the kidney to excrete phosphate leading to hyperphosphataemia. Serum calcium is usually very low but can be normal. Blood urea is invariably raised. The serum potassium is often increased. Radiologically the picture is that of rickets and dwarfism. In prolonged cases evidence of hyperparathyroidism may become prominent (page 206). Rickets should be treated with large doses of vitamin D, and it is especially important to monitor the serum calcium as there may be pre-existing hypercalcaemia. Hyperphosphataemia should be controlled with oral phosphate binders such as aluminium hydroxide, the use of iron exchange resins, correction of acidosis, haemodialysis and renal transplantation should be considered.

Hypophosphataemic vitamin D resistant rickets

Hypophosphataemic rickets is a specific defect of phosphate reabsorption by the renal tubules. It is inherited as an X-linked dominant disorder and manifests in males with hypophosphataemia, rickets and dwarfism. In countries where vitamin D deficiency has been eradicated by vitamin D supplementation of food, hypophosphataemic rickets is now the commonest (albeit rare) cause of rickets in children. Girls with the disease may manifest only hypophosphataemia while others may present with a classical rickets. The serum calcium is normal and the phosphate is very low. Treatment is with oral phosphate supplements (1.5–3 g/day) and vitamin D (2500–5000 i.u. daily) or 1,25-dihydroxycholecalciferol (0.5–1 μg/day) may be given. The dose of vitamin D should be reduced in the presence of hypercalcaemia.

In the *Fanconi syndrome* hypophosphataemic rickets is associated with amino-aciduria and glycosuria. It may be congenital or secondary to cystinosis or it may follow the administration of degraded tetracycline. Treatment is with large doses of phosphate, correction of acidosis and hypocalcaemia with sufficient vitamin D supplements to keep the serum calcium within normal limits.

3 Vitamin E

Deficiency of vitamin E is sometimes seen in pre-term babies in whom it causes oedema and a haemolytic anaemia. The haemolysis occurs usually between 6–10 weeks of age and is more prominent in infants fed on cows milk. It may be prevented by giving vitamin E 25 i.u./day. Vitamin E supplements have been shown to reduce the severity of retrolental fibroplasia in susceptible neonates. In older children the vitamin does not appear to have any place in therapy.

4 Vitamin B₁ (aneurine)

Deficiency of aneurine is liable to occur in infants fed on faddy diets and diets containing polished rice (leading to beri-beri). Anorexia, vomiting, constipation and oedema may occur early. Heart signs include enlargement of the heart and signs of congestive heart failure. CNS signs may predominate and include apathy, drowsiness, peripheral neuritis, absent deep reflexes, sensory nerve changes and convulsions. Hoarseness due to laryngeal nerve palsy occurs. Patients with beri-beri should be given 12 mg of aneurine per day, which is ten times the normal daily requirement. This should be combined with other vitamins in the B complex and a properly balanced diet.

5 Vitamin B₂ (riboflavine)

Riboflavine deficiency causes cheilosis, angular stomatitis, glossitis (smooth tongue), keratitis and seborrhoeic skin lesions. Photophobia may occur. Treatment consists of riboflavine 3–10 mg/day orally with vitamin B compound mixtures and a balanced diet.

6 Vitamin B₆ (pyridoxine)

The baby of a mother who has been treated with large doses of pyridoxine in early pregnancy may become pyridoxine-dependent and may require up to 1 g of the vitamin daily to prevent convulsions. Pyridoxine deficiency may result from isoniazid administration, which, in infancy, causes infantile convulsions and peripheral neuropathy. There may be cheilosis, glossitis and seborrhoeic dermatitis. To prevent these symptoms in patients on isoniazid 25 mg of pyridoxine daily is adequate.

7 Nicotinic acid (niacin)

Deficiency of niacin leads to *pellagra* ('rough skin') after a prolonged period of vague symptoms such as anorexia, weakness, burning feet, numbness and dizziness. The three 'D's' of pellagra are diarrhoea, dermatitis and dementia. Skin lesions occur in areas exposed to sunlight—the face, neck, hands and feet. They become thick, pigmented and rough and have the appearance of snake skin. Diarrhoea is often associated with stomatitis and glossitis. The dementia refers to the depression, disorientation, delirium and disturbances of sleep. Treatment is with nicotinamide in preference to nicotinic acid as it is free of the unpleasant vasodilating effects of the latter. The dose is 50–300 mg/day orally or, if diarrhoea is severe, 50–100 mg daily by injection.

8 Folic acid and vitamin B₁₂

See Blood Disorders (p. 96).

9 Vitamin C (ascorbic acid)

Deficiency of vitamin C causes *scurvy*, a rare disturbance of collagen formation. There is sufficient vitamin C in breast milk to prevent scurvy in the baby, provided that the mother is not herself deficient.

Scurvy occurs between six months and two years of age. It is characterised by progressive irritability and tenderness to the touch due to subperiosteal haemorrhage into the lower femur and tibia. Pain in the legs prevents movement (*pseudoparalysis*). Haemorrhages occur into the gums, skin, mucus membranes and internal organs. Anaemia is common.

X-rays show a white line at the ends of the long bones (Fig. 7.3). Subsequently an area of destruction occurs proximal to this white line. The periosteum is raised due to subperiosteal bleeding. The cortex becomes thinned and the trabeculae have a ground glass appearance. The epiphyseal centres are sharply outlined like 'signet-ring'. Epiphyseal separation may occur.

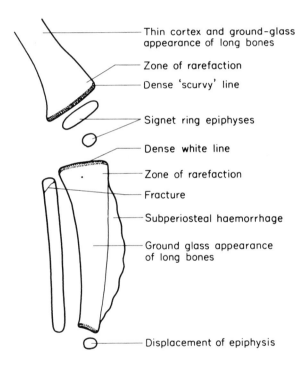

Thin cortex and ground-glass appearance of long bones

Zone of rarefaction

Dense 'scurvy' line

Signet ring epiphyses

Dense white line

Zone of rarefaction

Fracture

Subperiosteal haemorrhage

Ground glass appearance of long bones

Displacement of epiphysis

Fig. 7.3 Scurvy

The diagnosis is confirmed by injecting 100 mg of ascorbic acid in normal saline intravenously and measuring the amount excreted in the urine in the ensuing 3 hours. Patients with scurvy excrete less than 5 mg.

Scurvy is treated by giving vitamin C 100 mg daily. Recovery occurs within a few days. The subperiosteal haemorrhages calcify and may take months to disappear. Metaphyseal separation will correct itself.

metaphysis - wide part at end of shaft of a long bone adjacent to epiphysis

10 Vitamin K

Vitamin K in man is derived from food stuffs and is also synthesised in the intestine by bacteria. It depends on the presence of bile salts for proper absorption. Deficiency may result from inadequate dietary intake, poor intestinal absorption, severe liver disease, prolonged antibiotic therapy and anticoagulant therapy. Deficiency leads to hypoprothrombinaemia and spontaneous haemorrhages may occur into organ tissues. Vitamin K_1 (phytomenadione) is the least toxic form of vitamin K and should be given to all newborns to prevent *haemorrhagic disease of the newborn* due to hypoprothrombinaemia. The dose for small babies is 0.25–0.5 mg and for full-term babies 1 mg intramuscularly. In older children doses of between 5–20 mg may be used to prevent or treat vitamin K deficiency due to other causes. The prothrombin level should rise within 15 minutes and the clotting time should be shortened.

Iron deficiency

See page 95.

Protein-energy malnutrition (PEM)

Protein-energy malnutrition covers a spectrum of disorders in which there is protein deficiency, calorie (energy) deficiency or various combinations of these. Two forms are described here, kwashiorkor and marasmus, though it should be recognised that there may be considerable overlap between the two.

Kwashiorkor

Kwashiorkor is a severe form of protein-energy malnutrition in which deficiency of essential amino acids is associated with an adequate calorie intake provided mainly by starches. It is almost unknown in breast-fed infants. It commonly occurs in infants who have been weaned on to high carbohydrate low protein feeds, and occurs chiefly between four months and two years of age, sometimes later.

It is characterised by a 'sugar baby' face, failure to gain weight, irritability progressing to apathy, loss of appetite and the development of generalised oedema. The height and weight are below the third percentile for the age. Hypokalaemia leads to marked hypotonia and abdominal distension. The hair becomes thin, sparse and loses its normal black colour. It often has a light grey, brown or reddish colour. The 'flag sign' seen in some parts of the world, consists of alternating stripes of dark and light pigmentation of the hair due to varying periods of good and poor protein intake. Typical skin lesions consist of areas of increased pigmentation and depigmentation of the extremities. Large bullous lesions which burst are common, and should not be mistaken for burns. Hepatomegaly is common though cirrhosis does not usually occur. Ascites is not a feature.

Infection occurs frequently in kwashiorkor, particularly tuberculosis, otitis media, pneumonia, pyelonephritis and gastroenteritis. The latter commonly aggravates the oedema and one sometimes sees the curious anomaly of dehydration occurring at the same time as oedema of the lower extremities. It has been attributed to hypokalaemia of the tissues. Parasitic infections, notably roundworm and *Giardia lamblia* infestations occur.

There is usually some evidence of vitamin deficiencies. Vitamin B deficiency is probably the cause of the cheilosis, stomatitis and angular stomatitis which is commonly seen, though some authorities implicate amino acid deficiency. Vitamin A deficiency should be looked for as xerophthalmia may lead to blindness. Overt rickets is not usually seen as the patient is not actively growing. However it may develop when the patient recovers unless vitamin D supplements are given. Scurvy is rarely associated with PEM.

Laboratory findings
The serum albumin falls to below 25 g/l and sometimes to less than 10 g/l. Compensatory increase of gamma globulin occurs but the total protein remains low. The blood urea and cholesterol also remain low. The blood sedimentation is low during the acute illness but increases paradoxically with clinical improvement. The serum potassium and magnesium and the total body potassium and magnesium are low. Anaemia is common and may be normochromic or hypochromic; rarely macrocytic anaemia may occur.

Differential diagnosis
Kwashiorkor should be distinguished from the oedema of the *nephrotic syndrome* and *acute nephritis* by examination of the urine. In kwashiorkor there is rarely more than 1 + albumin, whereas in renal disease it is 2 + to 4 +. Ascites is common in nephrosis and almost never occurs in kwashiorkor even when oedema is severe. *Protein-losing enteropathy* may cause problems as it may develop in patients with kwashiorkor.

Congestive heart failure is characterised by engorged neck veins and liver, and marked dyspnoea. The oedema is not associated with a 'sugar baby' face.

Treatment
Initially fluid and electrolyte disturbances should be corrected. A diet containing adequate but not excessive protein and potassium should be given. Initially half-cream milk, which is a good source of both, may be used, especially if there is diarrhoea. Full-cream milk is introduced when the diarrhoea ceases. Skimmed milk is no longer recommended as some fat is required to produce formed stools. It may be used, however, to *prevent* kwashiorkor and 30–60 g daily, mixed in the diet, may be

sufficient. Other sources of protein such as meat, fish, eggs or cheese may be used. Pronutro is a suitable vegetable protein mixture. Supplementary vitamins should be given if the diet itself is deficient in these. Folic acid and iron may be necessary. Brewer's yeast is a good source of both vitamin B and protein. Milk of magnesia 2.5 ml once or twice daily will replace magnesium without aggravating the diarrhoea.

Secondary infections, particularly gastroenteritis, should be treated vigorously, parenteral fluids being given as required. Prolonged starvation is not recommended and feeds should begin within 12–24 hours even if the diarrhoea persists. If there is evidence of disaccharidase deficiency (sour smelling, acid stools) then lactose or other offending sugars should be omitted from the diet temporarily. Antibiotics are given when indicated for otitis media or other respiratory infection, isoniazid for tuberculosis. Parasites such as giardia and worms should be eliminated.

The patient may be expected to improve in the first week or ten days of treatment. The oedema disappears leaving behind a skinny, underweight infant. The patient becomes less irritable and is soon able to sit up and feed himself.

Marasmus

Marasmus is a form of protein-energy malnutrition due to starvation, *all* the elements in the diet being deficient. It may be due to inadequate calorie intake, faddy diets, chronic intestinal disease, metabolic disorders or chronic infection such as tuberculosis.

The clinical picture is that of emaciation, both weight and length being stunted. There is absence of subcutaneous fat so that the skin, especially on the inside of the thighs, hangs in folds. Peristaltic waves are easily seen through the thin abdominal wall. Oedema is characteristically absent. In marasmus the serum proteins are only moderately reduced whereas in kwashiorkor they are markedly reduced. Constipation is usual but small green 'hunger' stools may be present. In older children listlessness, poor school performance and recurrent infections are a feature. Retarded bone growth and delayed puberty are liable to occur.

Treatment
Underlying infections should be treated as this causes poor appetite and aggravates the disorder. A well-balanced diet should be provided with small snacks between meals if necessary. Social problems should be referred to the appropriate agency. Marasmus is not a condition which can be cured by a bottle of medicine.

Prevention
Protein-energy malnutrition thrives in areas of poverty and ignorance and its occurrence is a disgraceful reflection on the World Community.

The physician is morally bound to support all agencies such as family planning clinics, maternal and child welfare clinics, social welfare agencies and health and nutritional projects dealing with these problems. Both national and international efforts are required to eliminate what Hansen has called 'the biggest public health problem of our times'.

Rumination

Rumination is the rare habit of 'chewing the cud' developed by some babies. It begins with the regurgitation of small quantities of feed which are re-swallowed. The baby obviously enjoys the process, which has been attributed to emotional deprivation. Unfortunately the quantity brought up eventually exceeds that which is swallowed and the baby becomes progressively wasted (marasmus).

Treatment
It may be very difficult to break the habit of almost continuous regurgitation. Thickening milk feeds with Nestargel or feeding the baby with thick gruels may be helpful. His attention needs to be constantly distracted from the habit. Small doses of chlorpromazine, which acts as a tranquilliser and anti-emetic, may help some infants. When rumination is due to deprivation the baby needs love and attention.

CHAPTER 8

FLUID AND ELECTROLYTE DISTURBANCES

Infants are more susceptible to loss of water than older children because of their relatively greater metabolic rate and surface area. They also tend to lose more insensible water and heat from their skin surface, and their daily turnover of water is greater. Therefore an infant who loses excess water by diarrhoea and vomiting, or is deprived of water for even a short time, is liable to suffer more severely than an older child.

It is important to recognise the differences in composition between the intracellular and extracellular compartments. Inside the cell the most important cations are potassium (155 mmol/l) and magnesium (16 mmol/l), whereas outside the cell sodium (140 mmol/l) predominates. Of the anions phosphate, sulphate and protein are the most important intracellularly, whereas outside the cell chloride and bicarbonate are the most important. In each compartment the total sum of the cations equals that of the anions.

ELECTROLYTE DISORDERS

Hypokalaemia

Potassium loss in children may be due to:

1 Gastro-intestinal losses:
    (a) Diarrhoea and vomiting.
    (b) Gastro-intestinal fistulae or suctioning.
    (c) Laxative abuse.
    (d) Resins that exchange K^+ or Na^+.
2 Renal loss:
    (a) Associated with metabolic acidosis and alkalosis, and respiratory alkalosis.
    (b) Due to diuretics.
    (c) Renal-tubular disorders.
3 Endocrine factors:
    (a) Hyperadrenocorticalism.
    (b) Cushing's disease.
    (c) ACTH or corticosteroid therapy.
    (d) Primary aldosteronism.
    (e) Recovery from diabetic acidosis.

4 Reduced dietary intake:
   (a) Protein-energy malnutrition.
   (b) Prolonged intravenous feeding with inadequate K^+ replacement.

Clinical features
Hypokalaemia may be quite severe before symptoms develop. Classically generalised weakness, hypotonia, paralytic ileus and cardiac changes occur. It should be remembered that in *metabolic acidosis* there may be marked bodily depletion of potassium yet the serum potassium may be normal (3.5–5.5 mmol/l). In *metabolic alkalosis* the serum potassium is commonly below 3 mmol/l.
   ECG changes occur in the following order:

1 Slight prolongation of Q-T interval (in hypocalcaemia the S-T segment is longer).
2 Flattening, prolongation and inversion of T waves.
3 Depression of S-T segment.
4 Ventricular extrasystoles and A-V block may occur.

These changes are not specific unless confirmed by a low serum potassium level.

Treatment
The potassium deficit should be estimated and replaced slowly over 72 hours *or longer*. If renal function is satisfactory any excess will be excreted. If there is extrarenal uraemia due to dehydration, this should be corrected, and a good renal flow ensured before giving parenteral potassium. Up to 140 mmol/m²/day may be given safely parenterally. This may be given as half-strength Darrow's solution which contains about 18 mmol potassium per litre, or a concentrated solution of potassium chloride may be used for preparing 'home-made' solutions. However, the concentration of potassium should *never* exceed 40 mmol/l. As soon as the serum potassium level rises above 4 mmol/l the potassium should be reduced to maintenance levels. The best form for oral use is potassium chloride (KCl). It should be remembered that pure fruit juices (apple, orange, guava) and milk contain 30–40 mmol/l of potassium and this should be kept in mind in estimating daily requirements. In the presence of renal failure potassium intake should be sharply reduced unless dialysis is undertaken. This applies also to oliguria due to shock or dehydration. *Acidosis and alkalosis* should be corrected simultaneously with potassium replacement. In *diabetic acidosis* potassium phosphate salts are recommended because hypo-phosphataemia is usually present.

Potassium intoxication (Hyperkalaemia)

Hyperkalaemia means a serum potassium level of over 6 mmol/l. In premature babies 7 mmol/l is perhaps the danger level.

It is liable to occur in acute renal failure and in oliguric shock due to release of potassium from damaged cells. This may occur in drowning or haemolytic crises when large numbers of red cells break down in a short period. Renal failure may be associated with decreased potassium excretion.

Clinical features

There are no specific clinical features. The history should provide the early warning signals and the serum potassium level should be measured. Paraesthesia and mental confusion may occur. Slowing of the heart, a fall in blood pressure and cardiac arrest may occur.

Electrocardiogram

1 T waves become tall and peaked.
2 QRS lengthens.
3 P-R interval lengthens.
4 Gross irregularity and ventricular fibrillation.

Treatment

No potassium should be given by any route. Calcium gluconate 10% 2.5–5 mmol/m² may be given slowly intravenously under ECG control, to reduce the cardiac toxicity of potassium. The serum potassium level may be reduced by:

1 Peritoneal dialysis using potassium-free solutions
2 Haemodialysis
3 Exchange resins such as Resonium A (Kayexalate) orally or as an enema, repeated until the serum K^+ falls below 5 or 5.5 mmol/l. (Danger—hypernatraemia!) Resonium A 1 g/kg/day ÷ 4 will drop serum K^+ by ± 1 mmol/l
4 Intravenous glucose 10% with 1 unit of insulin per 2 g of glucose drives K^+ into the cell temporarily. It is important that a reliable i.v. line is available to continue i.v. therapy with glucose in the event of hypoglycaemia.

Hyponatraemia

Hyponatraemia may be classified into four groups:

1 Acute salt depletion.
2 Acute dilutional hyponatraemia.
3 Chronic dilutional hyponatraemia.
4 Inappropriate secretion of antidiuretic hormone.

1 Acute salt depletion

For example, gastro-intestinal losses, adrenal crisis, excess sweating in cystic fibrosis, or removal of too large a volume of ascitic fluid in cirrhotic patients. The common feature is hypotonic dehydration and shock. The serum sodium is less than 126 mmol/l and osmolality normal. It causes peripheral vascular collapse, hypothermia, weakness, thirst, behaviour changes and convulsions. There is evidence of dehydration.

Treatment
Intravenous sodium chloride 2–3 % if there are convulsions; otherwise normal saline until the serum sodium and chloride are normal. The dehydration should be corrected subsequently with a hypotonic solution such as half-strength Darrow's solution.

2 Acute dilutional hyponatraemia

Acute dilutional hyponatraemia or true water intoxication is due to overhydration with salt-free solutions, the use of large tap water enemas in Hirshprung's disease, to excess antidiuretic hormone formation following operations (in some patients, not all) or vasopressin overdose. Also morphine overdose may have this effect.

Clinical features
Water retention causes increase in weight, cerebral oedema, convulsions and coma. The serum sodium is less than 126 mmol/l and the plasma osmolality is *low* (less than 274 mOsmol/kg of serum). The urine osmolality is usually less than that of the plasma.

Treatment
If there are no symptoms, withholding water and the cautious use of a diuretic may solve the problem. If there are symptoms hypertonic saline 3 % may be given rapidly as the convulsions do not respond to anticonvulsants.
The dose of sodium required is calculated as follows:

$$(140 - X) \times 0.3 \times \text{weight in kg} = \text{mmol Na}^+ \text{ needed,}$$
where X = serum sodium of patient.

3 Chronic dilutional hyponatraemia

This occurs in nephrosis, oedematous glomerulonephritis, malnutrition and congestive heart failure. The condition is aggravated by a low salt diet and diuretics. Giving these patients hypertonic sodium chloride may *increase* the oedema. Water restriction may help some patients.

4 Inappropriate secretion of antidiuretic hormone

This can be due to meningitis, severe pulmonary tuberculosis, and other severe illnesses (see p. 194). These patients are normally hydrated but the serum sodium is low. They usually produce small volumes of urine, and the urine osmolality is commonly greater than that of the plasma.

Treatment

Treatment is by water restriction.

Hypernatraemia

Hypernatraemia means a serum sodium of more than 145 mmol/l and is associated with marked thirst. If the child has access to water there is no problem. If however he is unconscious, or if concentrated milk or excess salt is given, or if water is withheld for any reason, hypernatraemia may occur. It is liable to cause brain damage and if a lumbar puncture is done a marked increase in protein may be found. Subdural effusions occur. The commonest cause of hypernatraemia is gastroenteritis (*hypertonic dehydration*).

Treatment

Sodium chloride 0.3 % in 5 % dextrose-in-water should be given, the serum sodium being closely monitored. Too rapid rehydration may precipitate convulsions. Salt-free solutions should never be used. On the second or third days half-strength Darrow's solution is usually suitable, depending on the serum sodium and potassium levels. Calcium gluconate 10 % may be required in some patients.

The underlying cause of the hypernatraemia should be treated. Phenobarbitone or diazepam may be given to control convulsions.

ACID-BASE DISTURBANCES

Disturbances of acid-base equilibrium are common in infants and children and can be diagnosed by blood gas analysis. Arterial blood should be taken if an accurate Po_2 is required, otherwise free flowing capillary blood may be adequate (consult your laboratory on this matter). In newborns an arterial line may be placed in the umbilical or radial artery or blood may be taken from a radial artery stab. Some practitioners prefer the temporal or femoral artery in older children. The specimen in its syringe or capillary tubes should be packed in ice and tested as soon as possible.

The pH and Pco_2 are measured and the *base excess* is derived from special graphs. The following important information can be obtained from blood gas analysis:

1 If the Pco_2 is less than 35 a state of *respiratory alkalosis* exists. This is commonly due to overbreathing, as in anxiety states, overventilation with a respirator, or in head injury. It occurs in the early phase of aspirin poisoning. It indicates that pulmonary compensation is taking place.

2 If the Pco_2 is more than 55 a state of *respiratory acidosis* exists. This indicates CO_2 retention due to asphyxia, respiratory disease like

asthma, Cheyne-Stokes respiration, central or respiratory depression due to opiates.

3 If the base excess is more than 5 mmol/l a state of *metabolic alkalosis* exists. It may be due to loss of hydrogen ion by excess vomiting or due to excess intake of sodium bicarbonate. Initially the urine is alkaline, but depletion of chloride and potassium in the urine leads to *paradoxical aciduria.*

4 If there is a base deficit of 5 mmol/l (often expressed clumsily as a 'base excess of minus 5') a state of *metabolic acidosis* exists. It is due to loss of bicarbonate ions as in diarrhoea, or the retention of fixed acids as in diabetes mellitus, starvation ketosis, and late salicylate poisoning.

The normal pH of the blood is 7.35–7.45. Below this figure indicates *acidaemia* and in extreme cases of infantile gastroenteritis the pH may fall as low as 6.90. A pH above 7.45 indicates *alkalaemia.* It should be emphasised that acidosis and alkalosis may occur without change of pH because of compensatory mechanisms, mainly pulmonary. Should the pH fall as in acidaemia, or rise as in alkalaemia, then clearly these compensatory mechanisms have become exhausted and urgent therapy becomes necessary to prevent death.

Treatment
Respiratory alkalosis may be treated by re-breathing into a bag. For tetany, if re-breathing is inadequate, intravenous calcium may be infused.

Respiratory acidosis due to hypoventilation (pulmonary disease or respiratory depression) requires artificial ventilation to reduce carbon dioxide narcosis. Extreme care is required lest the patient be precipitated into alkalosis. It should be remembered that compensatory bicarbonate retention occurs in the kidney and chloride must be supplied to assist this adjustment.

Metabolic alkalosis due to vomiting should be treated by stopping the vomiting, e.g. by Rammstedt operation for congenital hypertrophic pyloric stenosis. Alkalis, especially bicarbonate, should be stopped. Sodium chloride and potassium chloride given together will supply the excess of chloride ions required to correct the alkalosis. It is rarely necessary to use ammonium chloride. Treatment should be aimed at correcting the underlying condition.

Metabolic acidosis due to loss of bicarbonate ions in severe diarrhoea requires urgent treatment if the pH falls below 7.1. The patient should be rehydrated and sodium bicarbonate given according to the formula:

Base deficit × 0.3 × weight in kg = mmol sodium bicarbonate required

The deficit should not be corrected too rapidly, as renal compensatory mechanisms are also at work for the patient and over-enthusiastic correction may cause a dangerous alkalosis. If half the deficit is corrected in the first 24 hours one can usually feel satisfied. Glucose should always be given to correct starvation ketosis. The serum electrolytes should also be controlled. For diabetic keto-acidosis see p. 213. For treatment of gastroenteritis see p. 250.

The anion gap

The concept of the anion gap is useful for understanding the relationship between electrolyte and metabolic disturbances.

$$\text{Anion gap} = Na^+ - (Cl^- + HCO_3^-)$$

Normal anion gap is 8–16 mmol/l (mean 12 mmol/l).

Sodium forms more than 90 % of the cations in the extracellular fluid while the sum of chloride and bicarbonate forms more than 85 % of the anions. Therefore these ions are the main ions needed to maintain electrical neutrality in the fluids outside the cell.

Increase in the anion gap occurs when acidosis is due to excess acid production. The excess hydrogen ions combine with bicarbonate to form carbonic acid $(H_2O + CO_2)$ and the excess carbon dioxide is blown off by the lungs. Thus sodium and chloride remain relatively unchanged and the anion gap increases.

Normal anion gap may occur in gastroenteritis or renal disease where acidosis is due to equimolar loss of both sodium and bicarbonate. There is thus an excess of chloride ions (hyperchloraemic metabolic acidosis).

Fall in the anion gap may occur due to excessive vomiting causing loss of hydrogen ions and chloride predominantly, with retention of bicarbonate. This results in metabolic hypochloraemic alkalosis.

PRINCIPLES OF FLUID AND ELECTROLYTE MANAGEMENT

Adults require approximately 2500–3000 ml of water daily to maintain homeostasis. Children may be given a suitable percentage of this using the percentage method for estimating doses (for example, a seven year old child requires 50 % of this dose, 1250–1500 ml daily). Infants on breast milk require less than infants fed cows' milk, albeit diluted, because breast milk contains less casein and far less electrolytes. In calculating fluid requirements one should remember that bottle-fed babies are on an entirely liquid diet. When they are put on to solids, though solids also contain a certain amount of liquid, extra water must be taken to cope with the solute load.

In disturbances of water and electrolytes balance, it requires fine judgement to decide whether an infant or child can be treated with oral fluids at home or whether parenteral feeding in hospital is required.

Determining the deficit

History

A 'guesstimate' of the fluid and electrolyte loss should be made from the type, severity and duration of the loss. It is of great help if the weight prior to the illness is known, as one can then estimate the weight loss with reasonable accuracy. The volume of urine is important. Loss due to fever and sweating should be included in the estimate.

Examination

The patient is often feverish (dehydration fever) and his eyes are hollow and sunken. In babies the fontanelle is usually depressed. The skin and subcutaneous tissues are dry and inelastic, so that when they are pinched between the index finger and thumb they do not spring back as in normal skin. In severe cases of dehydration, shock develops and the patient presents with tachycardia, weak thready pulse and low blood pressure. The urinary output is markedly reduced leading to extrarenal uraemia.

Degree of dehydration

1 *Severe* dehydration and shock = water deficit of 10 % of body-weight or more.
2 *Moderate* dehydration = water deficit of 5–10 % body-weight.
3 *Mild* dehydration = water deficit of less than 5 % of body-weight.

If deep rapid respiration of the Kussmaul type is present, *metabolic acidosis* is likely, but this should always be confirmed by blood gas analysis as alkalosis is sometimes indistinguishable clinically. Shallow respiration may be due to *central depression* as a result of overdose with opiates such as paregoric and codein and drugs such as diphenoxylate (Lomotil). *Tetany* is associated with alkalosis from any cause, including the over-enthusiastic use of intravenous sodium bicarbonate, for acidosis. *Convulsions* may be due to water intoxication, hypernatraemia or salmonellosis. Sclerematous changes in the skin are often associated with *hypertonic dehydration* but the serum sodium level should be measured for confirmation.

Laboratory tests that may be of value include:

1 Full blood count for evidence of anaemia or infection.
2 Haematocrit for haemoconcentration.
3 Serum electrolytes, blood urea and serum osmolality for type of electrolyte disturbance and evidence of extrarenal uraemia.
4 Urinary volume, specific gravity and microscopic examination for cells and casts in oliguria, and for assessing response to intravenous fluids. Acetone should be tested for.
5 Blood gas analysis for pH, P_{CO_2} and base excess to distinguish acidosis and alkalosis and to determine whether it is respiratory or metabolic in origin or both.

ESTIMATION OF FLUID REQUIREMENTS

There are three steps in estimating fluid requirements:

1 Replacement of deficit

One may either estimate the weight loss in kilograms and give this amount as litres of fluid, or one may use average losses as follows:

	Surface area dose	Adult dose*
Mild dehydration	850 ml/m²	1500 ml
Moderate dehydration	1100 ml/m²	2000 ml
Severe dehydration	1400 ml/m²	2500 ml
Shock with dehydration	1900 ml/m² or more	3250 ml

* Children may be given a suitable percentage of these doses using the percentage method.

Example
A baby weighing 8.5 kg (surface area approx. 0.44 m²) is severely dehydrated with shock. Estimate fluid replacement of this deficit:

$$\text{Assuming the baby has lost } 10/100 \text{ of } 8.5 \text{ kg} = 0.85 \text{ kg}$$
$$= 0.85 \text{ litres}$$
$$= 850 \text{ ml}$$

or 1900 ml × 0.44 = 836 ml
or 25 % of 3250 ml = 812 ml

One-half to one-third should be given within the first 4–6 hours as an isotonic or colloid solution, while the remainder should be given as a hypotonic solution. Although there are slight differences in these estimates, in practice one re-assesses the patient at frequent intervals and adjusts the dose according to the needs of the patient.

2 Maintenance

The normal maintenance requirements for fluid for an adult is ± 2500 ml/24 hours (1400 ml/m²/24 hours) best given as a *hypotonic* solution such as half-strength Darrow's solution. In tropical climates maintenance requirement may be based on an adult dose of 3000–4000 ml/24 hours (1700–2300 ml/m²/24 hours). To this should be added continuing losses.

3 Continuing losses

These are due to fever, vomiting, diarrhoea, burns, gastric suction and so on. These losses should be measured accurately where possible.
NB In all cases the child should be carefully re-assessed every 4–6

hours, day and night, and the rate of the infusion and its composition altered according to the needs of the patient. Formulae should be regarded only as rough guides to quantities; the response of the patient is what matters.

The virtues of hypotonic solutions

Throughout this book reference is made to the use of hypotonic solutions once the blood volume has been corrected by isotonic solutions such as normal saline, Ringer's Lactate Solution (Compound Sodium Lactate Injection, B.P.) or even blood and plasma. The current favourite 'all-round' hypotonic solution is half-strength Darrow's solution because it contains balanced electrolytes, including sodium, chloride, potassium and lactate ions, with an excess of water, to ensure adequate excretion of all obligatory solutes. It thus permits the body to titrate its own needs by excreting unwanted ions in the urine. It usually contains 2.5 % or 5 % dextrose to provide kilojoules and to counteract ketosis. The only real contra-indications to the use of this fluid are hyperkalaemia and persistent oliguria or anuria which could lead to hyperkalaemia. In such cases half-normal saline is usually satisfactory. Many other hypotonic solutions such as Dioralyte are available.

The treatment of fluid and electrolyte disturbances in common paediatric disorders are discussed under their appropriate headings.

Hyperalimentation

In patients with intractable diarrhoea, severe malabsorption, extensive bowel resection or intestinal fistulae, prolonged parenteral infusions may be required. It has also been used in pre-term babies when gastro-intestinal feeding has caused problems. As a patient cannot survive on water and electrolytes alone, hyperalimentation is practised. Amino acid mixtures such as Vamin and Aminosol may be given to reduce protein breakdown by the body. As amino acids and sugars only supply 4 kcal/g fat emulsions, notably Intralipid have been developed, which can be given by intravenous injection and supply 9 kcal/g. It is now possible, therefore, to nurture patients parenterally until the underlying condition can be corrected. Up to 1500 kcal/m^2/day can be given in this way. A careful aseptic technique should be used inserting and maintaining i.v. lines lest they become infected. Peripheral or central veins may be used. The supplementary use of plasma and whole blood should not be forgotten.

CHAPTER 9

DISEASES OF THE BLOOD AND RETICULO-ENDOTHELIAL SYSTEM

ANAEMIA

In children anaemia may be defined as any condition in which the quantity of haemoglobin per dl of blood is below the lower limit of normal. Usually the total number of red cells per mm^3 and the haematocrit are also reduced. The net result is a decreased oxygen carrying capacity of the blood. The type of anaemia should be determined by special investigation. Normal red cell values are shown in Table 9.1. An attempt should be made to find the cause of the anaemia before administering blood or haematinics lest the aetiology be obscured.

Table 9.1 Normal red cell values in infants and children (arrows indicate progressive change with age)

	Birth	*4 weeks*	*3 months*	*1 year*	*4 years*	*12 years*
Hb (g/dl)	19	14	11	12	13	14
	(16–22)	(11–17)	(10–13)	(11–15)	(12–15)	(13–15)
MCHC (%)	36	34	33	33	33	34
MCHb (pg)	35	30	29	28	29	31
MCV (fl)	110	100	90	84	90	92
PCV (%)	50	40	34	35	36	38

Note: MCHC = mean corpuscular haemoglobin concentration;
MCHb = mean corpuscular haemoglobin; MCV = mean corpuscular volume;
PCV = packed cell volume

A red blood cell count below 4 million per mm^3 may be regarded as abnormal at all ages. In the first four days of life the nucleated red cell count of up to 10 per 100 white cells may be found, and reticulocytes up to 6%. After four days the presence of nucleated red cells or reticulocytosis indicates haemolysis or active regeneration of red cells.

Physiological 'anaemia' of the newborn

In Table 9.1 it can be seen that by three months of age the haemoglobin of the newborn has fallen from 19 to 11 g/dl, and thereafter it slowly rises again. In small pre-term babies the haemo-globin may fall as low as 7 g/dl (see p. 37) and a 'top-up' transfusion may be necessary. In the very small pre-term baby folic acid and vitamin E should be given to prevent anaemia due to deficiency of these vitamins.

Classification of anaemias

Anaemia may be classified into four groups:

1 Deficiency anaemias, e.g. iron, vitamin B_{12}, folic acid, vitamin C and thyroxine deficiency.
2 Bone-marrow depression:
  (a) Primary, e.g. erythrogenesis imperfecta or Fanconi's anaemia
  (b) Secondary to drugs (chloramphenicol, sulphonamides, benzene, lead) neoplastic infiltration, ionising radiation, or infections.
3 Blood loss from trauma, bleeding disorders, hookworm, salicylate intoxication, gastro-intestinal haemorrhage.
4 Haemolytic disorders:
  (a) Congenital, e.g. hereditary spherocytosis, hereditary haemo-globinopathies and G-6-PD deficiency
  (b) Acquired, e.g. Rh and ABO incompatibility, auto-immune haemolytic anaemia, certain snake venoms and malaria.

A certain degree of overlap occurs, thus lead poisoning may cause anaemia by depressing the bone-marrow, by increasing haemolysis and perhaps by other mechanisms.

Deficiency anaemias

Normal iron requirements
In the first year of life the infant requires about 6–9 mg of elemental iron daily. After this age 10–15 mg is required daily, the larger figure being appropriate for girls after puberty.

Iron-deficiency anaemia

This is the commonest deficiency anaemia throughout the world. It is characterised by small (microcytic) poorly haemoglobinised (hypo-chromic) cells which are often distorted in shape (anisocytosis and poikilocytosis). The haematocrit, mean corpuscular haemoglobin, mean corpuscular haemoglobin concentration and mean corpuscular volume are all reduced. The serum iron is low but its ability to bind iron is increased.

Iron deficiency is common in infancy because cows' milk is deficient in this element. Breast feeding protects against anaemia because the small amount of iron present is more effectively absorbed and better utilised than that in cows' milk. A normal full-term baby has sufficient iron stores for at least six months, while small babies, especially if born pre-

anisocytosis → variation in size of RBC
poikilocytosis -   "   "   shape "   "

term, have reduced iron reserves. In older children anaemia may be due to an iron-poor diet, defective absorption (as occurs in coeliac disease or after bowel resection) or to poor utilisation of the iron. Chronic blood loss may be a factor. Rarely milk hypersensitivity may be associated with intestinal dysfunction and occult blood in the stools.

The patient with iron-deficiency anaemia is commonly between six and eighteen months of age with varying degrees of pallor (often disguised in cold weather by deceptively pink cheeks). The mother may complain that her child does not eat, but on inquiry one finds that he drinks excessive quantities of milk. Hepatosplenomegaly may be present. Koilonychia and glossitis are often found, if searched for, in chronic cases of iron-deficiency anaemia, while dyspnoea and haemic murmurs are manifestations of severe anaemia. Rarely heart failure may occur.

Treatment
All babies of low birth-weight should receive iron supplements from four weeks of age until about six months. Milk feeding should not be prolonged or excessive. Solids should be introduced from four months of age, meat broth and puréed green vegetables being good sources of iron. For treatment of overt iron deficiency, all soluble iron salts are satisfactory if given in adequate dose. Our personal favourite is Fersamal Liquid, which contains 140 mg ferrous fumarate supplying about 35 mg of elemental iron in 5 ml. Tablets of ferrous sulphate may be mistaken for sweets and have caused many cases of poisoning in children.

A rising haemoglobin and reticulocytosis indicate a satisfactory response to iron therapy.

Folic acid and vitamin B$_{12}$ deficiency

Folic acid deficiency is a factor in the anaemia of prematurity and is easily corrected. Goats' milk is deficient in folic acid and deficiency may also occur from malabsorption or from prolonged use of phenytoin (Epanutin) or certain other anticonvulsant drugs. It may be a factor in the anaemia of protein-energy malnutrition. It is expected during treatment with folic acid antagonists such as methotrexate. Folic acid deficiency should be suspected in the presence of a macrocytic anaemia and may be confirmed by measuring the red cell folate level. It may occur in small pre-term infants when they reach the age of six months or so. Both folic acid and vitamin C should be given.

Vitamin B$_{12}$ deficiency in children is even less common than folic acid deficiency. The clinical features are those of a macrocytic megaloblastic anaemia. Juvenile pernicious anaemia has been recorded as early as 8 years of age, associated with histamine fast achlorhydria. Congenital absence of intrinsic factor and other rare forms of vitamin B$_{12}$ deficiencies have also been described. Mothers on faddy diets during pregnancy may produce infants with temporary deficiency. Mothers with true pernicious anaemia may transfer intrinsic factor antibodies across the placenta but the baby's ability to absorb vitamin B_{12} corrects itself before 2–3 months of age.

Deficiency of erythropoietin may cause bone marrow depression, for example in chronic nephritis, thus causing a normochromic, normocytic anaemia.

Anaemia due to bone-marrow depression

Bone marrow depression may involve only one element, such as hypoplastic anaemia (red cells), agranulocytosis (granulocytes) or thrombocytopenia (platelets); or it may involve all three elements, i.e. aplastic anaemia (pancytopenia). Occasionally hypoplastic anaemia is congenital. Marrow depression may be due to infections or to infiltrations or neoplasms in the bone. It may also be caused by toxic chemicals (such as drugs) and irradiation. *Fanconi's syndrome* consists of aplastic anaemia with multiple congenital anomalies of the head, heart, kidneys and limbs.

Drug-induced aplastic anaemia

Chloramphenicol was the most frequent cause of aplastic anaemia in the USA between 1949 and 1952, and the incidence appeared to be directly related to the frequency with which this drug was prescribed. The disease was often fatal and occurred in conditions for which the chloramphenicol was not strongly indicated, for example colds, acne or mild infections. It is not possible to predict which patient will develop aplastic anaemia after chloramphenicol as it may occur weeks or months after the last dose has been given. Drugs like chloramphenicol and troxidone which can cause aplastic anaemia should only be used on the strongest indication.

Certain medicines regularly cause aplastic anaemia. They are the antileukaemic agents such as methotrexate, cyclophosphamide, busulphan, ionising radiation and many others. Usually the condition is reversible and the bone-marrow regenerates, one hopes without regeneration of the abnormal 'blast' cells for which the medicines were originally given.

Clinical features

Progressive, insidious anaemia leads to increasing pallor, anorexia, dyspnoea and weakness. Thrombocytopenia may cause bleeding into the skull, gums, bowel or kidneys, aggravating the anaemia. Agranulocytosis may present with sore throat and ulceration of the mouth and pharynx. Characteristically there is no hyperaemia around the lesions. It should be emphasised that the liver, spleen and lymph glands do *not* enlarge in aplastic and hypoplastic anaemias.

The diagnosis should be established by bone-marrow examination. As the distribution of aplastic marrow may be patchy, the diagnosis may require repeated bone-marrow examination or marrow biopsy.

aplasia- lack of development of organ or tissue or its cellular products

Treatment of aplastic and hypoplastic anaemias
Potentially myelotoxic drugs should be avoided where possible. If the patient is taking them, for epilepsy for example, weekly blood and reticulocyte counts should be done initially, then monthly for a few months, and then less frequently. The patient should report sore throats, bleeding gums or bruising. Unexplained fever may be an early warning symptom of aplasia of the marrow. The suspected drug should be withdrawn immediately before the aplasia becomes irreversible.

Anaemia is treated with packed whole human blood, agranulocytosis with repeated concentrated white cell transfusions. Infection is a serious hazard and antibiotics should be used in adequate dose. Anabolic steroids in large doses have been given for prolonged periods (more than a year on occasions) but their value is still uncertain. Haemorrhage due to thrombocytopenia should be treated with platelet-rich plasma. Occasionally splenectomy is considered if the condition is aggravated by hypersplenism. Bone-marrow transplantation may be considered in specialised centres.

Anaemia due to blood loss

Anaemia may be *acute* due to the rapid blood loss which occurs in accidents, peptic ulceration, oesophageal varices or bleeding disorders. In newborn infants surprisingly large volumes of blood may collect in a cephalhaematoma. Clinical signs are due to the rapid fall in blood pressure and blood volume, but may be masked for several hours by compensatory vasoconstriction and stasis. A fast thready pulse, pallor, rapid breathing and cold clammy skin may be noted. As renal shutdown may occur, the bleeding must be stopped and the blood volume should be expanded as soon as possible with whole blood to prevent this. If blood is not available then plasma, dextran or saline, in that order, may be given until whole blood can be obtained. Venous pressure should be monitored to prevent overloading.

Chronic haemorrhagic anaemia
This is due to small but repeated haemorrhages which may be due to the same causes as above. Chronic blood loss due to bleeding Meckel's diverticulum, polyps, hookworm and coagulation disorders should be remembered. Salicylates given for rheumatic diseases may cause anaemia from the combined effect of gastric irritation, reduced platelet stickiness and hypoprothrombinaemia. Full blood count reveals an iron-deficient anaemia with 4–5% reticulocytosis. The source of the bleeding in the bowel or genito-urinary tract should be sought. If the anaemia is severe, blood transfusion should be given, otherwise iron therapy for 2–3 months may be satisfactory.

Haemolytic anaemias

Haemolytic anaemias are anaemias due to the abnormal breakdown of red cells in the vascular system and spleen. This leads to an increase in serum unconjugated bilirubin and excretion of urobilinogen in the urine. The marrow activity increases, especially in thalassaemia, and there is a reticulocytosis. Erythrocytes labelled with ^{51}Cr are used to detect the rate and site of red cell destruction. *Haemolytic crises* may be due to a sudden increase in the breakdown of the red cells, or a failure of the bone-marrow to respond. They tend to recur and are associated with fever, nausea, vomiting and abdominal discomfort which may last 2–3 weeks. Pallor is always present, and the skin may have a yellowish tinge. The spleen is nearly always palpable.

When severe haemolysis occurs in the neonatal period it causes hyperbilirubinaemia which, if severe, may lead to kernicterus.

CONGENITAL ANOMALIES OF THE RED CELL

Hereditary spherocytosis (Congenital haemolytic anaemia)

Hereditary spherocytosis is characterised by rounded, fragile red blood cells called spherocytes, and the occurrence of aplastic crises. It is inherited as a dominant characteristic. In the neonate hyperbilirubinaemia is a feature and may be mistaken for ABO incompatibility since both may exhibit spherocytosis. Thereafter the clinical picture is very variable. Some children have no symptoms while others become jaundiced with each intercurrent infection. Many children develop a chronic transfusion-dependent haemolytic . anaemia. The red cells survive only 15 days in the circulation and are broken down in the spleen, which enlarges. Reticulocytosis of 10–50% may be found depending on the activity of the disease. The Coombs' test (direct) is invariably negative. In children gall-stones and pre-tibial ulcers, which are common in adults, rarely occur. Splenectomy ensures *symptomatic* cure but should be avoided before five years of age because of the increased tendency to infection which it may cause. Blood transfusions may be required at regular intervals for anaemia.

Sickle-cell anaemia

Sickle-cell anaemia is a form of haemolytic anaemia due to the presence of haemoglobin-S, characterised by sickling of the red cell when the oxygen tension is reduced. It is inherited as an autosomal recessive characteristic and is found amongst Negroes in the USA, the east coast of Africa and elsewhere. Heterozygous carriers can be detected by the presence of a sickle-cell trait, patients with the disease being homozygous. The trait appears to offer some protection against malaria, especially in children.

Sickle-cell anaemia can mimic many disorders. In addition to the usual features of chronic haemolytic anaemias there is a strong tendency to intravascular stasis and thrombosis. During such 'crises', children complain of tiredness, joint pains, abdominal pain, vomiting, fever and headaches. The plasma volume shrinks and the haemoglobin therefore may be deceptively high. Aplastic crises also occur in which reduced blood formation is present. Fatal crises due to massive splenic sequestration of sickled red cells may occur. Meningismus and convulsions may suggest meningitis. In infants dactylitis should lead one to consider this disease (hand-foot syndrome). Hepatosplenomegaly is usually present but repeated infarction and fibrosis lead to subsequent shrinking of the spleen. Enlargement of the heart and congestive failure may occur. *Salmonella osteitis* and pneumococcal infections may complicate the disease. Radiological examination reveals signs of bone-marrow hyperplasia (widened medullary spaces and 'hair-on-end' appearance of the skull).

Diagnosis

Diagnosis is established by finding sickling on sealed coverslip preparations and by haemoglobin electrophoresis. Anaemia, reticulocytosis, bilirubinaemia, decreased osmotic fragility and urobilinogenuria are present. In homozygotes there is more than 80 % haemoglobin-S while in heterozygotes there is less than 50 %.

Treatment

During crises intravenous 5 % dextrose-in-water, half-strength saline or plasma should be given to expand the plasma volume and improve stagnant circulation. Intravenous sodium bicarbonate may be helpful. Oxygen and hyperbaric oxygen may be given for cerebrovascular occlusions. Antibiotics are given for infection. Blood is given if anaemia is severe. Folic acid is required to prevent megaloblastic anaemia. Occasionally splenectomy may have to be considered.

Thalassaemia (Cooley's anaemia, Mediterranean anaemia)

Thalassaemia is a form of haemolytic anaemia, occurring along the Mediterranean coast in Italians, Greeks and Cypriots, characterised by the presence of excess fetal haemoglobin and deficient adult haemoglobin in the circulation. It was defined by Cooley in 1925 as an hereditary haemolytic anaemia, with characteristic 'frog-like' or 'Mongoloid' faces, skeletal changes and splenomegaly. A large number of normoblasts are found in the peripheral circulation, associated with an iron-resistant hypochromic microcytic anaemia. Target cells are commonly seen. The serum iron is normal or high thus distinguishing this disease from iron-deficiency anaemia. Mild disease (*Thalassaemia minor*) is associated with the heterozygous state, severe disease (*T. major*) with the homozygous state. Radiological changes are more marked than in sickle-cell disease due to the presence of a more active bone-marrow.

Diagnosis
Diagnosis can be confirmed by electrophoresis and the finding of 40 % or more fetal haemoglobin.

Treatment
Repeated blood transfusions should be given but lead eventually to haemosiderosis and haemochromatosis. Splenectomy should be considered when the size of the spleen becomes excessive, painful infarcts occur, and too many blood transfusions are required. A curious complication of splenectomy in these patients is a benign self-limiting pericarditis. More serious is the danger of overwhelming infection or cerebral thrombosis. The haemoglobin should be kept between 10 and 12 g/dl. Desferrioxamine, which chelates iron, is used to minimise haemosiderosis, but it may aggravate the hypochromic anaemia which is present, despite the presence of haemosiderosis. Bone narrow transplantation has been used successfully.

Prognosis
In *thalassaemia minor* the prognosis is good, but in the major form it is poor. Death may occur from heart failure, liver failure or infection.

Inborn red blood cell enzyme deficiencies

Glucose-6-phosphate dehydrogenase (G-6-PD) deficiency is the best known of these inherited enzyme deficiencies of the erythrocyte. It is commonest amongst Negroes, Sephardic Jews, the Mediterranean peoples and in the Far East. Nearly 100 variants of G-6-PD deficiency are known, many of which are asymptomatic. The most important are:

Congenital nonspherocytic haemolytic anaemia
Neonatal hyperbilirubinaemia often occurs in congenital nonspherocytic anaemia and the patient's life is shortened by recurrent or continuing haemolysis, splenomegaly, jaundice and aplastic crises. Transfusion haemosiderosis complicates the picture.

Favism
This refers to haemolytic episodes due to exposure to Fava beans, occurring in children with G-6-PD deficiency.

Drug-induced haemolysis
This occurs with varying intensity two to three days after exposure to primaquine, pamaquine, furazolidone, nitrofurantoin, certain sulphonamides and other oxidants. The anaemia may be mild or dangerously severe. Each episode is self-limited because newly formed red blood cells have higher G-6-PD levels than the older cells and are therefore resistant to haemolysis.

Pyruvate kinase deficiency
This is one of several red cell enzyme abnormalities involving the Embden-Myerhof pathway. It may present with neonatal jaundice which requires exchange transfusion to control the hyperbilirubinaemia. The subsequent progress depends on the intensity of the haemolysis. In mild cases the patient remains asymptomatic but severe haemolytic episodes may require repeated blood transfusions. In some cases splenectomy has proved of benefit by lengthening the life span of the red cell.

Acquired haemolytic anaemia

Haemolytic disease of the newborn
Haemolytic disease of the newborn due to Rh or ABO incompatability has been discussed in Chapter 5.

Auto-immune haemolytic anaemia
This is associated with a single or repeated episodes of haemolysis due to auto-antibody formation. The direct Coombs' test is strongly positive. It may be a primary disorder of unknown cause, or it may be secondary to other diseases such as chronic lymphocytic leukaemia, Hodgkin's disease, liver disease or various collagen diseases. The spleen enlarges and the haemoglobin may fall precipitously during acute episodes. Jaundice due to accumulation of indirect bilirubin may be noted. Up to 60 % reticulocytes may be found. Small numbers of normoblasts and spherocytes may be present. Erythrophagocytosis by white cells occurs in the peripheral circulation and can be detected in the incubated buffy coat of venous blood. Autoagglutinins, autohaemolysins and incomplete antibodies occur which may act specifically against the patient's own red blood cells, or they may be non-specific and affect any red blood cells.

Treatment
Severe anaemia is treated by blood transfusion. Corticosteroids usually suppress the symptoms. Initially large doses of prednisone (34 mg/m^2/24 hours) are given and the dose gradually tailed off to the minimum that will control symptoms. Splenectomy should be considered carefully in patients requiring too frequent blood transfusions. The prognosis is usually good.

Haemolytic disease due to infective and chemical agents

Streptococcal and *Clostridium welchii* infections have caused haemolytic anaemia but rarely. Malaria is constantly associated with haemolysis due to the multiplication of the parasite in the red blood cell. Blackwater fever is due to severe *falciparum* malaria causing acute haemolysis with haemoglobinuria. Of the drugs, primaquine, nitrofurantoin, griseofulvin and others cause haemolysis if G-6-PD is deficient in the red cell.

Sulphonamides, phenylbutazone and other drugs may sometimes cause haemolytic reactions. Certain snake venoms act by destroying red blood cells.

PURPURA

Purpura (Greek: purple) is a haemorrhagic rash of the skin and mucous membranes. When the lesions are pin-head in size the rash is called *petechial*; when they are large the rash is called a bruise or *ecchymosis*.

Purpura falls naturally into two main groups, those due to platelet deficiency and those due to other abnormalities of the clotting mechanism.

Platelet deficiency (thrombocytopenic purpura)

Thrombocytopenic purpura is classified as idiopathic or symptomatic.

1 Idiopathic thrombocytopenic purpura (ITP; Werlhof's disease)

This is a disorder characterised by a sudden marked reduction in thrombocytes (platelets) in the circulation, associated with normal or increased megakaryocytes in the bone-marrow, and haemorrhages into the skin and mucous membranes. Immune bodies which can cross the placenta, have been detected in mothers and their newborn infants. It is likely that the same antibody may also injure the capillary wall.

The patient presents with petechial lesions in the skin and mucous membranes. Slight trauma may produce extensive bruising. Nose-bleeds, haemorrhages into the gums, gastro-intestinal and genito-urinary tract may occur but fortunately brain haemorrhage is rare. The spleen is either not palpable or the tip can be felt. The cause is unknown but one sometimes obtains a history of a viral illness 2–4 weeks prior to the onset of the petechial rash. It is commonest between 2–8 years of age, occurring equally amongst boys and girls. This is in contrast to young adults in whom it is much commoner among females.

Investigation
The blood platelets are reduced in number, usually below 40 000/mm³. On blood smears few platelets are seen and these may be abnormal. Bone-marrow usually reveals an increased number of megakaryocytes, suggesting that the platelets either do not bud off (maturation arrest) or they are rapidly removed from the circulation by the spleen.

Bleeding time is prolonged, clotting time and prothrombin time normal but thromboplastin formation is impaired. Anaemia may be present, depending on the degree of bleeding. In all cases examination for LE cells is advised as *lupus erythematosus*, though very rare in children, may present initially with petechiae.

Prognosis
This is much better than in adults and 75% of children remit spontaneously usually in six weeks to three months. Sometimes the condition may smoulder for a year or more. Of those that persist for more than one year (chronic ITP) over 50% are cured by splenectomy.

Treatment
Fresh blood transfusions are given for anaemia or to stop bleeding. Platelet transfusions do not usually help as the transfused platelets are rapidly destroyed. Corticosteroids and azathioprine suppress the auto-immune mechanism with consequent increase in circulating platelets, but are rarely necessary. Splenectomy is considered in patients in whom megakaryocytes are plentiful but who do not respond to conservative therapy. Aspirin should not be used as it affects platelet 'stickiness'.

2 Symptomatic thrombocytopenic purpura

Thrombocytopenic purpura occurring in the newborn is nearly always secondary to other causes, such as anti-platelet antibodies (carried over from mother), the extended congenital rubella syndrome, toxoplasmosis or cytomegalosis. These may clear-up spontaneously but fatalities, due to the underlying disorder, may occur.

In older infants and children the following should be considered:

1 *Infections* such as septicaemia, glandular fever, scarlet fever and more rarely subacute bacterial endocarditis and typhus.
2 *Chemicals* (benzol derivatives), drugs, (sulphonamides, salicylates, chloramphenicol, antileukaemic drugs), and *physical agents* (X-rays and radioactive substances).
3 *Associated blood disorders*:
   (a) Aplastic anaemia and auto-immune haemolytic anaemia including Gasser's haemolytic-uraemic syndrome.
   (b) Hypersplenism secondary to other diseases.
   (c) Bone-marrow infiltration by leukaemia and neoplasms or displacement due to osteopetrosis. (dense bone)
   (d) Large haemangiomata may lead to recurrent thrombocytopenia.

In most of these patients both the platelets and the megakaryocytes in the bone-marrow are reduced. In all these disorders the primary cause should be eliminated where possible, and suspect drugs stopped. Treatment is mainly symptomatic.

Non-thrombocytopenic purpura

Anaphylactoid purpura
Anaphylactoid purpura is a disorder of childhood in which purpuric lesions due to a widespread angiitis are associated with a pleomorphic, urticaria-like eruption, and lesions in the bowel, kidney and joints.

angiitis - inflammation of vessel wall

When signs of an 'acute abdomen' dominate the clinical picture is called *Henoch's purpura*. The occurrence of vomiting, abdominal pain and bloody diarrhoea may suggest dysentery or even intussusception, and a barium enema may be required to exclude this possibility which is a rare complication of Henoch's purpura. In any 'acute abdomen' therefore the skin should be checked for a rash. In anaphylactoid purpura this may be confined to the buttocks or to the extensor surface of the elbows and ankles.

Schönlein's purpura is associated with painful swollen joints, especially the knees and ankles. The rash may appear simultaneously or some time later. A transitory nephritis is common but occasionally full blown acute glomerulonephritis occurs with anuria, uraemia and hypertensive crisis.

Investigations
The blood count is normal unless haemorrhage from the nose or bowel has caused an anaemia. The platelets are of course plentiful. Sometimes there may be haemolytic streptococci in the throat and the antistreptolysin titre may be raised. Other organisms and viruses have been implicated. Bleeding and clotting times are normal. Clot retraction is normal. The urine may reveal albumin, blood and casts. Renal biopsy reveals fibrinoid necrosis in the glomerulus with endothelial proliferation.

Treatment
The disease is usually self-limiting. Paracetamol may be used for joint pains. Streptococcal infection should be treated with benzylpenicillin for ten days to eliminate the organism. Corticosteroids have been used to alleviate abdominal pain.

Prognosis
The disorder usually clears up in 4–6 weeks but some cases pursue a chronic course lasting a year or more. Death may occur from cerebral or gastro-intestinal haemorrhage, or from renal failure.

DEFICIT OF CLOTTING FACTORS

In the newborn *hypoprothrombinaemia* is a common but transitory phenomenon. The plasma prothrombin reaches its lowest level on the fourth day, therefore circumcisions or other operations should not be done before the seventh day unless the patient has been given 0.5–1 mg of vitamin K_1 at least 12 hours prior to operation.

Rarely, congenital absence of fibrinogen has been described.

Haemophilia

The most important hereditary bleeding disorder after the neonatal period is *haemophilia* which is due to failure to synthesise antihaemophilic globulin (AHG or Factor VIII). It is transmitted as a sex-linked recessive trait and is quite rare (about 1 in 10 000 births). It gives the impression of being commoner than it is because one sees the same patient in dramatic circumstances over and over again. Characteristically the partial thromboplastin time is prolonged and the bleeding time normal. Clot retraction is poor. Platelets are normal, plasma AHG low. As the severity of AHG deficiency varies from patient to patient, so the incidence of bleeding and bruising also varies. Haemarthrosis leading to fibrosis and deformity of the affected joints is characteristic. Minor operations like circumcision, tonsillectomy or removal of teeth have led to fatal haemorrhages. Trivial trauma can cause persistent bleeding.

Treatment
Oozing can often be controlled by topical thrombin. Persistent or extensive bleeding should be treated by the immediate injection of fresh frozen plasma or AHG concentrate (human) in order to raise the plasma concentration of AHG to 20 % of normal. If anaemia is present fresh whole blood should be given. One school of opinion today favours preventative injections of AHG at regular intervals in order to keep the serum AHG level about 5 % to prevent haemarthrosis or other dangerous bleeds. In some centres the parents are taught to inject the plasma or AHG at home so that no time is wasted in stopping the bleed when it occurs. Each patient should wear a wrist bracelet stating that he is a haemophiliac and should belong to the appropriate National Society for Haemophiliacs. The co-operation of the whole family and the school staff should be sought in attaining optimum conditions for the child. Splinting of affected joints and physiotherapy aids recovery.

Factor IX deficiency (Christmas disease) resembles haemophilia except that *stored* plasma is effective for treatment. Factor IX is stable compared to AHG.

LEUKAEMIA

Acute leukaemia is a malignant disease of the white blood-forming tissues in which uncontrolled proliferation of one of the types of white blood cells occurs. Over 80 % of cases in children are lymphocytic in origin. A small percentage involve the myeloblasts while chronic granulocytic leukaemia is very rare. Acute leukaemia is commonest between three and five years of age, the sexes being equally affected. The risk of developing leukaemia in the general population is about 1 in 3000, if a sibling has had it the risk is 1 in 750, and in monozygotic twins 1 in 4.

Acute leukaemia is the commonest malignancy of childhood. It may be congenital, sometimes associated with Down's syndrome, but most cases are acquired. The causes are unknown but genetic factors, ionising radiation and viral particles may play a role. It is less common in Negroes.

Clinical features

Acute leukaemia may begin abruptly with anaemia and haemorrhagic manifestations, generalised lymphadenopathy and varying degrees of hepatosplenomegaly. Constitutional symptoms include anorexia, malaise, weakness and fever. Joint and bone pain may be present with or without sternal tenderness to percussion. Epistaxis, haematemesis, melaena or haematuria may occur. Sores in the mouth are common. Persistent bleeding after dental extraction may draw attention to the disease.

Meningeal leukaemia may occur during the course of the illness, *even after the patient attains haematological remission* with treatment. This is because the antileukaemic agents do not penetrate the blood-brain barrier. It presents with headache, vomiting, neck stiffness, drowsiness, cranial nerve palsies and other signs of raised intracranial pressure. The cerebrospinal fluid may show increased protein and 'blast' cells.

The peripheral blood usually reveals a severe anaemia and thrombocytopenia, while the white cell count is greatly increased, ranging from 20 000 to 200 000 white cells per mm^3. There is a marked increase in primitive cells ('blasts'). Sometimes the white cells are *decreased* initially (aleukaemic leukaemia) but bone-marrow puncture will confirm the presence of excessive 'blast' cells. *Leukaemoid reactions*, which are not malignant, occur in miliary tuberculosis, typhoid and some Gram-negative septicaemic states and may cause confusion on occasion. However, the absence of 'blasts' excludes leukaemia.

It is now possible to distinguish blast cells of thymic (T-cell) origin and those of bone-marrow (B-cell) origin by the presence of surface markers. However 75 % of lymphoblasts carry neither markers and are called 'null' cells. These differences may be important in assessing prognosis, T-cell leukaemia having the worst prognosis.

Treatment

By the time the acute leukaemia is diagnosed it is estimated that the patient has over 1 kg of leukaemic cells. There are four phases of treatment:

1 *Induction of remission.* The combination of vincristine (a plant alkaloid) and prednisolone seems to produce the highest remission rate (85–100 %). Sometimes daunorubicin is added. Other drugs of value, used in various combinations include methotrexate, mercapto-purine, cyclophosphamide, and cytosine arabinoside.

2 *CNS prophylaxis.* After remission there may still be 10 g of leukaemic cells scattered in the CNS, lungs, liver, spleen, gastro-intestinal tract and testes. These are known as sanctuary sites. Cranial irradiation plus intrathecal methotrexate are given (St Jude regimen).

3 *Maintenance therapy.* Intensive two, three and four drug regimens have been used. Daily mercaptopurine with weekly methotrexate is one of the best combinations and is given for two years or less.
4 *Post-chemotherapy phase.* Before stopping therapy a bone marrow puncture should be done, and repeated at intervals to determine 'cure' or recurrence. It should be emphasised that the treatment of leukaemia is not a field for amateurs and therapy should always be initiated and controlled by specialised centres. With modern therapy the number of 5-year and 10-year cures is steadily increasing.

SPLENOMEGALY IN CHILDREN

Enlargement of the spleen may be an isolated finding or part of some generalised disease. If the spleen is less than 2 cm below the left costal margin and there are no other symptoms or signs, it is unlikely to be of serious consequence. If the spleen is larger than this or other symptoms such as fever, pallor or malaise co-exist it should be fully investigated to exclude the following:

1 Infections:
   (a) Viral disorders such as glandular fever, common exanthemata (measles, rubella or roseola), coxsackie virus infection, cytomegalosis or infectious hepatitis. Recurrent upper respiratory infections are often associated with a palpable spleen in infants.
   (b) Bacterial infection especially septicaemia, brucellosis, typhoid, tuberculosis and syphilis.
   (c) Mycotic infections such as generalised moniliasis or coccidiomycosis.
   (d) Parasites such as malaria, bilharzia and congenial toxoplasmosis.
2 Blood disorders such as Rh incompatibility, congenital spherocytosis, thalassaemia and sickle-cell anaemia. Also moderate to severe iron-deficiency anaemia and thrombocytopenic purpura.
3 Malignancy such as Hodgkin's disease, leukaemia and lymphosarcoma often causes enlargement.
4 Metabolic disorders such as Gaucher's disease, amyloidosis, cystinosis, galactosaemia, mucopolysaccharidoses, porphyria and other rarities.
5 Congestive disorders such as heart failure (especially if recurrent), constrictive pericarditis or portal congestion.
6 Collagen diseases such as Still's rheumatoid arthritis, disseminated lupus erythematosus, sarcoidosis.

In many cases a thorough history and physical examination may provide sufficient clues to the diagnosis so that only one or two tests are needed to confirm the diagnosis. In other cases more extensive investigation is required and includes a full blood count and sedimen-

DISEASES OF THE BLOOD

tation rate, serum for Widal, Weil-Felix, Brucella complement fixation and Paul Bunnell tests, bacterial and viral cultures from blood, throat, urine and stools, tuberculin and Venereal Disease Research Laboratory (VDRL) tests, and biopsy of a suitable lymph node. Appropriate radiological investigation should be done. Even then some cases may defy elucidation for many weeks or months.

In the newborn the commonest causes of enlarged spleen include haemolytic disease of the newborn, rubella syndrome, cytomegalic disease and bacterial infection. Even a simple cold sometimes causes enlargement of the spleen in babies.

Splenectomy

Splenectomy is indicated in some cases of hereditary spherocytosis, auto-immune haemolytic anaemia and thrombocytopenic purpura. It may also be undertaken for gross splenic enlargement causing discomfort and pain, and for hypersplenism. The spleen is also removed for rupture, during porto-caval shunt operations and prior to renal transplantation.

Removal of the spleen carries a serious risk of septicaemia, especially in the under threes. The risk, if the spleen is removed for trauma, may be as low as $1-2\%$, but if it is done for thalassaemia major, the risk may be 25% or more. The commonest infection is pneumococcal septicaemia which may be fatal. Some degree of protection may be achieved with the use of prophylactic antibodies or polyvalent pneumococcal vaccine.

DISORDERS OF THE LYMPH NODES

Age-related changes in lymph nodes

Lymph nodes are present but not normally palpable at birth. The amount of lymph tissue in the body gradually increases until puberty and then tends to regress. In infants and children the inguinal nodes are usually palpable, being small and shotty. Like lymph nodes elsewhere they become large and tender in the presence of local pyogenic infection, and may suppurate. The following lymph nodes are of special interest when they enlarge:

Occipital nodes enlarge *symmetrically* in rubella. Unilateral or bilateral enlargement may occur in ringworm of the scalp, *pediculosis capitis and tick-bite.*

Post-auricular nodes may enlarge in infection of the posterior part of the pinna of the ear and in mastoiditis.

Pre-auricular nodes enlarge with infection of the lateral part of the eye-lids and in trachoma. The finding of enlarged pre-auricular nodes and conjunctivitis in the neonate suggests *inclusion conjunctivitis* and exludes gonococcal ophthalmia in which these nodes do not enlarge.

Submaxillary and submental nodes suggest infection inside the mouth, or skin of the lower jaw.

Cervical nodes most commonly enlarge in viral upper respiratory tract infections in which the nodes are soft and not tender, nor do they suppurate. Streptococcal infection of the tonsils causes bilateral enlargement of the jugulodigastric nodes. They often remain enlarged and firm after the primary infection has subsided. Sometimes the infection may spread to other nodes in the mid-cervical region, behind the sternomastoid muscle, with abscess formation. Diphtheria causes extensive swelling and brawny oedema of the upper cervical nodes ('Bull-neck'). In tuberculosis the nodes are characteristically fixed to the skin, matted and subsequently caseate. Hodgkin's Disease may begin as a localised cervical node swelling in which the nodes are painless and rubbery, later becoming matted.

Supraclavicular nodes: If the right-sided supraclavicular nodes enlarge the chest should be X-rayed to exclude a primary thoracic lesion, such as tuberculosis; left-sided enlargement calls for careful investigation for a primary lesion in the abdomen (via the thoracic duct).

Axillary and inguinal nodes usually enlarge as the result of a primary infection somewhere in the upper or lower limbs. Lymphangitis from the site of infection should be searched for. The infection may spread from the inguinal to the iliac glands which lie on the psoas muscle and may cause psoas spasm.

Abdominal nodes need to be very big or matted, or the abdominal wall very soft before these nodes can be palpated.

Epitrochlear nodes should lead one to think of secondary syphilis if they are bilaterally enlarged, and local infection if unilateral.

Generalised adenopathy

Generalised adenopathy may be due to the following causes:

1 Infections such as those listed for splenomegaly, notably rubella, syphilis, glandular fever, plague, toxoplasmosis and occasionally tuberculosis.
2 Haemolytic anaemias such as erythroblastosis, thalassaemia and sickle-cell anaemia.
3 Metabolic disease such as Gaucher's disease, cystinosis and reticuloendotheliosis.
4 Neoplastic diseases such as leukaemia, lymphosarcoma, Hodgkin's disease.
5 Drugs such as iodides (cough mixtures!), phenytoin, PAS, sulphonamides and antithyroid agents.
6 Generalised skin diseases such as infantile eczema and scabies.
7 Systemic lupus erythematosis and rheumatoid arthritis.

Diagnosis is usually confirmed by lymph node biopsy, especially when routine work-up fails to reveal the cause of the enlargement.

CHAPTER 10

ALLERGIC AND IMMUNOLOGICAL DISORDERS

Allergy (hypersensitivity) has been defined as an immune response that has gone wrong. It is an abnormal response of the patient to foreign antigens, usually proteins, such as contactants, ingestants (foods) or inhalants (pollens, animal dander). The term 'atopy' or 'atopic disease' is used when there is a strong familial or hereditary basis for the allergy, as in infantile eczema, hayfever and bronchial asthma. The characteristic features of atopic diseases include:

1 Eosinophilia of blood and tissue secretions.
2 Increased synthesis of immunoglobulin E (IgE) in response to exposure to certain allergens in the environment.
3 Tendency to bronchospasm.

It is important to distinguish *antigens* which produce a 'normal' antibody response and *allergens* which produce an 'abnormal' antibody reaction due to a state of 'altered sensitivity' (Von Pirquet).

Type I hypersensitivity (immediate hypersensitivity, anaphylaxis)

In type I reactions, the allergen reacts with IgE, a reagenic antibody bound to mast cells or to circulating basophils, and leads to degranulation of these cells with release of vasoactive amines such as histamine. The reaction to the allergen (e.g. bee-sting or penicillin) may occur with dramatic suddenness, leading to profound shock, laryngospasm, bronchospasm, pulmonary oedema and a precipitous fall in blood pressure. Less dramatic responses mediated by IgE include allergic rhinitis, extrinsic asthma, atopic dermatitis, urticaria, gastro-intestinal allergy and serum sickness.

Type II hypersensitivity (cytotoxic reactions)

In type II hypersensitivity the offending allergen becomes attached to the surface of the patient's own cells, especially his erythrocytes, thyroid or glomerulus. Complement is essential to this type of antigen/antibody reaction. Examples include Rhesus incompatibility and iso-immune reactions, auto-immune disease, bone marrow depression by drugs and thyrotoxicosis due to 'thyroid stimulating immunoglobulin' (TSI).

Type III hypersensitivity (immune complex)

In type III hypersensitivity there is a delay of 1–8 hours before symptoms appear. There is involvement of antibody, antigen and the C3 component of complement leading to aggregation of platelets and neutrophil involvement.

If there is an excess of antibodies the complexes tend to be large and are easily mopped up by phagocytes, as in the Arthus reaction.

If the antigen (allergen) is in excess the complexes are small, soluble and widely distributed, leading to immune complex disease or serum sickness (generalised). In post-streptococcal nephritis the complexes are deposited in the glomerular basement membrane.

Types I–III all involve humoral antibodies and cause immediate (up to 8 hours) reactions.

Type IV hypersensitivity (delayed, cell-mediated reactions)

Type IV hypersensitivity reactions are mediated by sensitised lymphocytes (T-cells or thymus derived lymphocytes) which specifically combine with allergens to release lymphokines. These reactions take about 24 hours to develop and it may take 2–5 days for a full response to occur (e.g. Mantoux test for tuberculin sensitivity, contact hypersensitivity and the rash of measles).

Anergy

Anergy is the inability to express cell-mediated immunity (CMI) and may be due to thymic aplasia, immunosuppression by drugs, infections such as measles, or Hodgkin's disease.

UNDERLYING FACTORS IN ALLERGIC DISEASES

Heredity
The risk of a child developing an allergy may be as high as 40 % if both parents have an allergy.

Infection
Viral infections of the upper respiratory tract may precipitate an attack of asthma. The runny nose of 'Coryza' should be distinguished carefully from that of allergic rhinitis which often precedes or accompanies an asthma attack.

Exercise
Running and bicycle riding often precipitate an attack of asthma in an asthmatic child. It may occur during or shortly after strenuous activity. Curiously enough swimming does not seem to precipitate asthma in atopic children and many authorities regard it as beneficial. Sometimes laughing and crying or breathing in cold air may precipitate an attack.

Environmental factors
High humidity, house dust, animal dander, pollens, various ingestants
(e.g. egg, milk, pork, fish, certain fruits, tomatoes and chocolate) and
contactants (e.g. soap, chemicals and wool) may cause allergic reactions.

FOOD ALLERGY

Food allergy may be responsible for the development of unexpected
reactions, not necessarily confined to the gastrointestinal tract. Cows
milk allergy in babies may be responsible for infantile colic, diarrhoea,
vomiting and on rare occasions gastrointestinal occult bleeding. The
role of cows milk in infantile eczema, bronchial asthma and the mucousy
baby syndrome remains controversial.

If a baby is thought to be allergic to any specific foodstuff, that food
should be withdrawn from the diet. If this relieves symptoms after a two
week trial period the substance should again be tested by giving a small
quantity to the baby. If he again develops symptoms then the food
should be withdrawn for a year before trying again.

Skin tests for food or other IgE-mediated allergy are not very reliable,
especially in early life. A more specific test is the radioallergosorbent test
(RAST) which is now available in many laboratories. Quantification of
total IgE can be achieved by a paper radioimmunosorbent test (PRIST)
though its value is limited by the fact that some patients with known
allergies have low or normal IgE levels.

RESPIRATORY ALLERGIES

Hay fever

Hay fever is an allergy to inhalants such as pollens (especially grass,
certain plants or trees), dusts or danders. The nasal mucosa swells, is
often paler than normal, with a bluish colour, and there is a profuse thin
discharge. Frequent sneezing is common, the eyes may swell and itch
and the patient feels miserable. Itching of the nose causes a characteristic
'allergic salute'. The condition may be seasonal or perennial. Parents
often say that the patient 'gets one cold after another'. Sometimes
rhinorrhoea precedes an attack of wheezing ('colds go to his chest').
Cough is commonly present. Chronic rhinitis may be associated with
blocked nasal passages, enlarged tonsils and adenoids, mouth-breathing
and a dull facial expression (adenoid facies).

Diagnosis
A nasal smear may reveal marked eosinophilia especially during the
acute attack. Circulating eosinophilia of more than 300 cells/mm^3 is
usual. The serum IgE is usually raised.

Treatment

If possible the offending allergen should be avoided. If inhalant sensitivity can be demonstrated, proper desensitisation by intradermal injection is successful in about two-thirds of patients. It acts by producing specific IgG blocking antibodies. Antihistamines provide temporary relief during acute attacks. Sodium cromoglycate by intranasal spray is effective in preventing attacks and may be tried.

Beclomethasone dipropionate nasal spray may be used three or four times daily continuously for prophylaxis. Decongestant nose drops such as ephedrine hydrochloride 0.25–0.5 % two or three times daily is effective for the relief of acute symptoms but should not be used for more than five or six days at a time as it may cause rebound congestion. The drops may be used 15 minutes before prophylaxis with sodium cromoglycate or beclomethasone during the first week, in order to improve the response of the patient to treatment.

Bronchial asthma

Bronchial or extrinsic asthma is an allergic disorder associated with repeated attacks of bronchospasm. There is a history of infantile eczema in about half the patients. Attacks may be precipitated by viral infection of the upper respiratory tract, by inhalants such as house dust, pollens, animal danders, strong odours (e.g. deodorants, hair sprays, paints), sudden laughing or crying, inhalation of cold air, certain ingestants and stress. Many attacks occur during the night and the parents may only be aware of a recurring nocturnal cough. The attacks may be attributed to feathers in the pillow or eiderdown, mites in the dust, woollen blankets or a pet animal. In fact it may be associated with the circadian rhythms of sleep itself. Emotional stress may be an important aggravating factor.

Clinical picture

The child may be constantly wheezy or have recurrent severe attacks of bronchospasm. He may simply present with attacks of night coughing. Abdominal pain is often present. He may become anxious and restless as his chest becomes increasingly tight. A short sharp inspiration is followed by a prolonged expiration as he tries to empty his over-distended lungs. Use of the accessory muscles of respiration is noted. Cyanosis is common. The attack may last a few hours or several days. If the attack does not respond to standard therapy or becomes worse, the term *status asthmaticus* is used.

Physical signs

The chest may be barrel-shaped. There is hyper-resonance to percussion over the distended lungs. On auscultation prolongation of the expiratory sound with poor air entry over both lungs may be heard. Sibilant rhonchi and wheezes are usually present while variable sonorous rhonchi due to plugs in the larger bronchi may be heard.

Diagnosis
One should try to distinguish true allergic bronchial asthma from asthmatic bronchitis. In the former a family history of allergy is usually present. The illness starts fairly suddenly with bronchospasm, sometimes preceded by a thin nasal discharge. In asthmatic bronchitis there is usually no history of allergy and the illness is preceded with a viral infection such as a cold 'which goes to the chest'. Fever over 38°C is usually present. In allergic asthma excess eosinophils are found in the nasal discharge as well as in the blood, whereas in bronchitis polymorphs are more likely to predominate. An X-ray of the chest may exclude underlying pathology. Respiratory function tests are of great interest in assessing the severity of the illness and response to therapy. The Wright Peak Flow Respirometer has been modified for use in children and the parents can learn to use it to assess their asthmatic child.

Therapy in asthma
Underlying causes should be eliminated. When a definite allergen is found, desensitisation by intradermal injection may be of value in many cases. The allergen should be eliminated if possible (e.g. by replacing feather cushions with sponge rubber, by oiling floors to retain the dust, or by daily vacuuming). Exercise should be encouraged and, if it precipitates attacks, it should be preceded by bronchodilator therapy or prolonged use of sodium cromoglycate. Physiotherapy is often of great benefit because it teaches the child breathing control and gives him confidence during the attack to expectorate viscid mucus.

Medicines in treatment
During the acute attack adrenaline injection is effective but specific beta-2-adrenergic stimulants such as orciprenaline (Alupent), salbutamol (Ventolin) and hexoprenaline (Ipradol) are finding increasing favour for breaking severe attacks, as they do not have the unpleasant side effects of adrenaline. They can be given orally, sublingually, intravenously and by inhalation. Of the xanthine derivatives, Choledyl is perhaps the best for children, and is given orally. As with aminophyllin, care must be taken not to overdose small children.

Corticosteroids: Intravenous corticosteroids should be given *early* in very severe cases as they take 4–8 hours to act. They should not be used as a last resort in difficult cases. In most cases their use can be stopped once the attack is under control. They should not be used for long-term control of asthma unless all other modes of therapy have been exhausted, as they result in marked growth disturbances. If possible, 10 mg of prednisolone on alternate days should not be exceeded.

In treating asthma it is not sufficient simply to relieve the bronchospasm. The patient must also cough up viscid sputum and the inflammatory oedema must subside. Increased fluid administration and the inhalation of water vapour may be helpful. The addition of mucolytics like bromhexine hydrochloride should be considered. Antihistamines play no role in asthma because they dry the mucosa. An excellent tranquilliser is hydroxyzine hydrochloride (Atarax) because it also has a slight bronchodilating effect.

Prevention of bronchial asthma

To minimise or prevent future attacks, bronchodilators may be administered periodically if attacks are mild, and continuously (three or four times daily) if attacks are frequent. Sodium cromoglycate is used between attacks to prevent the release of kinins by mast cells in the lung. It is inhaled three or four times daily. If the patient does not improve with this, beclamethasone dipropionate, a corticosteroid which is not absorbed into the systemic circulation, may be inhaled three or four times per 24 hours.

Löffler's syndrome (see p. 365)

INFANTILE ECZEMA

Infantile eczema is an allergic and inflammatory disorder of the skin. The onset is between two and six months of life and there is often a history of other allergies in the family. Allergy to milk and eggs can often be demonstrated on skin testing, but withdrawal of these foods has proved singularly unhelpful in therapy. There is little doubt however that breast feeding greatly reduces the incidence of atopic disorders and it has been suggested that in families with a history of allergy in both parents cows milk should be avoided. If necessary a soya bean milk may be substituted. Inhalants do not appear to play a role. Although the distribution may suggest a topical factor such as wool or nylon allergy, substitution with cotton does not often help. The curious association of eczema being replaced by asthma in nearly half these patients after the age of two years remains unexplained.

The clinical course of infantile eczema may begin with an unusually thick cradle cap (seborrhoeic eczema), or with redness and dryness of the cheeks followed by vesiculation, oozing and crusting. These lesions spread to the extensor surface of the limbs, especially elbows and knees, the upper trunk and buttocks, where itching leads to worsening of the lesion and secondary infection. The local lymph nodes frequently enlarge. The sufferers are utterly miserable and need urgent relief. Rubbing leads to thickening (lichenification) of the epidermis in the flexures of the elbow and knee (Besnier's prurigo, chronic eczema). By about two years of age the lesions tend to localise. *Kaposi's varicelliform eruption* is a serious complication of eczema, occurring when the patient is exposed to herpesvirus infection. The severity of infantile eczema waxes and wanes, and seldom disappears without treatment. This should be emphasised to the parents who should not expect the disease to be cured, only controlled.

The introduction of topical corticosteroids has revolutionised the management of infantile eczema. The acute weeping phase may be treated with betamethasone or fluocinolone lotions for a few days, followed by a suitable cream such as fluocinolone, or betamethasone which may be diluted up to ten times in aqueous cream B.P. and still remain effective. The danger of skin atrophy is also less. Simple 1 % hydrocortisone cream diluted three times is also suitable. Applications should never be stopped suddenly. In the presence of infection, oral antibiotics such as erythromycin or cloxacillin are advised until the infection is under control. For control of itch a corticosteroid lotion is usually effective but it may be worth giving oral antihistamines such as diphenhydramine (Benadryl) or promethazine (Phenergan) because they also have a useful sedating effect. Antihistamines and antibiotics should not be used topically because of their strong tendency to sensitise the skin. Seborrhoeic plaques on the scalp should be softened with oil and combed to remove them. The corticosteroid cream is then rubbed in.

SERUM SICKNESS

Serum sickness is a delayed allergic response to injections of horse-serum, penicillin and certain other drugs. Antigen-antibody complexes, complement and polymorphonuclear cells are involved in the pathological reactions which occur. Symptoms develop 6–10 days after the original injection, and the patient may develop urticaria, angioneurotic oedema, fever, generalised lymphadenopathy, bronchospasm, arthralgia and arthritis. In severe cases glomerulonephritis and peripheral neuritis may occur, and occasionally death. Usually however the condition clears in one to two weeks.

Treatment
Remove the antigen (e.g. penicillin) wherever possible. Adrenaline is the drug of choice for the acute illness. Corticosteroids may be given intravenously in severe cases. Milder symptoms may respond to antihistamines. Most patients recover within a week, though patients with peripheral neuritis are likely to take longer.

BEE STINGS

Allergy to the sting of insects is fairly common but bee stings are the most dangerous. The first time that the child is stung there is usually local swelling, redness and itch. Subsequent stings are likely to cause a serum-type reaction as described above. Anaphylactic shock may occur and cause death.

Treatment

Treatment is the same as for serum sickness in the acute phase. Topical steroids may reduce local itch and swelling. Any child who has had a severe response to bee stings should be desensitised by giving him carefully graduated doses of bee sting venom.

AUTO-IMMUNE DISEASES

Auto-immune diseases are disorders of the immune mechanism in which one or more normal constituents of the body behave like foreign antigens. These processes are sometimes initiated by local cellular destruction from trauma, infections (usually Gram-negative) and various toxins. The damaged cells release substances which are treated by the body as foreign antigens and they produce auto-antibodies against them. Many diverse diseases previously classified as collagen diseases appear to have an auto-immune basis. It does not necessarily follow that this is the cause of these diseases.

These disorders may be organ specific, involving a particular organ such as the thyroid gland in Hashimoto's disease, or they may be widely disseminated as in systemic lupus erythematosis (non-organ specific).

CLASSIFICATION OF AUTO-IMMUNE DISEASES

Organ Specific:

> Hashimoto's thyroiditis
> Primary myxoedema
> Thyrotoxicosis
> Addison's Disease
> Juvenile onset diabetes Type IB
> Auto-immune haemolytic anaemia
> Idiopathic thrombocytopenic purpura
> Active chronic hepatitis
> Ulcerative colitis

Non-Organ Specific:

> Systemic lupus erythematosus
> Dermatomyositis
> Scleroderma
> Rheumatoid arthritis

Sometimes auto-antibodies (e.g. cold agglutinins) are detected without accompanying disease. In certain infections such as syphilis, glandular fever and hepatitis B, humoral antibodies are detected which form the basis of diagnostic tests.

DISORDERS OF HUMORAL IMMUNITY
(immunoglobulin deficiency)

Human immunoglobulins are synthesised by B-cells (plasma cells) formed in the germinal centres of the lymphoid tissue of the body. They include immunoglobulins IgG, IgM, IgA, IgD and IgE. They are all concerned with immunity except IgD. IgA is chiefly responsible for providing protection of the mucous membranes and is found in tears, colostrum and secretions of the respiratory tract. It is also found in breast milk and helps to protect the infant against enteral infection. IgM can be synthesised by the infant antenatally in the presence of transplacental infection. IgM can successfully combat multivalent antigen such as bacteria. IgG is transferred passively across the placenta to the mother.

Immunoglobulin deficiency may be partial (dysgammaglobulinaemia) or complete (agammaglobulinaemia), general or selective and congenital or acquired. *Transient hypogammaglobulinaemia of infancy* is not uncommon and is due to low levels of IgG which may persist for up to 24 months. Such infants may develop recurrent otitis media and asthmatic bronchitis. Treatment is the same as for X-linked agammaglobulinaemia until recovery occurs (see below). *Immunoglobulin A deficiency* is an example of congenital selective immunoglobulin deficiency. It occurs in 0.5 % of the population and may be asymptomatic but may present with steatorrhoea, recurrent respiratory infections or collagen disease.

Combined IgG and IgA deficiency associated with increased IgM produces a syndrome of susceptibility to pyogenic infection, recurrent neutropenia and various auto-immune phenomena. It may be X-linked or acquired.

Combined B-cell deficiency may result from nephrotic syndrome, enteric protein loss or drug therapy. Such patients are especially susceptible to infections with streptococci and *Haemophilus influenzae*. *X-linked agammaglobulinaemia* is rare and is due to complete deficiency of immunoglobulin synthesis in which B-cells are deficient in the male. The infant is well until humoral antibodies carried over from mother disappear from his circulation and he fails to make his own. As a result he is subject to repeated attacks of bacterial infection including conjunctivitis, sinusitis, otitis media, pneumonia and skin infections. The microbes responsible are often *Haemophilus influenzae*, meningococcus and *Pseudomonas aeruginosa*. The tonsils and lymph glands may be very small. Complications include empyema, lung abscess and bronchiectasis. Rheumatoid arthritis-like illness may develop. Viral immunity is not affected and the patient responds normally to vaccination. Diagnosis is confirmed by finding that the total immunoglobulins are less than 5 % of the normal, i.e. 0.4–0.6 g/l (normal 8–10 g/l). Specific antibodies to diphtheria, tetanus and typhoid vaccines are not formed. The Schick test remains positive despite repeated injections of diphtheria vaccine. Plasma cells are absent from the circulation and germinal centres are absent in lymph nodes.

Treatment
Antibiotics are given to clear up all current infections. Normal Human Immunoglobulin Injections B.P. which contains about 145 mg protein/ml is given in sufficient quantities to raise the serum concentration of immunoglobulin to about 2 g/l. A dose of 100 mg/kg of body weight intramuscularly per month usually provides adequate protection against infection. A loading dose of three times this dose needs to be given, divided as necessary over several sites.

DISORDERS OF CELL MEDIATED IMMUNITY

The cells which are responsible for recognising antigen and which mediate cellular immunity are derived from the thymus and are called T-cells. Deficiencies are rare and form a heterogenous group of diseases. *Congenital thymic hypoplasia* (Di Georges syndrome) results from maldevelopment of the third and fourth pharyngeal pouches. The thymus and parathyroid glands do not develop and there are also malformations of the ear, nose and jaw as well as a right-sided aortic arch. In addition to hypoparathyroidism the patient has defective cellular immunity and is likely to develop chronic monilial infection of the mouth and skin, chronic diarrhoea and pneumonia with unusual organisms such as *Pneumocystis carinii*. Viral infections pose a serious threat to life. Measles is accompanied by giant cell pneumonia and chickenpox can be fatal. Herpetic and slow virus infection may occur.

Diagnosis
Diagnosis is confirmed by finding less than 3000 lymphocytes per mm^3, failure of lymphocytes to respond to phytohaemagglutinin stimulation and absent skin response to standard antigens (monilia, streptokinase and others). There is no contact sensitivity to 5 % dinitrofluorobenzene (DNF). Lymph node biopsy reveals absence of T-cells. Skin grafts from unrelated donors are rejected. B-cell function is normal. The immune defect has responded to fetal thymus grafts.

Hereditary forms of thymic dysplasia also occur but in practice disorders of cellular immunity are most often seen in association with infections such as tuberculosis, influenza and measles. T-cell dysfunction also occurs with neoplasms, for example leukaemia and during treatment with cytotoxic drugs, steroids and radiation.

Combined immuno-deficiency

This is a rare familial disorder resulting from a deficiency of both B- and T-cells. Patients present in early infancy with recurrent bacterial and viral infections. They have chronic diarrhoea and fail to thrive. There are signs of combined B- and T-cell deficiency with absent tonsils, thymus and small lymph nodes. There is agammaglobulinaemia and lymphopenia. The disorder is fatal within the first year and unless treatment can be given with a compatible bone marrow graft.

LEUCOCYTE DISORDERS

Neutrophils can fail to respond to infection in a variety of ways. In *the lazy leucocyte syndrome* neutrophils fail to migrate to the site of infection. Neutrophil migration may also be impaired with certain general disease states such as diabetes mellitus. The actual ingestion of microbes at the site of infection may be suppressed by drugs (cytotoxics) and by *defects of opsonisation* which may occur in IgG deficiency and complement deficiency. In these cases patients are liable to develop pyogenic infections. Impaired killing of ingested microbes occurs in *chronic granulomatous disease*. This is usually an X-linked recessive disorder and is due to enzyme deficiency. During phagocytosis diminished degradation and vacuole formation occurs. Infection occurs in skin, lymph nodes, bone, liver and lung, particularly with *Staphylococcus pyogenes* and *E. coli*. The tissues become infiltrated with granulomas containing histocytes.

SERUM COMPLEMENT

Serum complement consists of a chain of enzymes which are activated in 'cascade' fashion in antigen-antibody reactions. Activation leads to various enhanced inflammatory responses such as chemotaxis, phagocytosis and bacterolysis. Peptide fragments released during the process increase vascular permeability, release histamine and cause smooth muscle to contract.

The most abundant complement is C3, but reduced amounts of C3 are found in some cases of the nephritic and the nephrotic syndrome indicating an immunological problem.

Absent serum inhibitor of activated C1-esterase occurs in *hereditary angioneurotic oedema*. It is a rare Mendelian autosomal dominant disease characterised by recurrent episodes of circumscribed oedema in the subcutaneous tissues, throat and gastro-intestinal tract. Attacks are provoked by trauma, anxiety, menstruation and extremes of temperature. The occurrence of erythema marginata-like rash usually heralds an attack. The area of oedema does not itch, pit, or become red. Involvement of the bowel causes colic, watery diarrhoea and vomiting. Surgery is not indicated. *Oedema glottidis* occurs and is often fatal. Hereditary angioneurotic oedema can be distinguished from *allergic angio-oedema* by absence of eosinophilia and absent Cl-esterase inhibitor activity.

Treatment
The acute attack can be abated by giving fresh frozen plasma which replaces the missing serum inhibitor. Danazol can be given on a long-term basis to prevent attacks occurring.

[handwritten at top: hypoxia - reduced O₂ supply to tissues despite adequate perfusion of tissue]

CHAPTER 11

DISEASES OF THE HEART AND CIRCULATION

Probably 70–75 % of all heart disease in childhood can be diagnosed by taking a careful history and doing a careful clinical examination. A further 20 % require an electrocardiogram, phonocardiogram and appropriate X-ray studies. To elucidate the final 5–10 %, cardiac catheterisation, cineangiocardiography, dye dilution studies, radioisotope techniques and echocardiography may be required.

[handwritten: cyanosis. bluish discoloration due to reduced Hb]

SYMPTOMS AND SIGNS OF CARDIOVASCULAR DISEASE

Dyspnoea on exertion may be due to heart failure or to severe lung disease, and is often associated with cyanosis and clubbing of the fingers and toes.

Cyanosis is a bluish discoloration of the body surface. *Peripheral cyanosis* is limited to the extremities which are usually cold to the touch due to sluggish circulation. *Central cyanosis* is noted on the mucous membranes as well as the nailbeds and is often associated with clubbing of the fingers. It is usually due to cardiac or pulmonary causes, and occasionally due to methaemoglobin. Oxygen administration may relieve pulmonary cyanosis but not that due to intracardiac shunts. Cyanosis is usually present when the oxygen saturation of the blood is less than 85 %. *Cyanotic spells* are attacks of hypoxia occurring in Fallot's tetralogy. The spells consist of sudden attacks of cyanosis, dyspnoea and irritability which may lead to convulsions and coma. Another feature of Fallot's tetralogy is the tendency to squat after mild exertion and to sleep in the knee-chest position.

Fatiguability may be due to heart or lung disease, but can also be due to unrelated causes like tuberculosis. *Excessive sweating* frequently occurs in heart failure and in left-to-right shunts.

Recurrent respiratory infection may be a feature of large left-to-right shunts, but may also be associated with chronic lung disease, allergy or immunoglobulin deficiency states.

Fainting spells due to heart disease are rare; they may however be a sign of tight aortic stenosis, especially when associated with angina or exertional dyspnoea.

Growth disturbances usually occur with severe left-to-right shunts and in cyanotic patients. Children with Down's syndrome are small whether a heart lesion is present or not. In Marfan's syndrome the patient is often long and thin, despite mitral or aortic lesions. Turner's syndrome is a form of dwarfism associated with ovarian dysgenesis and coarctation of the aorta. Many other growth disturbances are associated with heart defects.

Alterations in the pulse rate occur normally in children during breathing (sinus arrhythmia), the pulse increasing with inspiration and slowing down during expiration. Fever, crying, exercise or nervousness can increase the pulse by 30 beats per minute or more. In febrile infants a pulse of 160–180 beats per minute may occur, which settles when the fever returns to normal. A persistently high or low pulse should be regarded as significant, particularly during sleep.

There is a wide range in the normal pulse and respiratory rate, as well as in the blood pressure readings. Table 11.1 therefore is intended only as a guide.

Table 11.1 Normal pulse, respiration and blood pressure

Age	Sleeping pulse rate/min	Sleeping respiration rate/min	Blood pressure mmHg
Fetus	120–160		
1st week	120 ±20	30–60	80/50
2–8 weeks	110 ±20	40 ±10	90/55
3–12 months	100 ±20	30 ±10	100/60
1–6 years	90 ±15	24 ±5	110/65
7–12 years	80 ±10	20 ±5	120/70

In infants the pulse is most easily felt at the temporal, brachial or femoral arteries. Absence of the femoral pulse suggests coarctation of the aorta. In older children, as in adults, the radial artery may be palpated to estimate the rate, rhythm, volume and tension of the pulse.

The blood pressure should be taken with a cuff that is two-thirds the length of the upper arm or thigh. Three or four different cuff widths should be available. Cuffs may be folded to make them narrower. If a cuff is too narrow it tends to increase the blood pressure reading.

The cuff for measuring the blood pressure in the lower limb should be twice as long as that for the upper, otherwise it will not sit snugly when blown up. The systolic blood pressure in the lower limb is about 10 mmHg higher than in the upper limb; the diastolic pressure may be lower.

The blood pressure can be measured in the upper and lower limbs in infants using the *flush method*. The limb is elevated and firmly bandaged from the top proximally in order to squeeze the superficial blood out of the skin. An infant blood pressure cuff is applied above the bandage and blown up to any figure *above* the estimated systolic blood pressure. The bandage is removed and the limb will be found to be blanched. The pressure in the sphygmanometer cuff is slowly released until the limb suddenly flushes. This measures the *mean* blood pressure.

In older children the blood pressure is measured in the same way as for adults. Methods based on ultrasound techniques can be used simply and accurately on children of all ages.

The electrocardiogram in the neonate normally reveals a right axis deviation and right ventricular dominance. In infancy and childhood the left side gradually increases its dominance over the right. The interested reader should refer to larger texts for details, e.g. A. J. Moss and G. C. Emmanouilides' *Practical Pediatric Electrocardiography* (Lippincott, 1973).

The normal chest X-ray appearances are shown in Fig. 11.1.

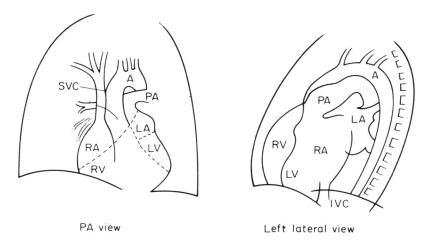

PA view   Left lateral view

Fig. 11.1 X-ray appearance of the normal heart

Differences in clinical signs in children and adults

In infants the normal apex beat is usually one space higher than in adults, i.e. it is in the fourth space slightly inside the nipple line. Before puberty the position of the nipple in both boys and girls is reasonably constant, and it is easier to find than the mid-clavicular line.

Right ventricular hypertrophy may cause a sternal heave on palpation while left ventricular hypertrophy causes an apical heave. If enlargement develops in infancy, bulging of the praecordium may be seen.

To detect enlargement of the heart percussion should be very light in infants and young children. The 'feel' is more important than the sound.

On auscultation in infants the pulmonary second sound is usually louder than the aortic second sound. It is usually single at birth but splits in the first 24 hours. The aortic and pulmonary sounds are of about equal intensity after the age of about 7 years, and by 12 years the adult relationship exists in which the aortic sound is much louder.

The heart beats faster in infants and children giving the sound a 'tic-tac' rhythm rather than a 'lub-dup lub-dup' sound. A third heart sound is often heard at the apex especially if the child lies on his left side. This must not be confused with the opening snap of mitral disease. It is due to the rapid flow of blood into the ventricles in early diastole and is accentuated by increased flow into the left ventricle, for example in ventricular septal defect, patent ductus arteriosus, aortic insufficiency and high output states. It is also a constant feature of the functional vibratory systolic murmur.

The fourth heart sound is due to sudden dilatation of the ventricle during atrial contraction and it is heard just before the first heart sound, especially if the atrial pressure is increased.

Venous pressure is not usually detectable in infants because of their short fat necks. Older children lie propped up on cushions at a 45° angle, and the height of the distended jugular vein above the suprasternal notch can easily be measured. If measured directly by means of an intra-atrial manometer, the mean venous pressure under ten years of age is 4 mmHg or about 50 mmH$_2$O (0.5 kPa).

Oedema

In right heart failure in adults and children oedema is gravity-dependent and appears over the lower extremities. In infants, however, it may first accumulate around the orbit, and later become generalised. The liver usually enlarges at the same time.

HEART FAILURE

The following symptoms and signs are common to all forms of heart failure in children. There is irritability, anorexia, gallop rhythm, tachycardia and enlargement of the heart. *Left-sided failure* is associated with cough, dyspnoea, orthopnoea, and crepitations at the bases of the lungs due to pulmonary congestion. Heaving of the apex beat may be felt outside the mid-clavicular line. *Right-sided failure* is associated with oedema, congestion of the neck veins and swelling of the liver which may be tender and rounded. There is a tapping beat or substernal heave at the left of the lower part of the sternum.

Combined right and left failure has features of both.

Treatment
The underlying cause of heart failure should be treated wherever

possible. Surgery should be undertaken when indicated. The use of penicillin in rheumatic fever is mandatory. Heart failure often improves if the patient is put to rest in an oxygen tent, with sufficient oxygen flow to overcome cyanosis. A sedative such as chloral hydrate 600 mg/m² may be used for restlessness. For 'cardiac asthma' aminophylline intravenously or morphine subcutaneously has a good reputation. In congestive heart failure considerable relief can be gained by use of a rapidly acting diuretic such as frusemide (Lasix) 12 mg/m² by injection or 24 mg/m² orally. This may be repeated in 4–6 hours if necessary and then given once or twice daily. As potassium is lost in the urine it should be replaced in the form of potassium chloride orally. With this regime it is rarely necessary to use large doses of digoxin. In fact 0.15 mg/m² twice daily may be adequate in many patients. However, others may require this dose three or even four times daily. Indications for reducing dosage include clinical improvement, bradycardia, anorexia, nausea, vomiting and cardiac irregularities.

Full details concerning the use of digoxin will be found in P. Catzel's *The Paediatric Prescriber* (Blackwell Scientific Publications, 1981). The use of drugs acting on cardiac arrhythmias are also described. For the cyanotic spells of Fallot, propanolol 0.1 mg/kg intravenously is recommended.

CARDIAC ARREST

Heart arrest may occur during the course of an anaesthetic, from electric shock, poisoning, severe arrhythmias or electrolyte disturbances. As a result the pulse cannot be felt, the heart cannot be heard and the pupils dilate. The practitioner has only two or three minutes to get the heart going again.

Management
The infant or child should be placed on a firm surface. Quickly squeeze the heart between sternum and spine. In an infant two fingers sharply pressed against the sternum may be sufficient; in older children pressure from the whole hand on the sternum may be necessary. At the same time one should yell for help, check the time and make sure that the airway is open.

Mouth-to-mouth breathing and external cardiac massage should be instituted at once. If a second person is available he should pump the sternum 60–100 times per minute while air is blown into the lung at least four times per minute.

This should be continued until mechanical respiration can be instituted, and an ECG done to distinguish between fibrillation and cardiac arrest. Intravenous sodium bicarbonate 30–40 mmol/m² (approximately 2 mmol/kg) may be given immediately. It is an advantage to treat these problems in an intensive care unit where defibrillators, monitors and other apparatus are available. The energy dose for defibrillation in a child is 2 J/kg of body weight, doubling if the response is not adequate (*Adult range*: 300–400 J).

HEART SOUNDS

Grades of systolic murmurs

1 Very soft, one must strain to hear it.
2 Easily heard without strain.
3 Very loud but thrill not palpable.
4 Very loud with palpable thrill.
5 So loud that it can be heard if only the edge of the stethoscope touches the chest.
6 So loud it can be heard with a stethoscope 1 cm from the chest.

Thus a very loud murmur without a thrill would be designated grade 3/6. Diastolic murmurs are never louder than grade 4.

The innocent murmur

An innocent or 'functional' murmur is one which can be heard over the heart in the absence of anatomical or pathological changes. The history, physical signs, ECG and X-rays are normal.
There are four important innocent murmurs in childhood:

1 Vibratory systolic murmur.
2 Pulmonic systolic murmur.
3 Supraclavicular systolic murmur.
4 Venous hum.

1 Vibratory systolic mumurs

These are grade 1–2, short mid-systolic murmurs best heard in the third or fourth interspace at the sternal edge, or just inside the apex. A bell stethoscope is required to pick up the vibratory, buzzing or 'twanging string' quality. It is maximum in the supine position and intensified by exercise or fever. It is commonly heard before 7 years of age. Intracardiac phonocardiographic studies have established that the murmur arises from within the left ventricular outflow tract.

2 Pulmonic murmurs

These are grade 2, short, mid-systolic murmurs best heard in the second left intercostal space at the sternal edge. It is blowing in character, often musical, higher pitched than the vibratory murmur and best heard with the diaphragm of the stethoscope. It is also best heard in the supine position, varies with posture and respiration, and is intensified by fever and by exercise. The murmur seems to originate from within the pulmonary artery and not from the valves. These murmurs are particularly common in children with flat chests (*the straight back syndrome*), the heart being close to the anterior chest wall. The murmur can be accentuated by pressing the stethoscope firmly against the chest wall.

3 Supraclavicular innocent systolic murmurs

These are arterial murmurs often heard above both clavicles in children, as well as in the suprasternal notch. They are mid-systolic with a coarse crescendo-decrescendo character. They are louder above the right clavicle. They are best heard with the child sitting up and looking straight ahead. They disappear if the child slowly pulls his elbows back to obliterate the subclavian artery.

4 The venous hum

This is a continuous murmur best heard above the inner end of the clavicles. It may be a low-toned musical murmur or it may be rough and roaring. There may be accentuation in diastole and when the patient sits up. It disappears when the ipsilateral internal jugular vein in compressed or if the head is rotated to left or right. It commonly disappears on lying down.

In children it is important to distinguish between the above innocent murmurs and murmurs due to organic disease (see Fig. 11.2). The latter will also be described under the individual disorders.

CONGENITAL HEART DISEASE

It is incumbent on the general practitioner and school health officer to have sufficient knowledge of heart disease in children to separate the innocent murmurs from the organic and to determine which children need investigation and which do not. He should avoid creating cardiac neurosis!

The incidence of congenital heart disease varies between 6 and 10 per 1000 live births. Of these up to one-third may die in the first year of life. In the neonate there may be no symptoms at all, or the patient may present early with congestive heart failure. Puffiness of the eyes and a swollen liver are cardinal signs of this; generalised oedema develops later. Attacks of pallor and sighing occur which may be regarded as the equivalent of 'fainting' in the older child. Respiratory distress and noisy respiration, cyanosis and opisthotonos may be found. In older children squatting and clubbing of the fingers may accompany cyanosis.

opisthotonos - spasm in which head + heels are bent back + body curved forward

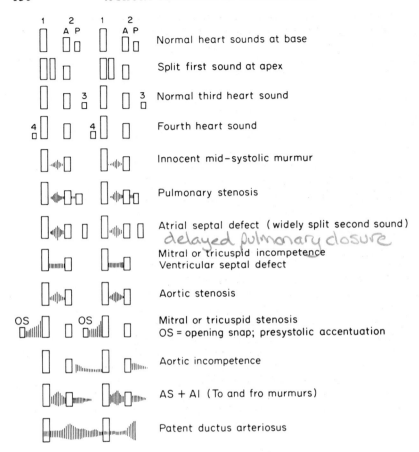

Fig. 11.2 Some normal and abnormal heart sounds. (1 = first heart sound; 2 = second heart sound; OS = opening snap; A = aortic component of second sound; P = pulmonary component of second sound)

In taking a history one should emphasise the early pregnancy when the mother may have had rubella or taken drugs for excessive vomiting, or other causes. A few conditions are hereditary.

The fetal circulation

In the fetus the placenta acts as both source of nutrition and source of gas exchange. The fetal bowel and lung are, for all practical purposes, non-functioning. The unexpanded lungs offer greater resistance to blood flow and therefore the right heart pressure *in utero* is the same as that on the left. Three shunts are necessary *in utero* to maintain the fetal circulation. They are the foramen ovale, the ductus arteriosus and the ductus venosus (see Fig. 11.3).

At birth the first cry and the clamping of the umbilical cord are followed within minutes, sometimes hours or days, by extensive readjustment to the circulation. As the lungs fill with air there is a fall in pulmonary vascular resistance and the pulmonary blood flow increases. At the same time the systemic vascular resistance increases. Functionally the foramen ovale, the ductus venosus and the ductus arteriosus close. Constriction of the ductus arteriosus is favoured by a high oxygen concentration. Many congenital heart lesions can be explained by failure of these adjustments to occur, for example persistence of the ductus arteriosus, septal defects and perhaps coarctation of the aorta. Other congenital anomalies are due to persistent fetal

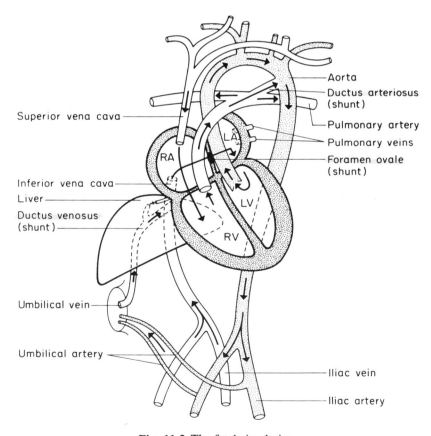

Fig. 11.3 The fetal circulation

malformations such as right-sided aorta or other anatomical disorders. It is stated that the foramen ovale can be probed open in about 50 % of children under five years of age. In any condition where the right atrial pressure rises, a right-to-left shunt may occur through the foramen ovale.

CYANOTIC CONGENITAL HEART DISEASE

Transposition of the great vessels

In transposition of the great arteries, the aorta rises from the right ventricle and the pulmonary trunk from the left. Thus the aorta lies in front of the pulmonary trunk or a little to one side. The mitral and tricuspid valves lie in their normal position so that pulmonary valve tissue may be continuous with the anterior mitral leaflet. Pulmonary stenosis may be present.

Life can be maintained postnatally only if communications between the systemic and pulmonary circulations exist. Thus there may be an atrial septal defect (ASD), ventricular septal defect (VSD), patent ductus arteriosus (PDA) or collateral circulation between the aorta and pulmonary bed via large bronchial arteries. Three factors determine the final picture:

1 The type of communication between the systemic and pulmonary circulations.
2 Pressure gradients between these communications.
3 Pulmonary bed resistance.

Clinical features

Severe cyanosis and congestive heart failure commonly occur in early infancy. The heart is always enlarged and the occurrence of murmurs depends on the type of communication present. The pulses are often bounding in character. Clubbing develops in the first few months of life. Boys are affected up to four times more commonly than girls.

The classic X-ray picture is the 'egg on its side' appearance of the heart, with a narrow pedicle due to a hypoplastic thymus, and plethoric lung fields. In the presence of pulmonary stenosis the picture may resemble the boot-shaped heart seen in Fallot's tetralogy (Fig. 11.4). Cardiac enlargement of variable degree is present. The diagnosis should be confirmed by echocardiography, cardiac catheterisation and angiography as soon as possible. Palliation may be achieved by a Rashkind septostomy which creates an artificial atrial septal defect. Further procedures can be done when the infant is older. The Mustard operation corrects the defects in some cases.

plethoric - excess of blood

The tetralogy of Fallot

This consists of four anomalies, listed in order of their importance:

1 Subpulmonary or infundibular stenosis.
2 Interventricular septal defect (VSD).
3 Dextroposition (over-riding) of the aorta.
4 Hypertrophy of the right ventricle.

Haemodynamically, the severity of the lesion is determined by the degree of pulmonary stenosis and the size of the VSD. The degree of cyanosis depends on the quantity of blood shunted from the right to the left side of the heart.

Clinical features
Cyanosis and dyspnoea appear early and get steadily worse. Clubbing of the fingers usually occurs after about two years of age. Babies may have 'fainting spells' due to pulmonary infundibular spasm. After four months of age these become clarified as spells of paroxysmal dyspnoea. After two years of age cerebral abscess may occur. A harsh grade 4/6 systolic murmur and thrill may be felt over the second or third left intercostal space next to the sternum. However, the severest grades of Fallot's tetralogy often have soft murmurs. Blood count reveals a polycythaemia. X-ray reveals a small boot-shaped heart, the tip of the 'boot' being turned up due to right ventricular hypertrophy and small pulmonary conus. There is reduced blood flow to the lung in most cases (Fig. 11.4). If increased vascularity is seen this is likely to be due to collateral bronchial vessels. The ECG shows right ventricular hypertrophy with peaked P waves.

Treatment
Open heart surgery with closure of the septal defect and repair of the subpulmonary stenosis may be attempted when feasible. Alternatively an artificial ductus is created by anastomosis of the left pulmonary and left subclavian arteries (Blalock-Taussig operation) or pulmonary

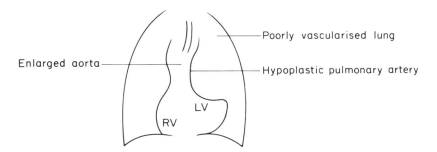

Fig. 11.4 X-ray of the boot-shaped heart in Fallot's tetralogy

artery and ascending aorta (Waterston operation). In Pott's operation a ductus is created between the descending aorta and left pulmonary artery.

Two conditions which may resemble Fallot's tetralogy clinically are Eisenmenger's complex and pulmonary stenosis with patent foramen ovale.

Eisenmenger's syndrome

This consists of increased pulmonary vascular resistance combined with a shunt such as a septal defect or PDA. The pulmonary valve itself is normal but the haemodynamic effects of this condition are similar to that of severe Fallot's tetralogy. Thus cyanosis, dyspnoea and congestive heart failure may occur early. The murmur is rarely louder than grade 3/6 and the pulmonary second sound may boom.

Pure pulmonary stenosis

Narrowing of the pulmonary outflow tract may be due to fusion of the pulmonary cusps, supravalvular or infundibular stenosis. The pulmonary pressure may exceed the systemic and become great enough to reopen the foramen ovale.

Clinical features

The clinical findings depend on the degree of stenosis. A mild degree of stenosis may be asymptomatic. Severe degrees may lead to cyanosis and right heart failure. These patients may have high cheek bones, moon face and hypertelorism. Clubbing is associated with chronic cyanosis. There may be a heaving right ventricle and a systolic thrill may be present over the pulmonary area and suprasternal notch. A rough, ejection grade 4/6 murmur is heard. In mild cases a pulmonary ejection click which varies with respiration is usually heard over the second intercostal space. In severe stenosis the click may merge with the first sound giving it a high-pitched, clicking quality. The second sound also varies with the degree of stenosis. In mild stenosis it may be widely split and clicking whereas in severe cases it is single as the pulmonary component cannot be heard. A prominent A wave is seen in the jugular pulse.

The ECG shows right ventricular hypertrophy. In severe cases P pulmonale is found. On X-ray the heart may be normal or right ventricular enlargement, with or without right atrial enlargement, may be present. Post-stenotic dilatation of the pulmonary artery may occur (Fig. 11.5). In cyanotic patients there is reduced vascularity of the lungs. Catheterisation may be required to determine the degree and type of stenosis.

hypertelorism- wide spaced eyes

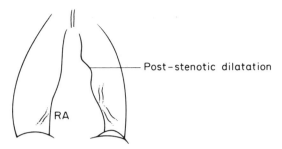

Post-stenotic dilatation

RA

Fig. 11.5 X-ray of pulmonary stenosis (valvular)

Treatment
The greater the obstruction, the earlier surgical correction should be attempted.

Ebstein's anomaly

Ebstein's anomaly consists of downward displacement of the posterior and septal leaflets of the tricuspid valve. This results in a small right ventricle and a very large, dilated right atrium. Some degree of tricuspid regurgitation is usually present. Cyanosis and congestive heart failure may occur in infancy but improves with increasing age. In children cyanosis may be slight unless an atrial septal defect is also present.

On auscultation a triple rhythm is associated with a soft systolic murmur and a characteristic soft scratchy mid-diastolic murmur at the lower left sternal border. These may be due to tricuspid incompetence and stenosis due to an abnormally attached tricuspid valve. The first sound is widely split due to late closure of the abnormally large tricuspid valve. The second sound is also widely split due to an associated right bundle branch block. Attacks of paroxysmal tachycardia often occur.

X-ray of the heart shows the organ to be enlarged with a massive right atrium and decreased pulmonary vascular markings (Fig. 11.6). The

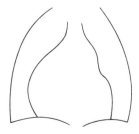

Fig. 11.6 X-ray of cardiomegaly in Ebstein's anomaly

electrocardiogram reveals a giant P wave (right atrial hypertrophy) and some degree of right bundle branch block. Paroxysmal supraventricular tachycardia is commonly seen on ECG.

Cardiac catheterisation should be avoided as fatal arrhythmia may occur. Angiography may confirm the 'atrialisation' of part of the right ventricle.

Prognosis depends on the severity of the malformation. Death usually occurs in early infancy or in the third decade of congestive heart failure or cardiac arrhythmia. The use of cardiac glycosides, anti-arrhythmic drugs and diuretics prolong life. Palliative surgery carries a high mortality. An ASD, if present, can be closed. Tricuspid valve replacement or annuloplastic repair of the valve may be attempted.

Tricuspid atresia

There is a complete obstruction of blood flow from the right atrium to the right ventricle (the 'right heart by-pass syndrome'). To keep the patient alive there is a large atrial septal defect so that an extra volume of blood reaches the left ventricle. Blood can only reach the pulmonary artery through a VSD, a patent ductus arteriosus or bronchial collaterals. In some patients transposition of the great vessels is found.

As a result of these abnormalities cyanosis is marked from birth and congestive heart failure occurs in early infancy. Treatment is by palliative surgery, which attempts to increase pulmonary blood flow, or by atrial septostomy.

Total anomalous pulmonary venous return

Instead of entering the left atrium, the pulmonary venous blood drains into the left superior vena cava (persistent anterior cardinal vein), the right atrium, the coronary sinus or into the portal veins below the diaphragm (Fig. 11.7). Thus blood in the right atrium contains a mixture of oxygenated pulmonary and deoxygenated systemic blood. An ASD is always present, so that part of this blood shunts into the left atrium. If

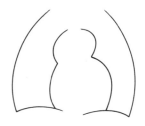

Fig. 11.7 X-ray of total anomalous pulmonary venous drainage ('figure-of-eight')

pulmonary vascular resistance is normal these patients are less disabled. If the pulmonary vascular resistance is increased, the patient becomes cyanotic and develops right heart failure. Surgical treatment is often possible, provided that the pulmonary arterial pressure is normal.

NON-CYANOTIC CONGENITAL HEART DISEASE

The non-cyanotic congenital heart lesions include:

1 Atrial septal defect (ASD)
2 Ventricular septal defect (VSD)
3 Patent ductus arteriosus (PDA)
4 Dextrocardia
5 Lesions of the aorta (aortic stenosis, coarctation).

Atrial septal defects (ASD)

There are three types:

1 High ASD (ostium secundum type)
2 Low ASD (ostium primum-associated with endocardial cushion defects)
3 Complete ASD (common atrioventricular canal or AV communis).

To understand atrial septal defects one should remember that during fetal development two septa and three openings are formed (Fig. 11.8).

The septum primum is a thin wall which grows down towards the endocardial cushion to separate the two atria. A connection between the right and left atrium, the *ostium primum*, is formed at the lower end of the *septum primum*. When this seals off, an *ostium secundum* forms in the upper part of the septum. A second septum, the *septum secundum*, is formed to the right of the *septum primum* leaving an opening at its lower portion (foramen ovale). This septum forms a flap across the ostium secundum but, under certain conditions, blood can pass through the foramen ovale, to the ostium secundum and into the left atrium (see p. 138).

1 Ostium secundum defects

Absent or incomplete formation of the septum secundum produces an opening high up between the two atria. The atrioventricular valves are not affected because the endocardial cushion is not involved.

Clinical features
These children are usually small but otherwise without symptoms. If the atrial septal opening is large, the volume of the shunt increases with age, the right atrium and ventricle enlarge and increased flow occurs through

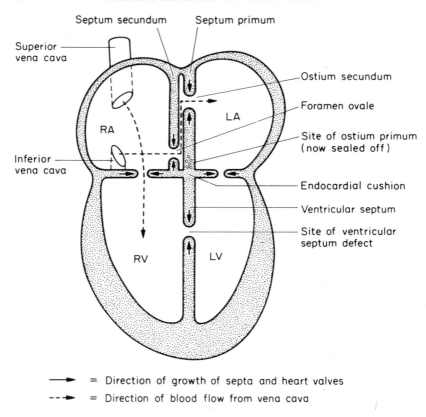

Superior vena cava

Septum secundum

Septum primum

Ostium secundum

Foramen ovale

RA

LA

Site of ostium primum (now sealed off)

Inferior vena cava

Endocardial cushion

Ventricular septum

Site of ventricular septum defect

RV LV

⟶ = Direction of growth of septa and heart valves

--⟶ = Direction of blood flow from vena cava

Fig. 11.8 Diagram of the origin of the septa and valves of the heart

the lungs. Sometimes this is associated with repeated respiratory infections and some reduction of exercise tolerance.

There is a grade 1–3/6 ejection systolic murmur over the pulmonary area usually associated with a widely split and fixed P_2. It is unaffected by the Valsalva manoeuvre. If there is increased flow across the tricuspid valve a rumbling early or mid-diastolic murmur may be heard in this area. Rarely pulmonary artery pressure increases early; it is usually delayed to the third decade. This increases the pressure in the right ventricle and hence the right atrium. This may halt or even reverse the shunt. Cyanosis becomes apparent in these patients. Such reversal may also be precipitated by an attack of bronchitis or pneumonia. When this occurs the diastolic murmur disappears and the split of the second pulmonary sound becomes less.

The electrocardiogram reveals right axis deviation with an rsR′

pattern over lead V_1 and deep s wave over lead V_6. A right bundle branch block pattern may be present. X-ray confirms right atrial and ventricular enlargement with increased pulmonary vascular markings. On fluoroscopic screening pulsation of the hilar vessels ('hilar dance') may be present.

Treatment
Surgery to close the defect may be offered between five and ten years of age if the blood flow is large enough to enlarge the right ventricle and increase the pulmonary vascularity.

Prognosis
It is possible to live an entirely normal life with a small or even medium-sized secundum defect. Often, however, pulmonary hypertension with reversal of the shunt, cyanosis and congestive heart failure may occur after the third decade.

2 Ostium primum defects

The septal opening is *low* and is associated with lesions of the endocardial cushion. Haemodynamically this produces changes similar to secundum defects (due to the atrial opening) but in addition there may be congenital mitral or tricuspid insufficiency, high ventricular septal defects or various combinations of these endocardial cushion defects. These are the types of defect commonly noted in Down's Syndrome. The severest form of defect is AV communis.

Infants with ostium primum defects may develop congestive heart failure or pulmonary hypertension early in life. The ECG is unusual in showing *left* axis deviation with right ventricular hypertrophy. Operative repair of as many of the defects as possible has been undertaken in some centres.

Ventricular septal defect (VSD)

The opening in a VSD may be high or low, but symptoms depend on whether the opening is large or small. Owing to the dominance of the left ventricle in childhood, the flow is from left to right. In the first few days of life, however, the pressures in the two ventricles are similar and therefore no flow occurs across the opening, and no murmur is heard.

Clinical features
The majority of children with VSD have no symptoms but they may have very loud and alarming murmurs. Alarm is transmitted from doctor to parent and may cause unnecessary cardiac neurosis.

The murmur is usually a grade 2–4/6 pansystolic murmur, maximum in the third or fourth left intercostal space. A thrill is often palpable. With *large* left-to-right flow enlargement of the heart may occur, leading to congestive heart failure in infancy. Increased blood flow across the pulmonary artery may be associated with pulmonary hypertension in many patients. The second pulmonary sound is normally split until pulmonary pressure increases and the split becomes narrow and accentuation of the pulmonary component occurs. Bulging of the praecordium may develop.

Ventricular septal defect may be associated with other defects such as pulmonary stenosis (see p. 133), Eisenmenger's syndrome (p. 134), ASD, transposition of the great vessels, coarctation of the aorta and others.

Recurrent respiratory infections are common with large defects. Dyspnoea and easy fatiguability are associated with slow weight-gain.

With small shunts the ECG is normal. Large shunts may be associated with pure left ventricular hypertrophy, but with the development of pulmonary hypertension the right ventricle also hypertrophies. X-ray shows a large left-to-right shunt (Fig. 11.9).

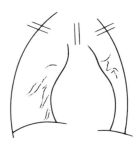

Fig. 11.9 X-ray of ventricular septal defect (large left-to-right shunt)

Therapy
Congestive heart failure is treated with digoxin and diuretics until surgical correction is possible. In small infants a band has been placed around the pulmonary artery in order to reduce pulmonary blood flow and pressure. However, most authorities prefer to attempt immediate corrective surgery. This should be done before permanent pulmonary vascular damage develops.

Prognosis
Small defects are usually asymptomatic and 25 % close spontaneously by two years of age, 66 % by eight years and 75 % by ten years. Some even close in adulthood. Large defects can lead to early heart failure. Pulmonary hypertension may occur in infancy.

Patent ductus arteriosus (PDA)

Shortly after birth the pressures in the aorta and pulmonary artery are nearly equal so that very little flow occurs through the ductus arteriosus.

Thus no murmur is heard in the first few weeks of life. With growth the pressure in the pulmonary artery gets less and a systolic murmur may be heard in the second left intercostal space during the first year. Gradually the typical continuous 'machinery murmur' of the patent ductus arteriosus develops.

Children may remain completely asymptomatic but if the shunt is very large dyspnoea on exertion may develop. Ten per cent of patients develop pulmonary hypertension which may lead to progressive heart failure in the third decade of life. The pulmonary component of the second heart sound may become accentuated. The pulses bound owing to a large pulse pressure. Some patients have increased pulmonary vascular resistance which may lead to a reversal of the shunt. This may be precipitated by a respiratory infection. Differential cyanosis in which only the left arm and both feet are affected, but not the right arm and head, may be present. The murmur may disappear or be insignificant.

X-rays may be normal. A large shunt may lead to biventricular enlargement. The aorta is prominent. Pulmonary vascular engorgement depends on the size of the shunt. The pulmonary artery may be dilated. The ECG may be normal or show mild ventricular hypertrophy. Deep Q waves may be found in the left ventricular leads.

Diagnosis

The typical machinery murmur must not be confused with a venous hum; the latter disappears on pressing on the jugular vein. Patent ductus arteriosus with pulmonary hypertension must be distinguished from PDA with pulmonary vascular obstruction. In the latter the oxygen content of the ductus is not increased while systemic arterial saturation is decreased.

Treatment

Surgical correction is usually advised on diagnosis. If pulmonary hypertension is present immediate operation is essential but if pulmonary pressure is normal no harm comes of delaying operation. Patients with irreversible pulmonary vascular obstruction should be left alone.

In the pre-term baby PDA is common but most close within a few weeks. Indomethacin, a prostaglandin inhibitor, can be used to close the duct if there is heart failure. Spontaneous closure of a simple PDA may occur up to the age of two years, rarely after.

Dextrocardia

Dextrocardia, in which the apex of the heart points to the right, may be associated with *situs inversus* in which the positions of all the organs are reversed. One can then percuss the normal liver in the left hypochondrium and a gastric gas bubble on the right. With complete reversal of all the organs the heart is haemodynamically normal. The parents should be warned always to notify their doctor should the patient ever develop an acute abdomen—there may be a left-sided appendix! 'Pure' dextrocardia (i.e. without *situs inversus*) is always associated with other intracardiac anomalies.

Diagnosis is confirmed by X-ray and by ECG. P waves are inverted in lead I. Lead II resembles lead III and vice versa. In lead I the QRS wave is mainly a negative deflection.

Congenital aortic stenosis (AS)

Congenital aortic stenosis is a condition in which a systolic pressure gradient of more than 10 mmHg is found between the left ventricle and the aorta. Most are due to a bicuspid aortic valve, a few to a membranous ring, to subaortic hypertrophy of the muscle or to supra-valvular stenosis.

Clinical features

The majority of patients have no symptoms during childhood, though they may be small and have a delicate 'Dresden china' appearance. Severe stenosis may lead to dizziness and syncope. Occasionally sudden death from heart failure or coronary insufficiency may occur.

Most children have a heaving left ventricle and a systolic thrill over the aortic area and in the suprasternal notch. A grade 4/6 rough ejection murmur is heard in the second right interspace and is transmitted along the subclavian arteries and carotids, and towards the apex. Sometimes there may be a short blowing diastolic murmur due to aortic in-sufficiency. This is associated with a pulsus bisferiens. An ejection click may be heard at the apex or over the aortic area. It occurs shortly after the first sound. If the click is absent one must suspect one of the rarer types of aortic stenosis. A plateau pulse is usual in aortic stenosis.

The ECG may be normal in mild stenosis. Increasing stenosis is associated with left ventricular hypertrophy and strain pattern. X-ray reveals that initially the heart may be normal. With severe stenosis left ventricular hypertrophy may be found. Post-stenotic dilation of the aorta may be present. The gradient across the aortic valve is measured during left heart catheterisation.

Treatment

Surgery is indicated early if symptoms occur or the ECG shows a strain pattern. If there are no symptoms, operation may be deferred to any time after the age of ten years. The main danger of aortic stenosis in children is angina pectoris or sudden death after exertion. Therefore competitive sports should be forbidden.

Coarctation of the aorta

Coarctation means 'contracted', 'tightened' or 'narrowed'. It usually occurs in the thoracic aorta, very rarely in the abdominal. It is at least

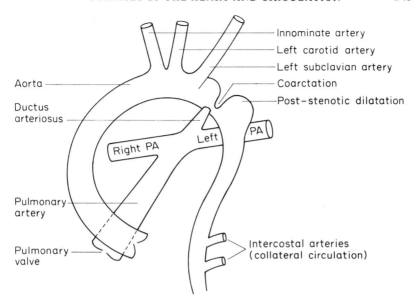

Innominate artery
Left carotid artery
Left subclavian artery
Coarctation
Post-stenotic dilatation
Aorta
Ductus arteriosus
Right PA
Left
PA
Pulmonary artery
Pulmonary valve
Intercostal arteries (collateral circulation)

Fig. 11.10 Coarctation of the aorta

three times more common in boys than girls, and may be found in Turner's XO syndrome. In 98 % of patients the narrowing occurs just below the origin of the left subclavian artery (Fig. 11.10). It is characterised by progressive hypertension of the vessels proximal to the coarctation, reduced blood pressure in the distal vessels and the development of a collateral circulation. In children it may be entirely asymptomatic or it may present with nose bleeds, headache and very rarely with pain in the limbs on walking (intermittent claudication). Palpation of the femoral pulses, which should be a routine exercise, reveals that they are weak or absent, whereas the brachial pulses are strong and arterial pulsation is present in the suprasternal notch. The systolic pressure in the arms may be normal or it may be raised. An ejection grade 2/6 systolic murmur may be heard over the site of the coarctation, both front and back, and down the left sternal border. The ECG is not characteristic. The X-ray may show an aorta shaped like a '3'. The first arc of the '3' is due to dilation of the proximal part of the aorta, the middle line of the '3' is the coarctation and the second arc is due to post-stenotic dilation. On barium swallow the 'E' sign may be found (see Fig. 11.11). Notching of the ribs usually occurs after the age of eight years and is due to pressure by the dilated collateral arteries.

Treatment
Surgical correction should usually be undertaken between 10 and 15 years of age. Earlier operation is indicated if symptoms are present, in

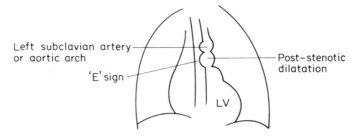

Left subclavian artery
or aortic arch

'E' sign

Post-stenotic
dilatation

LV

Fig. 11.11 X-ray of barium swallow showing the 'E' sign in coarctation of the
aorta

order to prevent permanent hypertension. If necessary the operation can
be done between 3 and 6 years of age. Congestive heart failure is treated
medically.

Congenital hypoplasia of the left heart

The 'hypoplastic left heart syndrome' involves the aortic tract complex
including an underdeveloped left atrium, atresia of the mitral valve,
small left ventricle and aortic atresia, singly or together, complete or
incomplete, causing obstruction of flow through the left heart. It causes
a low output state with a small heart. Cyanosis is usual and congestive
heart failure commonly occurs in the first 4–6 weeks of life, depending
on the site and severity of the lesion and the existence of various
intracardiac shunts. The elucidation of most of these lesions requires the
full resources of a cardiac unit. The prognosis is uniformly bad.

Aortic vascular rings

Although rare, persistent double aortic arch may press on the oesophagus causing dysphagia, or on the trachea causing dyspnoea and
stridor from birth. Diagnosis is made by barium swallow. Treatment is
surgical.

PRIMARY MYOCARDIAL DISEASE

Endocardial fibroelastosis is characterised by congestive cardiac failure
occurring usually before one year of age, occasionally later. The cause is
unknown. At autopsy the endocardium, the subendothelial layer of the
left ventricle and the left atrium are thick and milky white. There are no
shunts but mitral incompetence is common. Treatment requires prolonged treatment with digitalis and diuretics, for congestive heart
failure. Life is thus prolonged for a few years but the ultimate prognosis
is bad.

 The disease should be suspected in infants and young children with
mitral disease in whom no evidence of rheumatic fever is found.

ACQUIRED HEART DISEASE

Acute myocarditis

In the neonate *coxsackie group B virus* has caused epidemics of acute myocarditis in the nursery. The infection may be subclinical or the baby may present with congestive heart failure. Puffiness of the eyes may precede oedema elsewhere by several days. The liver is enlarged to the umbilicus and tachycardia and tachypnoea are usually obvious. Diagnosis is confirmed by virus studies. Therapy consists of cautious digitalisation and diuretics.

In the older child myocarditis may be caused by acute rheumatic fever (p. 315) where it forms part of a pancarditis. In diphtheria (p. 317) myocarditis is a dangerous complication which carries a 50 % mortality. Viral infections such as measles, mumps and poliomyelitis may sometimes show ECG signs of myocarditis but this is rarely of serious import.

Pericarditis

Pericarditis may be due to acute rheumatic fever. Coxsackie group B virus, which causes serious neonatal myocarditis, can also cause an acute, benign, self-limiting pericarditis in older children. It begins suddenly with fever and precordial pain, and a pericardial friction rub is heard. A pericardial effusion may develop (see Fig. 11.12). The majority of children recover without sequelae, treatment consisting of bed rest, good nursing and symptomatic therapy. There is no specific therapy and the value of corticosteroids is doubtful. The same syndrome can also be caused by influenza virus but often no cause can be found.

Purulent pericarditis may be due to *Staphylococcus aureus*, *Haemophilus influenzae* or meningococcus infection. It may be due to septicaemia, or to direct extension from an empyema or a liver abscess. Tamponade requires urgent relief. Antibiotics are given according to the sensitivity of the organism. Constrictive pericarditis may develop with surprising speed.

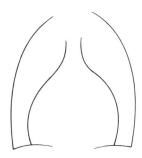

Fig. 11.12 X-ray of the pear-shaped heart in pericardial effusion

Tuberculous pericarditis

This is probably due to direct extension from infected mediastinal glands. Its onset is very insidious and it is rarely diagnosed before evidence of constrictive pericarditis is obvious. Prognosis has improved with antituberculous therapy and surgery.

Post-pericardiotomy syndrome

This has come to the fore since heart surgery has become an everyday procedure. It occurs as a complication of opening the pericardium and is characterised by fever, chest pain and pericardial friction rub which develops usually 14–21 days after the operation. It may occur as early as three days postoperatively to six months after the operation. The cause is unknown but viral infection, sterile inflammation and auto-immunity have been suggested. The condition usually clears on conservative therapy in 2–3 weeks and may recur at 2–3 week intervals.

Pericarditis may also occur in rheumatoid arthritis, thalassaemia and renal failure. Trauma may cause pericardial bleeding and tamponade.

Bacterial endocarditis

Subacute bacterial endocarditis (SBE) is an uncommon but important complication of heart disease in children. About two-thirds are associated with congenital heart disease and the rest with rheumatic endocarditis. It is caused by bacteria colonising a damaged endocardium, either rheumatic valves or endocardium traumatised by a jet of blood. This should be distinguished from acute bacterial endocarditis in which the heart is healthy but the valves are colonised by *Staphylococcus aureus* during the course of an acute septicaemia. The commonest organism cultured in SBE is *Streptococcus viridans*, but on occasion *E. coli*, *Staphylococcus albus*, *Pseudomonas aeruginosa* and *Aspergillus* have been found.

The onset is insidious with fever, malaise, rigors, joint and chest pains. There is usually evidence of an underlying heart lesion. Petechiae, Osler's nodes and flame-shaped haemorrhages under the nails may be present. Many but not all patients have splenomegaly. Microscopic haematuria, leucocytosis and a raised sedimentation rate are usual. The picture may be obscured by congestive heart failure.

Diagnosis

The disease should be suspected in any cardiac patient who does not do well or who unexpectedly deteriorates. Blood cultures are usually positive but may have to be repeated several times if the first culture is negative.

Therapy

Penicillin G in large intravenous doses of 5–10 million units/m²/day, is the drug of choice for *Streptococcus viridans* infection. In resistant cases streptomycin, or gentamicin in full doses should be given. For

Osler's nodes – small raised tender swollen areas, bluish, pink or red in pads of fingers or toes or hypo / thenar eminences of soles of feet

staphylococci, isoxazole penicillins like cloxacillin are advised. In selected cases erythromycin, cephaloridines, lincomycin or chloramphenicol may be required.

If the endocarditis is due to an infected prosthesis, this may have to be removed before success can be achieved.

Prevention

Before teeth or tonsils are removed in children with heart disease, or before any operation (including heart operations) are undertaken, prophylactic antibiotics should be given. Fortified procaine penicillin injection 700 mg/m^2 may be given 1–2 hours prior to surgery, followed by procaine penicillin injection 700 mg/m^2 daily for 3 days after operation. In the case of appendicectomy or genito-urinary instrumentation, the use of a broad spectrum antibiotic active against Gram-negative organisms, such as gentamicin should be given.

Hypertension

Hypertension in childhood may be defined as a blood pressure of 130/90 mmHg or more on *three* successive occasions. It has been estimated that on these criteria 1–2 % of children are hypertensive. In children a raised blood pressure is nearly always secondary to some underlying cause, usually renal. It may be caused by acute glomerulonephritis, hypoplastic kidneys, hydronephrosis, pyelonephritis or polycystic kidneys. However, if the plasma renin activity is normal a renal cause is excluded in most cases. Extrarenal causes include coarctation of the aorta, patent ductus arteriosus, prolonged increase in intracranial pressure, lead poisoning and phaeochromocytoma. In these conditions if the underlying condition is cured, then the hypertension will settle by itself. The treatment of hypertension and hypertensive crises is dealt with on pp. 287–288.

Mitral valve prolapse (the billowing mitral leaflet syndrome; Barlow's syndrome)

It is now well recognised that mitral valve prolapse is a common entity in children as well as adults. The condition is recognised on auscultation by the presence of an apical non-ejection systolic click which may be accompanied by a late systolic murmur. Most children are asymptomatic but some complain of palpitations, dyspnoea, chest pain or fatigue. Conduction defects, arrhythmias and electrocardiographic T wave changes may be associated features. Echocardiography is a useful non-invasive technique for confirming the diagnosis.

The prognosis is excellent. Where a late systolic murmur is constantly present, denoting mild mitral regurgitation, prophylaxis against infective endocarditis is recommended at times of risk.

Rheumatic heart disease

Acute rheumatic fever is rare in Western countries (p. 315). During the course of the disease the heart may be relatively unaffected, or the child may develop an endocarditis, myocarditis, pericarditis or pancarditis. Recovery may be complete or the patient may develop chronic valvular disease. During the acute attack, there may be tachycardia *out of proportion to the fever*, which persists when the patient sleeps. Hence the importance of recording the sleeping pulse.

The first heart sound becomes muffled and an increased P-R interval may be found on the ECG, suggesting the presence of a first degree heart block.

The development of a pansystolic murmur at the apex, which transmits to the axilla or the left sternal border, indicates the presence of mitral valvulitis with incompetence. A low-pitched mid-diastolic murmur means that there is increased flow across the mitral valve, from atrium to ventricle, during ventricular diastole (Carey-Coombs' murmur). These murmurs may disappear entirely on recovery from acute rheumatic fever, although it may take many months or even years for this to happen. In other patients there is increasing damage to the mitral valve resulting in chronic mitral regurgitation, mitral stenosis or mitral regurgitation *and* stenosis.

Less commonly the aortic valve is affected during acute rheumatic fever. The murmur may be very soft initially and consists of a soft blowing diastolic murmur of aortic incompetence. This is usually irreversible and *chronic aortic insufficiency* becomes established with or without the development of aortic stenosis.

Treatment

In acute rheumatic heart disease bed rest is advised. Penicillin (or erythromycin in penicillin-sensitive patients) should be given in full doses for at least 10 days to eradicate the haemolytic streptococcus. Heart failure is treated in the usual way with sedatives, oxygen, digoxin and diuretics. Some authorities believe that heart failure in rheumatic fever is an indication for steroid therapy.

Recurrence of rheumatic fever should be prevented by the regular administration of penicillin V 250 mg twice daily or by 600 mg/m^2 of benzathine penicillin by deep intramuscular injection every four weeks for life. Erythromycin 250 mg twice daily may be used for patients allergic to penicillin. Full doses of antibiotics should be given for sore throats and for dental extraction to prevent subacute bacterial endocarditis. Surgical treatment for chronic rheumatic valve disease may occasionally be required in childhood.

DISORDERS OF CARDIAC RHYTHM

Sinus arrhythmia

The heart speeds up on inspiration and slows down with expiration. It is very common in children but is sometimes so marked as to cause concern. An electrocardiograph is diagnostic—a long lead II should be taken in both deep inspiration and expiration for best results.

Gallop rhythm sounds like a galloping horse on auscultation. It may be a protodiastolic gallop (lub-dup-dup lub-dup-dup) or a presystolic gallop (lub-lub-dup lub-lub-dup). When these two sounds fuse, it is called a summation gallop. The appearance of a gallop rhythm during the course of heart disease or heart failure is usually a bad sign.

Paroxysmal tachycardia is a condition in which an abrupt acceleration of the heart to 180 or more beats per minute occurs. It lasts for a variable time and then as abruptly ceases. It is accompanied by pallor, sweating, restlessness, laboured respiration and a frightening sensation of impending death. It may occur in an otherwise apparently normal heart, or it may accompany heart disease. If the attack is severe and prolonged it may lead to congestive heart failure and death. The attacks tend to recur. In those patients in whom the heart is normal between attacks, the attacks become less and less severe and eventually disappear.

Electrocardiogram

The rate varies from 180–400 beats per minute. The stimulus for contraction is outside the SA node. In the supraventricular type the QRS complexes are normal but very close together. In ventricular tachycardia the QRS complexes have a bizarre shape and occur independently of the P wave. After the attack the ECG may be normal or the child may have a short PR interval as in the Wolff-Parkinson-White syndrome.

Treatment

The attack may be aborted by change of posture such as squatting, drinking iced water or by vagal stimulation such as eye-ball or carotid pressure. Oxygen may be helpful even if the child is not obviously cyanosed. A sedative such as morphine or pethidine may be required. For patients not responding to the above a beta-adrenergic blocking agent such as propranolol may be effective. If this does not work the child should be digitalised. Rarely cardioversion may be required.

Fibrillation

Atrial fibrillation

This is a grossly irregular heart rhythm associated with dropped beats. It may precipitate heart failure. The patient should be digitalised to slow the heart and then given a suitable anti-arrhythmic agent to revert the rhythm to normal. If the patient has mitral stenosis this therapy may have to be continued for prolonged periods.

Ventricular fibrillation
Ventricular fibrillation in children may be a complication of cardiac surgery or of intravenous drug therapy. It is a sign of impending death. For emergency external cardiac massage should be performed until an ECG can be done to confirm the diagnosis. Electrical defibrillation should then be carried out.

Heart block

First-degree heart block
This is diagnosed by the occurrence of prolongation of the P-R interval on ECG. It is common in acute rheumatic fever and may be suspected when the first heart sound at the apex becomes softer.

Second-degree heart block
This is associated with dropped beats. Thus there may be a 2 : 1 or 3 : 1 partial AV block. In the *Wenckebach phenomenon* there is a progressive lengthening of the P-R interval until a ventricular beat is dropped.

Complete heart block
This means that the atrium and ventricle beat independently. It may be congenital or it may result from disease of the AV node. The ventricle beats below 80 in infants, below 50 in older children and about 40 per minute in adults. Exercise and atropine do not increase the heart rate in adults but may produce a slight increase in children. The prognosis is usually good but some patients develop Stokes-Adams' attacks in which they have short convulsive attacks and syncope due to temporary ventricular asystole. In such patients a pacemaker may have to be implanted.

CHAPTER 12

DISEASES OF THE CENTRAL NERVOUS SYSTEM

CONGENITAL MALFORMATIONS

Neural tube defects

Disturbances of mid-line fusion of the skull and spine may lead to certain well-defined disorders. Their aetiology is multifactorially determined.

1 Dermal depression and dermal sinus

These usually occur in the lower lumbar or sacral region and may simply consist of a dimple, or it may form a dermal sinus which may extend from the skin to the meninges (pilonidal sinus). Infection along this tract should be considered in any patient who has repeated attacks of meningitis. The sinus should be eradicated surgically.

2 Spina bifida occulta

Spina bifida occulta refers to the finding of unfused vertebral arches, commonly in the lumbo-sacral region (Fig. 12.1 A). The defect may be palpable, or it may be an incidental X-ray finding of no significance. There is often a capillary naevus, a tuft of hair or a lipoma superficial to the legion, pointing to its presence.

3 Spina bifida cystica (meningocele)

This is a form of neural tube defect in which a meningeal sac protrudes through the opening (Fig. 12.1 B). The skin over the swelling is usually thin and the mass transilluminates. Pressure on the sac causes the fontanelle to bulge.

4 Meningomyelocele

This is a form of neural tube defect in which a sac containing neural elements protrudes through the spinal defect (Fig. 12.1 C). The overlying skin is very thin and often leaks spinal fluid. Secondary infection is commonly present. There are always neurological and orthopaedic defects present and about 80 % of these patients have an *Arnold-Chiari malformation*. This is an elongation of the cerebellar tonsils into the foramen magnum, associated with internal hydrocephalus. The legs are commonly weak or paralysed, reflexes are absent and deformities such as

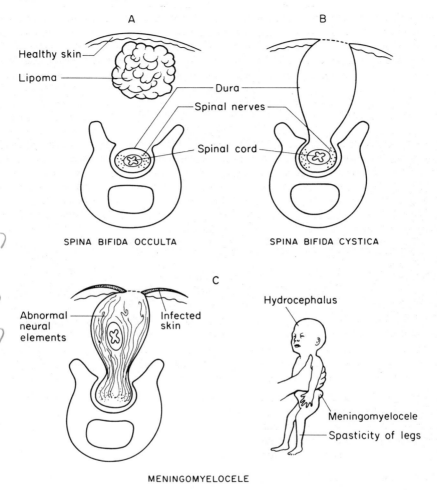

Fig. 12.1 Varieties of spina bifida

clubfoot or pes cavus may be present. Anal and urinary incontinence are a particularly unfortunate problem with these patients. Sensory changes are common but difficult to estimate accurately in young babies.

Complications

Urinary infection is very common in incontinent patients. Meningitis with mixed organisms is common if the skin is infected or a sinus is present. In some cases the *filum terminale* of the spinal cord is tethered or it is split by a bony spur (diastematomyelia) which may lead to progressive weakness of the legs with growth. Charcot's joint may occur with painless disorganisation of the ankle, knee or hip. Hydrocephalus due to the Arnold-Chiari malformation is common.

Diagnosis
Antenatal diagnosis may be made, provided that the neural tube defect is open, by a raised alphafetoprotein level in the amniotic fluid. Ultrasonic examination may reveal large lesions. Postnatal diagnosis is usually clinical, but in difficult cases, or prior to surgery, X-rays of the spine to determine the extent of the lesion, tomograms, myelography and air studies may be required. An IVP and renal function tests are advised to determine the extent of the urinary tract problem.

Treatment
Asymptomatic spina bifida occulta requires no therapy. It is often blamed for nocturnal enuresis but there is unlikely to be any causal relationship between the two conditions. Meningoceles should be repaired early to prevent the sac becoming infected, and a tethered *filum terminale* requires surgical release. Bony spurs or cystic masses pressing on the cord should be excised. In patients with more extensive lesions highly specialised teams are performing remarkable feats of rehabilitation by means of surgery, orthopaedic appliances, correction of deformities, reduction of hip dislocations, re-routing of urinary and faecal discharges, the insertion of drainage valves for hydrocephalus and the use of sophisticated electronic devices. The end result can be viewed as a triumph or tragedy, depending on one's viewpoint.

Hydrocephalus

Hydrocephalus ('water-head') is an excessive accumulation of cerebro-spinal fluid in the ventricles, resulting in enlargement of the ventricles, thinning of the cerebral cortex and widening of the sutures of the skull. In infants the majority are due to obstruction to the flow of CSF in the aqueduct of Sylvius or in the foramina of Luschka and Magendie. The obstruction may be due to inflammatory products or clotted blood causing gliosis, to intracranial masses, brain tumour or abscess, to arteriovenous malformations in the region of the foramina or to the Arnold-Chiari malformation in which a tongue of cerebellum projects through the foramen magnum. Deformity of the base of the skull in achondroplasia or platybasia may be a cause. Rarely it may be due to excess formation of CSF due to choroid plexus papilloma, or it may be due to reduction in absorption caused by arachnoiditis. In the last two conditions there is no obstruction within the ventricular system, therefore it is referred to as a *communicating hydrocephalus*.

Clinical features
Signs and symptoms depend on the age of onset, the site of the obstruction and the speed at which the fluid accumulates.

gliosis - excess of astroglia in damaged areas of CNS

In infants the first indication of hydrocephalus is enlargement of the head. The sutures become widened and the fontanelles feel tense. The forehead becomes rounded and the eyes tend to look downwards (the 'setting sun' sign). The skin over the skull is stretched and shining and the veins are prominent. Percussion may reveal a rather flat sound like percussing a watermelon, and the head transilluminates. If the hydrocephalus develops slowly in infants there may be no symptoms at all. Rapid onset of hydrocephalus may be associated with irritability, vomiting, a shrill cry and stupor. In older children in whom the fontanelles have already closed, there is an increase in intracranial pressure which causes springing of the sutures, a cracked pot sound on percussion, multiple cranial nerve palsies, spasticity and papilloedema. Optic atrophy is common. Nutrition is usually affected and infants who survive may have enormous heads with thin wasted bodies. Death may occur from respiratory failure due to medullary cone formation. The insertion of modern shunts and valves has changed the picture in that reasonable cortical function may be preserved. It should be pointed out that if the accumulation of fluid is very slow cortical function of the brain may remain intact. In some cases there is spontaneous arrest of the disease and these children may grow up with normal intelligence. Their milestones, however, may be retarded because there is mechanical difficulty in lifting a heavy fluid-filled head.

Diagnosis
Prenatally the size of the fetal head can be monitored by serial sonar investigations. After birth the head circumference of every baby should be measured and thereafter every time the baby is examined. Hydrocephalus can then be anticipated although the cause of the disorder may create difficulties. Serological tests for syphilis, toxoplasmosis, rubella and cytomegalovirus should be done.

X-ray of the skull may show flecks of calcification suggesting toxoplasmosis as a cause. In the newborn and in early infancy ventricular size can be measured using real-time ultrasound. Computerised axial tomography will show the size of the ventricles, the thickness of the cerebral cortex and the site of the obstruction. Sometimes air encephalography is required. CSF should be taken for examination.

Differential diagnosis
In *familial macrocephaly* several members of the family have large but normal heads. In these patients the *rate of growth* of the head is normal. *Subdural haematoma* may cause enlargement of the skull and is easily excluded by subdural taps. Blood or a xanthochromic fluid may be found. *Hydrancephaly* is a large fluid-filled sac which replaces the cerebral cortex. The head transilluminates brilliantly but is not necessarily enlarged. Benign increase in intracranial pressure (*pseudotumor cerebri*) should be excluded.

Management
A small percentage of hydrocephalics may arrest spontaneously, therefore one should observe the patient carefully, measure his head daily and chart its percentile growth. Rapid crossing from one percentile line to the next is an indication for active therapy. Where an underlying lesion such as syphilis can be treated, this should be done. Most patients will require some sort of shunting operation to preserve as much cortical function as possible and to prevent excessive growth of the head. These shunts must be checked regularly as they easily become blocked or infected. Also the tubes may become too short when the patient grows. The size of the ventricle and the CSF pressure should be checked periodically. It should be emphasised that the width of the cortex is not a good guide to brain function. A cortex which thins very slowly may have good function.

Prognosis
Without operation less than one-third of patients survives ten years. Of these only a small percentage can look after themselves. With operation perhaps two-thirds survive ten years and many children remain asymptomatic despite blocked valves. However a minor head injury may lead to renewal of symptoms. An appreciable number of patients have normal or near normal intelligence.

Craniosynostosis

Premature closure of one or more cranial sutures leads to distortion in the growth of the skull; for example, premature closure of the coronal suture leads to brachycephaly (boat-shaped head) and of all the sutures to oxycephaly (turret head). In Apert's disease acrocephaly (peaked head) is associated with syndactyly while Crouzon's disease consists of oxycephaly, beaked nose, exophthalmos and hypertelorism.

About one-third of patients develop symptoms due to increasing intracranial pressure, such as headache, vomiting, cerebral cry, squint, optic atrophy, mental retardation and convulsions. In such cases the affected sutures should be excised and replaced by an inert material to prevent re-fusion. The aim of the operation is to permit the brain to expand, and to prevent mental retardation.

Microcephaly

The head is small, usually under the third percentile for the age, and the forehead low. The fontanelles are small but open at birth, as are the sutures. The face is of normal size, contrasting with the tiny head. The limbs are often hypertonic or spastic, and there is always marked mental retardation present.

Aetiology
Microcephaly may be genetically determined, or it may be due to various environmental causes such as rubella, toxoplasmosis, cytomegalosis or

possibly congenital syphilis in the antenatal period. Hypoxia, the antenatal use of medicines or maternal disease may be factors. Irradiation has been implicated, and in animal experiments certain vitamin deficiencies.

Management
These patients may be difficult to manage because of their destructive habits and eventually most survivors need to be cared for in an institution. As the brain is congenitally small the prognosis is poor. Microcephaly must not be confused with craniosynostosis (see above) which is treatable.

MENTAL DISORDER

The terms used by professionals to describe various aspects of mental health have lead to some confusion and much criticism. In the UK the Mental Health Act 1983 defines *mental disorder* as 'mental illness, arrested or incomplete development of mind, psychopathic disorder and any other disability of mind'. The term *subnormality* is replaced by *impairment*, which is associated with 'abnormally aggressive or seriously irresponsible conduct'.

Mental handicap is a permanent disability which is detectable from an early age and is often associated with genetic or perinatal damage. This term is now used to describe retarded intellectual and cognitive development (which is usually also associated with social and emotional retardation) and should not be confused with *mental impairment*, which implies mental handicap with serious behaviour disorder. Most mentally handicapped people do not come under the Mental Health Act 1983 (UK).

Elsewhere, *mental retardation* is sometimes used to describe intelligence which is below normal in some people. Intelligence cannot be measured *per se*. Intelligence quotient (IQ) tests are often used as a convenient measure of intellectual level, but may be unreliable in mentally handicapped people, depending on the motivation of the person and the particular test used. However, a useful grading of mental handicap is: slight (IQ between 50 and 70), moderate (IQ between 30 and 50) and severe (IQ below 30).

The World Health Organisation has also used intelligence quotients to classify mentally handicapped people into ranges of 'subnormality' from mild to moderate, severe or profound.

In educational terms, all mentally handicapped pupils in the UK are now described as 'children with special needs' and the intellectual level of each is assessed individually. All factors, not just IQ, are taken into consideration.

There are two medical terms which must also be defined: *amentia*, in which a mental defect is present from birth, and *dementia*, in which the

mental disorder develops in a child (or adult) who was previously normal.
Mental handicap will now be considered.

CAUSES OF MENTAL HANDICAP

Mental handicap may be due to hereditary or environmental causes. The following are a selection of the more important ones.

Hereditary disorders

1 Chromosomal abnormalities such as Down's syndrome, cat-cry syndrome and Klinefelter's syndrome.
2 Single gene metabolic diseases, many of which can be diagnosed antenatally:
    (a) Amino acid disorders, e.g. phenylketonuria (PKU), maple syrup disease, Wilson's disease.
    (b) Lipoidoses, e.g. A-Beta-lipoproteinaemia, Tay Sachs' disease.
    (c) Metabolic sugar disorders, e.g. hereditary fructosuria and galactosaemia.
    (d) Mucopolysaccharidosis, e.g. Hurler's disease ('gargoylism').
3 X-linked mental disorder.
4 Congenital anomalies, such as microcephaly, hydrocephaly and craniosynostosis.

Environmental disorders

Antenatal
1 Antenatal infections such as rubella, syphilis, toxoplasmosis and cytomegalovirus (CMV) inclusion diseases.
2 Placental dysfunction and maternal disease such as toxaemia may possibly play a role.
3 Prematurity, twins and light-for-dates infants (the smaller the baby at birth, the greater the likelihood of mental handicap).
4 Birth trauma and anoxia. Subdural haematoma should never be forgotten.

Postnatal
1 Infections picked up during or shortly after birth, notably *E. coli* meningitis.
2 Cerebral haemorrhages due to any cause.
3 Kernicterus due to hyperbilirubinaemia.
4 Hypothyroidism.
5 Metabolic disorders, such as severe hypoglycaemia, hypocalcaemia and severe electrolyte disturbances.
6 Cultural factors.

toxemia - metabolic disturbances leading to preeclampsia + eclampsia
eclampsia - hypertension edema proteinuria + neurological disorders (convulsions + coma)

It should be emphasised that the cause of mental handicap in a large number of people is unknown. Many such cases occur in families. Many are multifactorial in origin.

Dementia (i.e. mental disorder occurring in a previously normal child) may be due to brain infection (meningitis, encephalitis, brain abscess), trauma from any cause (usually household or motor accidents), poisoning (heavy metals, carbon monoxide), brain tumours, vascular accidents (haemorrhage, thrombosis or embolus), degenerative diseases (Schilder's disease) and metabolic disorders (e.g. Tay Sachs' disease). [subacute or chronic leukoencephalo-pathy (destruction of white cerebrum)]

Signs of mental handicap

Some features such as those of Down's syndrome are obvious at birth; others like cretinism may take six weeks or longer to be recognised, while others may be so mild as to escape notice until the child enters school. High degrees of mental handicap can exist in children who appear outwardly normal. The combination of mental handicap and hepatosplenomegaly suggests one of the lipoidoses, such as Tay Sachs' disease (p. 226) or gargoylism.

If a baby pays no attention to its environment by eight weeks, or does not respond to light or sound, he should be investigated for blindness, deafness or mental handicap. Careful analysis of the baby's milestones of development are compared with those of normal babies. It should be remembered that social adaptation and speech may be impaired whereas motor development may be normal. In cases of doubt expert opinion should be called in as soon as possible. A 'wait and see' attitude can no longer be condoned, as there are a number of patients in whom a useful intelligence can be attained if they are treated early enough, as in cretinism, phenylketonuria and some of the rare metabolic disorders.

Diagnosis

The history of the patient should place emphasis on antenatal, natal and postnatal disturbances in mother or fetus. The milestones of development should be carefully assessed. The examination should elicit the characteristic syndromes such as Down's or Klinefelter's syndromes. The child's response to his environment is important and obvious visual, auditory or motor defects should be noted.

Diagnostic tests:

1 X-ray of the skull to exclude intracranial calcifications, anatomical defects such as microcephaly, or signs of increased intracranial pressure.
2 EEG in suspected epilepsy.
3 Blood thyroxine and thyroid stimulating hormone for hypothyroidism.

4 Serum and urine for amino acid chromatography in suspected hereditary metabolic disorders such as phenylketonuria.
5 Blood for sugars (glucose, fructose, galactose), serum calcium, electrolyte and blood gas analysis.
6 Serological tests for rubella, cytomegalic virus, toxoplasmosis and syphilis.
7 CAT scan for hydrocephalus and cerebral atrophy.
8 Skull scintogram or echo-sounding for localising tumours.
9 Carotid angiogram when necessary.
10 Chromosome analysis.

A few of the recognisable forms of mental handicap will now be described.

Down's syndrome

Down's syndrome is a form of mental handicap associated with 47 chromosomes due to non-disjunction (trisomy-21) or with 46 chromosomes due to translocation of chromosomes 14 or 21. Clinically there are a number of features which combine to form an easily recognisable picture (see Fig. 12.2). All affected children look as though they belong to a single family. The IQ ranges from 20–70, the average being about 45. They rarely walk before three years of age and speech is delayed and simple. Their mental development is rarely greater than eight years of age, but they are adaptable and can often be trained within the family unit.

The head is small and round. The occiput is flattened when the cerebellum is small (brachycephalic). The *face* is flat with slanted eyes (hence the old term 'Mongolian idiot') and an inner and outer epicanthic fold. The nose is short due to underdeveloped nasal bones. Small white (Brushfield) spots are sometimes noted on the iris. The tongue is often protruded from the mouth and becomes furrowed as the child grows older ('scrotal tongue'). External ears are small and simple and often low set. The *neck* is short and broad. The *hands* are also short and broad with incurved little fingers due to a small middle phalanx. The palmar crease is transverse and often single. Proximal triradii subtend an angle of more than 60° with the triradii at the base of the second and fifth fingers, confirming the presence of a squat hand. The *foot* has a wide space between the big toe and second toe, often with a deep groove between them extending on to the sole.

Neuromusculature
Generalised hypotonia is present. A small percentage can be educated to perform simple tasks. Speech is limited. The voice is raucous. The patient is usually pleasant, friendly and is fond of music and rhythmic activity.

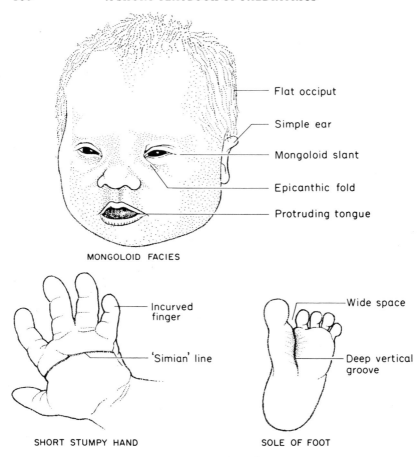

Flat occiput

Simple ear

Mongoloid slant

Epicanthic fold

Protruding tongue

MONGOLOID FACIES

Incurved finger

'Simian' line

SHORT STUMPY HAND

Wide space

Deep vertical groove

SOLE OF FOOT

Fig. 12.2 Down's syndrome

Associated defects
These babies have a T-cell deficiency and are more likely to develop acute leukaemia than the normal child population. If a newborn baby with Down's syndrome develops intestinal obstruction it is usually due to duodenal atresia. About 40 % of patients have congenital heart lesion such as atrial septal defect with endocardial cushion defects.

Incidence
About 1 in 700 live births. More than 5 % of all mentally handicapped people in institutions suffer from Down's syndrome.

Genetic counselling
The child with Down's syndrome who is born to elderly parents nearly always has a trisomy-21 as this type is maternal age-related. In young

parents the condition is sometimes associated with a translocation. The mother and father may be phenotypically normal. Their karyotypes may be normal or one of them may have 45 chromosomes with a balanced translocation. The offspring may have 46 chromosomes with an unbalanced translocation defect resulting in Down's syndrome. Sometimes mosaicism occurs due to an error in early mitotic division.

The risk of recurrence of trisomy-21 in future pregnancies where both parents' karyotypes are normal is about 1 in 100, irrespective of age. In women over the age of 45 years the risk of producing a baby with Down's syndrome is 1 in 30 to 1 in 40.

In translocation, if the mother is a carrier there is a high risk of recurrence of abnormal offspring (1 in 10 to 1 in 20). If the father is a carrier and the mother normal, there is a lower risk (1 in 40) with less risk of unbalanced offspring.

Diagnosis
Diagnosis is made on the clinical picture and confirmed by chromosomal studies.

Prognosis
The feature that used to shorten life in Down's syndrome in the past was recurrent respiratory infection. Today that is controlled by antibacterial agents. If cyanotic congenital heart disease is present then the prognosis worsens.

Numerous other chromosomal anomalies associated with mental handicap have been described; most of them are extremely rare, e.g. trisomy-13 and trisomy-18.

Sex chromosome abnormalities

These are often associated with mild degrees of mental handicap, though many of these patients may be entirely normal mentally. Examples include Klinefelter's syndrome (XXY), Turner's syndrome (XO), 'superfemale' syndrome (XXXX) and 'double male' syndrome (YY, XYY or XXYY). X-linked mental disorder may be chromosomally detectable in some affected families.

Mental handicap due to inherited abnormalities of metabolism

Several inborn errors of metabolism are associated with mental handicap, for example phenylketonuria, maple syrup urine disease, galactosaemia, and certain mucopolysaccharidoses. These, and others, are described in Chapter 14.

Mental handicap due to degenerative disease in white matter

There are many causes of degenerative disease of white matter in children but fortunately they are all rare. Such disease leads to progressive dementia and premature death. The age of onset of symptoms varies from disease to disease, e.g. Alexander's disease begins at birth, Krabbe's globoid cell leukodystrophy in early infancy, Metachromatic leukodystrophy at 1–2 years and Schilder's disease at 5–10 years. Some degenerations are familial. Special investigations are required to make an accurate diagnosis. Subacute sclerosing panencephalitis is described on p. 179.

NEUROMUSCULAR DISEASES

A check list of some of the causes:

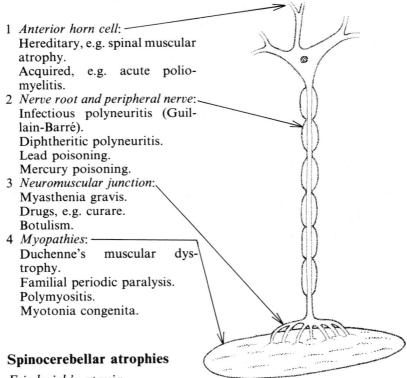

1 *Anterior horn cell*:
  Hereditary, e.g. spinal muscular atrophy.
  Acquired, e.g. acute poliomyelitis.
2 *Nerve root and peripheral nerve*:
  Infectious polyneuritis (Guillain-Barré).
  Diphtheritic polyneuritis.
  Lead poisoning.
  Mercury poisoning.
3 *Neuromuscular junction*:
  Myasthenia gravis.
  Drugs, e.g. curare.
  Botulism.
4 *Myopathies*:
  Duchenne's muscular dystrophy.
  Familial periodic paralysis.
  Polymyositis.
  Myotonia congenita.

Spinocerebellar atrophies

Friedreich's ataxia

This is a familial form of ataxia, genetically transmitted as a dominant or recessive, characterised by atrophy of the spinocerebellar, pyramidal and dorsal tracts. The disease begins insidiously, at about ten years of age, with ataxia which gets steadily worse. The foot is noted to have a high arch (*pes cavus*) and kyphoscoliosis is common. Deep reflexes may be absent due to posterior column involvement while an extensor plantar response is evidence of pyramidal tract damage. The abdominal reflexes are usually normal. Nystagmus and dysarthria are of cerebellar origin. Generalised weakness is common. Intellectual deterioration usually occurs due to cortical involvement. Cardiac involvement may be noted on ECG and the patient may terminate in heart failure. The average patient survives for about 15 years after diagnosis is made and is usually bed-ridden during the last 10 years of life.

Peroneal muscular atrophy (Charcot-Marie Tooth disease)

This may be familial or sporadic, and inheritance may be dominant or recessive. It begins shortly after the age of six years with slowly progressive atrophy of the muscles of the feet and lower legs, producing a 'stork leg' appearance. The hands and forearms may become involved. Peroneal atrophy causes foot-drop resulting in a typical high-stepping gait. The proximal muscles of the thighs and arms are spared. The ankle reflexes are absent but the knee jerk and biceps jerk are usually normal. Rarely ataxia and other features found in Friedreich's ataxia occur, suggesting a relationship between these diseases, but the intelligence is usually unaffected.

The floppy infant syndrome

Some babies appear floppy at birth and it is important to decide whether this is due to primary neuromuscular disease or some other cause.

Primary neuromuscular hypotonia

This may be due to a congenital myopathy, myotonic dystrophy, muscular dystrophy or spinal muscular atrophy (Werdnig-Hoffman's disease, see below). The hypotonia is usually generalised and the baby feels 'limp' on handling. It is associated with a variable degree of weakness. Many of these disorders are familial so every effort should be made to establish an accurate diagnosis so that genetic counselling and a prognosis can be given. A careful family history should be taken and the records of any previous stillbirth or neonatal death should be perused. Affected babies can be investigated using nerve conduction studies, electromyography, muscle biopsy histology and histochemistry, serum enzyme studies and muscle ultrasound. In some cases no definite diagnosis can be made.

Secondary hypotonia

This may be due to Down's syndrome, cretinism, Ehlers-Danlos syndrome and osteogenesis imperfecta, all of which are either obvious at birth or become so within a few weeks. Cerebral palsy may often present with hypotonia, but eventually these patients become increasingly spastic. In Tay Sachs' disease the infant is initially normal and hypotonia may not develop for several months. In myasthenia gravis, ptosis and impairment of eye-movement and weakness after exercise are characteristic.

Werdnig-Hoffman's disease

This disorder is characterised by progressive lower motor neuron atrophy of the muscles of the neck, shoulder and pelvis which eventually involves the muscles of respiration. Fasciculation of the tongue may be present. It is uniformly fatal before two years of age. Variations of this disease in which symptoms start later in life and are more slowly progressive have been described.

Muscular dystrophy

Muscular dystrophy is a progressive disease of muscle characterised by weakness and atrophy of muscle groups and increasing disability and deformity. The commonest type is Duchenne's pseudohypertrophic form but several variations are described.

The prevalence of Duchenne's muscular dystrophy in the United Kingdom is 3 in 100 000 of the population. It is inherited as an X-linked recessive trait affecting males and transmitted by females as in haemophilia. The carrier can be detected by the occurrence of raised creatine phosphokinase (CPK) levels. It begins in infancy or early childhood with difficulty in walking, rising from the floor (Gower's sign) and climbing steps. The gait is waddling due to weak gluteal muscles. Weakness of the shoulder girdle makes it difficult for the child to raise his arms or comb his hair. Pseudohypertrophy may involve the calf muscles, the supraspinatus, deltoids and triceps, and is due to large subcutaneous fat deposits. The tendon reflexes progressively disappear. There is no fasciculation or degeneration of the muscles. Cardiomyopathy is frequently present.

Prognosis
The prognosis is poor, death occurring in 5–10 years after onset due to intercurrent infection.

Treatment
Physiotherapy to prevent deformity may be helpful. Obesity should be avoided. Orthopaedic consultation is essential to keep the patient ambulant for as long as possible.

A milder dystrophy which starts later and is more benign has been described by P. E. Becker. By 30 years of age most of these patients are confined to wheelchairs.

In all cases the CPK is markedly increased and can be used to pick up pre-clinical cases and to identify carriers. Muscle biopsy is diagnostic and separates these patients from Kugelberg-Welander's benign spinal muscular atrophy which resembles Becker's disease clinically.

Facioscapulohumeral muscular dystrophy (Landouzy-Dejerine) begins after six years of age and affects the face and shoulder girdle. The eyes droop and the face becomes expressionless. It spreads downwards over many years. It is inherited as a dominant trait.

NEUROCUTANEOUS SYNDROMES

The skin and nervous system both derive from the ectoderm and the following are some of the disease of ectodermal origin.

Tuberose sclerosis

Tuberose sclerosis (adenoma sebaceum; epiloia) is a dominant autosomal disease with marked variability of expression. The full syndrome includes:

Skin
1 Depigmented patches (achromic naevi, best seen under Wood's light).
2 Shagreen patches (raised leathery patches seen mainly on the back).
3 Adenoma sebaceum, which consists of a pink, papular rash over the nose and cheeks and nasolabial folds. They are fibro-angiomatous naevi and are not usually obvious before five years of age.
4 Subungual fibromas are sessile growths which protrude from the groove of the nail-bed.

Central nervous system
1 Mental retardation is common, but some patients may be normal.
2 Convulsions due to the presence of tubera (sclerotic nodules) in the brain are common.
3 Intracranial calcification may be demonstrated by CAT scan. Air encephalogram may reveal nodules projecting into the ventricles ('candle-wax dripping'). Hydrocephalus may occur.
4 Small retinal lesions near the disc or raised clusters of translucent white tissue may be seen more peripherally. Other lesions sometimes associated with the disease are rhabdomyoma of the heart, honeycomb lung and angiofibroids of the kidneys.

Diagnosis
In infants the association of infantile spasms and patches of depigmentation is suggestive of this disease. In older children the triad of grand mal epilepsy, mental retardation and adenoma sebaceum on the face is diagnostic. In many cases only one or two features may be present and the diagnosis may be very difficult if there is no confirmatory family history.

Treatment
Treatment is symptomatic.

Neurofibromatosis

Neurofibromatosis (von Recklinghausen's disease) is also a dominant autosomal disease with marked variability of expression. The earliest lesions are oval 'café-au-lait' (light brown) patches and numerous pigmented naevi. Depigmented patches also occur and soft lipoma-like tumours may sometimes be felt in the subcutaneous tissues of older children.

Neurofibromata occur along the peripheral nerves and nerve trunks. A neurofibroma situated on the auditory nerve (*acoustic neuroma*) may be the sole evidence of the disease. It causes signs of increased intracranial pressure and localising signs such as deafness, tinnitus and facial palsy. Convulsions are common and resistant to treatment.

The tumours may press on bone causing local rarefaction and sometimes abnormal growth. In the spine it may cause kyphoscoliosis and signs of pressure on the spinal cord.

Diagnosis
In adenoma sebaceum the lesions are mainly in the brain and cord whereas neurofibromas grow from the nerve.

Treatment
Treatment is symptomatic. Epilepsy should be treated and one may have to be satisfied with partial control. Surgical removal of those tumours causing symptoms may be required, but is not always successful.

Sturge-Weber's disease

This is a *trigeminal angiomatosis* in which a port-wine stain is found in the distribution of one or more divisions of the trigeminal nerve. Focal convulsions occur on the opposite side but may become generalised. Hemiplegia and varying degrees of mental retardation occur. An angioma of the meninges is present on the same side as the port-wine stain, and it causes pressure atrophy of the underlying brain. Calcification over the affected meninges occurs producing the typical 'train-line' appearance on X-ray, limited to the convexity of the brain in the parietal or occipital area. A CAT scan may demonstrate cortical atrophy and dilatation of the affected ventricle.

EXTRAPYRAMIDAL SYNDROMES

These are syndromes characterised by involuntary movements which may be choreiform, athetotic or dystonic. Tremors may be a feature. Paucity of spontaneous movement and rigidity of the lead-pipe type may be present. Both Parkinsonism and Huntington's chorea have been described in children but are too rare to warrant discussion. Sydenham's chorea is discussed under 'Rheumatic Fever' (p. 315).

Hepatolenticular degeneration (Wilson's disease)

See page 227.

Familial tremor

A fine action tremor of the hands, with or without an accompanying tremor of the head, runs in certain families. It may start in early childhood or adolescence. The family history will usually determine the diagnosis and whether or not it is necessary to exclude other extrapyramidal syndromes.

EPILEPTIC SEIZURES

Gibbs and Lennox define epilepsy as a *paroxysmal cerebral dysrhythmia*. The manifestations of epilepsy depend on the site of the abnormal focus and the manner in which the discharge spreads through the brain. It is one of the common disorders of childhood and an incidence of 1 % of children affected has been quoted. Fortunately the stigma once attached to epilepsy has been minimised in many parts of the world by educational programmes and the formation of Epilepsy Leagues. As a result many of these children are able to attend normal schools. A sensible explanation by the teacher (preferably *before* the child has an attack) will do much to reassure other children in the class.

Classification of epilepsy

1 *Grand mal*—generalised tonic-clonic convulsions.
2 *Petit mal*—fleeting 'absences'.
3 *Minor motor*—akinetic attacks, myoclonic attacks, infantile spasms (salaam attacks).
4 *Focal seizures* (Jacksonian seizures)—auras, temporal lobe epilepsy.
5 *Extra-cerebral conditions stimulating epilepsy.*

Epilepsy can also be classified anatomically, for example centrencephalic, diencephalic or focal cortical seizures, or it may be classified according to EEG patterns, such as the three-per-second 'spike and wave' dysrhythmia characteristic of petit mal attacks.

Causes of epilepsy

1 *Antenatal*—genetic, inborn errors of metabolism such as glycogen storage disease and phenylketonuria, congenital anomalies of the brain such as porencephaly or neurocutaneous syndromes, intra-uterine infections such as rubella, cytomegalovirus disease, meningo-encephalitis and toxoplasmosis.
2 *Perinatal*—birth injury, infections, hyperbilirubinaemia, hypoglycaemia and hypocalcaemia.
3 *Postnatal*—trauma, meningitis, encephalitis, encephalopathies (e.g. lead poisoning), hypertensive crises, acute infections, exanthemata,

poisoning with central stimulants (e.g. amphetamines, imipramine), severe electrolyte disturbances, piridoxine deficiency or dependency, neoplasms and degenerative disorders of the CNS.

Grand mal seizures

Most attacks of grand mal epilepsy are sudden in onset. The eyes roll up, the patient becomes pale and loses consciousness. The child falls if he has been standing, and often injures himself. The whole body is seized by a tonic spasm (the tonic phase) which, by causing compression of the chest and larynx, may lead to an 'unearthly' cry. Cyanosis is due to temporary respiratory arrest lasting 15–20 seconds. This is followed by a clonic phase in which the limbs jerk violently but rhythmically, breathing is stertorous and the tongue may be bitten. Autonomic discharge causes profuse sweating, salivation (foaming at the mouth), involuntary urination and defaecation. The clonic phase usually lasts a minute or two but may last hours (*status epilepticus*). It decreases in severity and the patient recovers with little or no after-effect, or he falls asleep. He may waken feeling tired and head-achey. Recurrent seizures may occur frequently or infrequently.

Most cases of recurrent epilepsy of unknown cause (idiopathic) are genetic in origin and are described as *centrencephalic*. The discharge starts in the mid-brain and spreads peripherally. There is no preceding aura or warning. *Symptomatic epilepsy* on the other hand usually begins cortically and may produce an initial warning (aura), such as a strange smell or the sound of voices. The discharge then spreads and becomes generalised. Often the child does not remember the aura on recovering from the attack. He may be left with a temporary (Todd's) paralysis.

Diagnosis
Grand mal epilepsy is basically a clinical diagnosis. There is often a family history of similar seizures and a careful history reveals the typical tonic and clonic phases and the autonomic discharges. An EEG may confirm the presence of abnormal foci but in at least 10 % of cases the EEG may be normal. In symptomatic epilepsy a detailed neurologic examination, X-ray studies of the skull and appropriate laboratory studies may be required to elucidate the underlying causes of the disorder.

Management of idiopathic grand mal epilepsy
The first attack may occur any time after infancy and cause tremendous emotional upset within the family circle. The practitioner must therefore counsel the whole family and gradually wean them from the idea of the patient having an 'unspeakable affliction'. Constant reassurance to child and family are basic to the management of the disorder. Solutions must be found for educational, social and economic problems as they arise.

There are considerable differences of opinion with regard to the participation of the child in sport, riding, skating or swimming. A seizure at a critical time may lead to a serious accident or to drowning. Nevertheless this has happened so rarely that many authorities feel that these activities may be permitted *provided that the patient's seizures are under perfect control.* The more cautious practitioner would insist on supervision at all times, particularly during swimming and riding. Staircases and heaters should be guarded and locks should be removed from the bedroom and bathroom so that the epileptic is not locked in should he have a fit.

A large number of drugs are available for the treatment of grand mal epilepsy. These include phenytoin, carbamazepine, phenobarbitone (or primidone), sodium valporate and clonazepam. Recent work has shown that if phenytoin or carbamazepine are given in optimum therapeutic doses, as judged clinically and by serum levels of these drugs, then only *one* drug is required to control seizures in 70 % of cases. It is usual to start with a small dose of phenytoin and then slowly increase the dose to maximum tolerance, i.e. the point at which side-effects such as drowsiness or ataxia become excessive. The dose is then slightly reduced. If despite adequate phenytoin blood levels seizures persist, then a *second* drug, of a different type, such as carbamazepine, valproate or phenobarbitone, is added in gradually increasing doses. If the patient does not respond to two drugs he should be referred for neurological consultation. Sometimes a patient may be controlled for prolonged periods and then have seizures again. It should be remembered that phenobarbitone is an enzyme inducer and may increase the metabolic breakdown of phenytoin so that larger doses of the latter become necessary to control seizures. Also the dose of medication may need to be increased because of the growth of the patient. By using phenytoin in suspension form, the insoluble drug sinks to the bottom of the bottle and, unless it is well shaken, the doses at the bottom of the bottle may become excessive. The patient develops signs of toxicity such as nausea, vomiting and ataxia.

Phenobarbitone often causes behaviour disorders in children, and is no longer the drug of first choice in grand mal epilepsy for this reason.

In many cases failure of medication to control seizures is due to failure of compliance. Assessment of the blood levels of the anticonvulsant will readily determine whether or not this is so.

Medication should never be stopped suddenly, otherwise status epilepticus may be precipitated.

Treatment of status epilepticus

Persistence of seizures for more than half an hour, or frequent seizures, may produce harmful effects on the brain in the form of structural changes leading to personality disturbances, intellectual impairment, physical difficulties and subsequently more difficult control of seizures. It is important therefore to control the seizures as soon as possible. The airway should be kept open by continuous suction of the throat and the use of an oropharyngeal airway. Oxygen may be administered and diazepam is given intravenously, the doses being 0.5 mg every minute until the seizure stops. As the action of diazepam lasts only three or four hours, it should be followed by a suitable dose of phenobarbitone, 50–100 mg/m^2 intramuscularly, followed by oral maintenance doses of phenytoin when the patient recovers from the seizure. In unresponsive cases a general anaesthetic quickly controls convulsions and permits control of respiration until the patient recovers.

The maintenance treatment of grand mal epilepsy should continue for two to three years after the last attack. The dose of the drugs is then very slowly tapered off over a further period of six months.

Petit mal epilepsy

Petit mal attacks consist of momentary impairment of consciousness, associated with flickering of the eyelids or twitching of the mouth. Characteristically the attack occurs during a voluntary movement. The patient may be lifting a spoon to his mouth when he stops half way, stares blankly into space for a second or two, and then carries on as if nothing has happened.

Single attacks rarely cause problems, but frequently repeated seizures may cause confusion and the patient seems to be in a continuous daze (*petit mal status*). Often there is concomitant evidence of grand mal.

Prognosis
About half the cases gradually clear up without treatment. About one-third also have grand mal seizures.

Diagnosis
The EEG shows three-per-second 'spike and wave' complexes which are diagnostic. Such bursts of activity are not accompanied by clinical seizures unless they last longer than four or five seconds. Many patients have accompanying changes compatible with grand mal epilepsy.

Treatment
The drug of choice in petit mal seizures is ethosuximide (Zarontin). It is given in increasing doses until the seizures are controlled (maximum 1.2 g/m^2/day). In severe cases it may be combined with valproate or clonazepam. The most effective drug, but also the most toxic, is troxidone (Tridione). If it is given it must be used in full dosage to get optimum results. However it can cause agranulocytosis in sensitive patients, therefore blood counts should be done monthly.

In some children, if the petit mal seizures have been controlled for six months, the drug may be withdrawn without recurrence of symptoms.

Minor motor seizures

Minor motor seizures are commonly associated with underlying brain damage and with symptomatic epilepsy. They may, however, occur as isolated phenomena.

Akinetic attacks (drop seizures)
Akinetic attacks are due to a sudden loss of postural tone of the head (bobbing attacks) or the whole body in which the patient suddenly drops to the ground. He may injure himself in the attack. Mental disorder and neurological signs are often detected. The EEG may show continuous runs of generalised slow spike and 1.5–2 per second slow waves.

Myoclonic seizures
Myoclonic seizures may occur in association with grand mal or petit mal seizures, or as isolated attacks of clonic spasms of a group of muscles. They may be associated with diffuse brain damage. They may consist of rhythmic jerking of the eyelids, neck or arms. They may cause the patient to drop things or to cause attacks of shuddering.

Infantile spasms
Infantile spasms (massive myoclonic spasms, salaam attacks, jack-knife seizures, lightning seizures) are seizures which occur only in infants and are usually associated with extensive brain damage and mental disorder. When attacks occur singly parents rarely seem to realise the significance of the attack and may in fact be amused at the unexpected 'salaam' or 'jack-knife' spasm. The attacks usually last a few seconds and dozens of attacks may occur daily. The attacks gradually become less or may change character to become grand mal or focal in type. The course is usually one of progressive deterioration.

Treatment
Minor motor seizures may respond to nitrazepam (Mogadon), a sedative related to diazepam. Severe cases of infantile spasms sometimes respond to ACTH, the usual dose for an infant being 40 i.u. daily for two weeks, and then tailing off over the next three weeks. Side-effects nearly always occur at this dosage. Other anti-epileptic drugs such as ethosuximide and diazepam help the occasional patient and sometimes a stimulant of the dexamphetamine class has a place in therapy. Often a ketogenic diet has been successful but is difficult to persist with for any length of time.

Focal epilepsy

In focal or Jacksonian epilepsy there is a 'march of events' in which the attack starts on one side of the body, for instance the face or fingers, and then spreads in an orderly fashion until the whole side undergoes clonic movements. Consciousness may be retained and the child may watch the jerking of his own limbs with interest. However, the convulsion usually spreads to the opposite side and consciousness is then lost. The attack is then indistinguishable from grand mal seizures. On recovery there is amnesia for the event.

Focal epilepsy may be limited to a small area of the cortex. It may produce auditory, visual or other hallucinations of short duration. A variety is *temporal lobe* (psychomotor) epilepsy in which the child may perform stereotyped movements such as smacking the lips or plucking at a garment. It may be accompanied by flushing, sweating, pallor or attacks of abdominal pain. It may be limited to hallucinatory experiences which may be very frightening. Whereas in adults a focal seizure calls to mind an expanding intracerebral lesion, in children atrophic lesions are more usual.

Recurrent migraine-like headaches or abdominal pain has been attributed to an 'epileptic equivalent' but the diagnosis may be difficult to prove in the absence of an abnormal EEG.

Treatment
Focal seizures usually respond to the same drugs that are effective in grand mal seizures. Phenytoin is usually effective but carbamazepine, valproate and clonazepam may be as good in some cases.

It is often stated that infants and children tolerate large doses of anti-epileptic drugs. This is only true if the dose is related to body weight. Thus if an adult requires 1 mg/kg of a particular drug, the infant will require 2–2.5 mg/kg of that drug. For this reason we believe that a better relationship between dose and size of patient is obtained by the use of surface area methods for estimating doses. See *The Paediatric Prescriber* (Blackwell Scientific Publications, 1981).

Disorders simulating epilepsy

Breath-holding attacks
These usually occur between 6 and 36 months of age. They are very frightening to witness. They are usually precipitated by pain, fright or frustration. The baby cries until all the air is forced out of his chest and he rapidly becomes cyanosed. The attack may proceed to unconsciousness with or without convulsions. The cyanosis is usually terminated by the patient taking a deep breath. The patient then sinks into a normal sleep. The whole attack is over within a minute or two and may be repeated several times during the day. Parents usually panic when an attack occurs. They shake the affected child, scream or throw cold water over him. They need reassurance that infants do not die of the disorder and that anoxia forces them to breathe again before cerebral damage can occur. The attacks are often thought to be 'fits' and attributed to 'naughtiness' for which anti-epileptic treatment or tranquillisers are given. This usually aggravates the disorder.

Pallid syncope
Like breath-holding attacks, pallid syncope may be precipitated by sudden pain and fright, but not usually by frustration. The child becomes pale, faints and may have a convulsion. It may be associated with a brief cardiac arrest. If attacks occur too frequently they can be prevented by giving small doses of atropine two or three times daily.

Cerebral anoxia
Cerebral anoxia may be caused by fainting spells due to congenital heart disease, for example Fallot's tetralogy, intermittent heart block or vasomotor instability. The blood pressure should be measured in both lying and standing positions to detect a sudden drop on change of posture.

Hypoglycaemia
Hypoglycaemia can occur at any age. It is common on the second or third day of life in pre-term babies and light-for-dates babies. It may be associated with jitteriness and convulsions. In older children the attacks are preceded by weakness, pallor, sweating and a gnawing 'hunger pain'. Blood should be taken immediately to confirm the presence of hypoglycaemia and sugar administered orally or intravenously.

Hypertensive encephalopathy
This should be excluded by measuring the blood pressure and examination of the urine for albumen and cells. The commonest cause in small children is acute nephritis.

Fainting spells
Fainting spells are common at puberty and during adolescence. Closely related is the fainting of orthostatic hypotension. It occurs on jumping up from the supine to the erect position.

Masturbation
Masturbation may take bizarre forms in childhood. It is often associated with rhythmic rocking, flushing of the face and a look of intense concentration. On reaching a climax the child becomes limp and dazed. He or she resents any interruption of the pleasure. The parents should be reassured that no harm comes of the habit. Should it embarrass them, the incidence can be reduced by keeping the child busy.

Narcolepsy
Narcolepsy is an overwhelming desire to sleep occurring in children who are bored, never when they are active. It is helped by methylphenidate or dexedrine, made worse by phenobarbitone.

Hysteria
Hysteria produces bizarre attacks which should not be confused with true epilepsy. They must be differentiated carefully from the bizarre extrapyramidal attacks of dystonia due to phenothiazine overdosage.

Occasionally a child may copy a sibling's attack of epilepsy quite closely in order to gain his mother's attention.

The Pickwickian syndrome
This syndrome is the association of obesity, hypoventilation and carbon dioxide narcosis. It is relieved by losing weight and consciously breathing more deeply.

Miscellaneous
Acute labyrinthitis and hiatus hernia may cause atypical 'fits'. In hiatus hernia the child may assume bizarre postures in order to aid his swallowing.

FEBRILE CONVULSIONS

Febrile convulsions are acute sporadic seizures associated with fever. They occur in about 5 % of children. There may be a single attack or the attack may recur with each febrile illness. The majority occur in the first three years of life. There is often a familial incidence but its relationship to epilepsy is obscure. Many epileptics have a history of febrile convulsions in infancy. A few infants who have several febrile convulsions in infancy develop epilepsy later, perhaps less than 8 %.

Aetiology
The commonest cause of this common disorder is an acute upper respiratory infection, but it may occur in any illness associated with a temperature of over 39°C. It may thus occur in tonsillitis, pyelonephritis or pneumonia. The duration of the seizure is short-lived and leaves no sequelae.

Diagnosis
Practitioners soon learn that certain families are prone to these benign febrile convulsions and treat accordingly. In many cases it is necessary to determine whether or not there is some more serious underlying condition such as hypoglycaemia, uraemia, intracranial infection or true epilepsy which has been precipitated by the fever, and the appropriate laboratory tests should be done to exclude these.

Management
In the majority of cases of febrile convulsions, the seizure has ended by the time the practitioner sees the patients. He should then treat the underlying infection. In patients who are still convulsing or who show sequelae such as paralysis (Todd type) or mental change, admission to hospital for observation and fuller investigation is advised.

High fever is aggravated by dehydration and often an intravenous drip of normal saline or half-strength saline in 5 % dextrose-in-water is sufficient to reduce the temperature. Tepid sponging is helpful but its effect is negated if the patient develops rigors. It is wise therefore to precede the sponging with an intramuscular injection of chlorpromazine (15 mg/m^2). Salicylates and paracetamol are commonly used antipyretic drugs. If the patient has had three simple febrile convulsions further attacks can be prevented with prophylactic phenobarbitone or valproate.

MENINGITIS

The commonest organisms causing meningitis in children are *H. influenzae*, pneumococcus and meningococcus. The illness commences with fever, irritability, vomiting and headache. Convulsions may occur, sometimes associated with cranial nerve palsies. On examination there is neck-stiffness with a positive Brudzinski and Kernig's sign.

If a petechial rash is found meningococcal infection should be assumed, as the illness can progress with startling rapidity and the patient may die within a few hours. However, the rash may also be found with pneumococcal meningitis, influenza type B and certain viral infections. In many patients meningitic signs may be overwhelmed by signs of septicaemia and shock (Waterhouse-Friderichsen syndrome).

Neonatal meningitis is usually due to *E. coli* or other Gram-negative organisms. It is often preceded by prolonged labour, premature rupture of the membranes or maternal sepsis. It should be suspected in any newborn with the above history who goes off his food, vomits and develops expiratory grunting, bulging of the fontanelle and a high-pitched cerebral cry. The temperature may be raised, but more often is low, and convulsions may occur. One must never hesitate to do a lumbar puncture, even in the smallest baby, if there is the slightest suspicion of meningitis.

Diagnosis
Diagnosis is established by lumbar puncture. The cerebrospinal fluid is usually under pressure and may appear to be turbid or clear on inspection. The glucose is greatly reduced, usually below 2 mmol/l, the protein is increased (over 0.45 g/l) and the cell count, mainly polymorphonuclear leucocytes, is increased. Culture should reveal an organism if the patient has not previously had antibiotics in the initial stages of the illness. A blood culture should always be done at the same time, as one sometimes cultures organisms from the blood when the CSF is sterile. Haemophilus or meningococcal antigen can be detected in CSF or serum by countercurrent immunoelectrophoresis.

Therapy
Until an organism has been isolated initial treatment should begin with intravenous chloramphenicol 1000–2000 mg/m^2/day in four divided doses despite the remote possibility of aplastic anaemia. It may be used for all three organisms commonly occurring in children. *H. influenzae*

resistance to chloramphenicol has been repeated but it is much rarer than resistance to ampicillin. Cefuroxime 1000–2000 mg/m²/day in three divided doses has been used as an alternative to chloramphenicol but should be used cautiously in patients allergic to penicillin.

In the neonate treatment should begin with chloramphenicol and gentamicin as the number of different organisms causing meningitis in this age group is much greater (see p. 43). The dose of chloramphenicol should not exceed 25 mg/kg/day for the first week of life, especially in the pre-term baby. The dose of gentamicin for the newborn is 5 mg/kg/day (50 mg/m²/day) in two divided doses.

Once the organism has been identified and the sensitivity determined then the most appropriate drug is given, e.g. penicillin for meningococcus and β-haemolytic streptococcus, carbenicillin for *Pseudomonas* infection. Treatment should be given for at least seven days, longer in neonates.

Supportive therapy
Extremes of body temperature should be controlled. Nutrition, fluid and electrolyte balance should be maintained. Convulsions may be controlled with diazepam (Valium), phenytoin or phenobarbitone. Change in posture 4-hourly helps to prevent pneumonia. For reducing increased intracranial pressure dexamethasone (Decadron) may be given orally or by injection, the dose being 30 mg/m² immediately, followed by 3 mg/m² every six hours for three days. Oxygen and assisted ventilation may be required. Subdural effusion should be suspected if the fontanelle bulges and subdural taps should be done, if necessary, every day.

Waterhouse-Friderichsen syndrome is a form of peripheral vascular collapse due to meningococcaemia. Disseminated intravascular coagulation is usually also present. Plasma or plasma protein fraction should be given, followed by 0.9 % sodium chloride in 5 % dextrose. A high rate of infusion is required initially but this should be adjusted according to the central venous pressure and the blood pressure. Any metabolic acidosis should be corrected with sodium bicarbonate. Large doses of hydrocortisone (600–1200 mg/m²) should be given for three or four doses, then reduced to 300 mg/m² per 24 hours. Disseminated intravascular coagulation is treated with heparin, 500–750 units/m²/hour.

Complications
In meningitis the dose of antibiotics should *not* be reduced for at least three or four days after the temperature falls, because clinical improvement may be associated with reduced penetrability of the blood-CSF barrier. Only large doses of antibiotic overcomes this. Subdural effusion and brain abscess require surgical drainage. Hydrocephalus, optic atrophy, eighth nerve damage and rectus externus paralysis may be permanent.

Tuberculous meningitis
See page 327.

Benign aseptic meningitis syndrome

The benign aseptic meningitis syndrome is characterised by all the signs of meningeal irritation, the CSF may contain hundreds of cells, but the sugar is normal and no bacteria are cultured. The infant or child with benign aseptic meningitis may present with a clinical picture identical to meningitis or encephalitis. In infants irritability, fever, vomiting or refusal of feeds may or may not be associated with bulging of the fontanelle. In older children fever, headache and vomiting are associated with neck stiffness and a positive Kernig's sign.

Lumbar puncture reveals fluid under pressure. It may seem clear or turbid on inspection and there may be hundreds of cells per mm³ present. Initially polymorphs, but later lymphocytes, predominate. The CSF protein level may be raised but characteristically the glucose is normal. No organisms are seen with Gram staining but in some cases enteroviruses can be cultured, usually coxsackie, ECHO, arbo and even poliovirus. Most viruses which can cause encephalitis (e.g. measles, mumps, rubella or herpes virus) can also cause an aseptic meningitic picture. The same syndrome may occur with fungi, parasites and rickettsiae.

An accurate diagnosis is important because the course of acute aseptic meningitis is usually benign and self-limiting, even in the presence of thousands of cells in the CSF. Problems in diagnosis may arise in incompletely treated bacterial infections such as *H. influenzae* or tuberculous meningitis. However, in these conditions the CSF glucose level is reduced, despite an absence of organisms.

Treatment
Treatment is symptomatic and antibiotics are not indicated. Repeated lumbar puncture may be required to relieve headache and to assess progress.

Viral encephalitides

Invasion of the central nervous system by viruses may produce the following syndromes:

1 *Meningeal syndrome.* This is identical to the aseptic meningitis syndrome described above. The disease is self-limiting, the prognosis excellent.
2 *Encephalitic syndrome.* Headache and drowsiness which may proceed to coma occur. Fever, delirium, muscular paralyses and autonomic disturbances may be present. Recovery is usual but permanent

sequelae such as hemiplegia, behaviour disturbances and mental handicap may occur. Measles tend to cause severe disease, mumps and varicella are mild. The CSF is usually under increased pressure, the protein may be slightly increased and the glucose is always normal. In the first 24–48 hours many polymorphs may be found, but after this lymphocytes predominate.

3 *Myelitic syndrome.* The spinal cord is predominantly involved by the virus. Paraesthesia and weakness of the limbs may occur, commonly associated with disturbances of the bladder sphincters. Permanent sequelae are common.

4 *Radicular syndrome.* This may involve a single nerve root as in herpes zoster, or it may be extensive and symmetrical as in the *Guillain-Barré syndrome.* In the latter there is characteristically an increase in CSF protein *without* pleocytosis. The muscles are weak, the proximal muscles often being more affected than the distal ones. Sensory loss is usually present. In *Landry's paralysis* there is an ascending paralysis which may terminate in respiratory failure.

Encephalitis may be caused by the following viruses:

1 Arbo (arthropod-borne) viruses including equine and West Nile viruses.
2 Enteroviruses including ECHO, coxsackie A and B and polioviruses.
3 Paramyxoviruses (mumps).
4 Herpesviruses.
5 Rabies virus.

In addition there is a large variety of diseases which are probably of viral origin but in which no virus has been isolated. These include:

1 Reye's syndrome (encephalohepatitis)

Severe vomiting is followed by convulsions and coma. Delirium and screaming, resembling a patient on a 'trip', may occur. Marked hypoglycaemia, not responding to intravenous glucose solutions, is common and is associated with fatty degeneration of the liver and other organs. Liver function tests are abnormal. A raised serum ammonia carries a bad prognosis. Thirty per cent of patients die.

2 Postinfectious encephalitis

This term is used to cover a number of diseases which follow on viral diseases such as measles and mumps or after rabies vaccination or other immunisation procedures. The symptoms of encephalitis may occur up to ten days *after* the primary illness, distinguishing it from the acute illness which accompanies viral disease. In infants under one year of age encephalitis after yellow-fever vaccination may occur on rare occasions.

3 Subacute sclerosing panencephalitis (SSPE)

Also known as *Dawson's inclusion encephalitis*, SSPE is a late complication of measles, occurring five to seven years after the initial illness. Its incidence is greatly reduced by vaccination against measles. In the first stage there are personality changes. In the second stage apathy, loss of memory, myoclonic seizures, choreo-athetosis and dystonia may occur. Finally the patient deteriorates until decorticate rigidity sets in. There is no specific treatment.

Diagnosis of encephalitides
Diagnosis is made on the history and development of the illness. Very high measles antibody titres in the serum and CSF are diagnostic.

Treatment
Treatment is symptomatic; careful nursing, attention to nutrition, fluid and electrolyte balance, bladder and bowel care are all important. Pooling of secretions in the throat require repeated suction. Tracheotomy and assisted respiration may be required. Repeated lumbar puncture may relieve headaches. If the pressure is very high there is danger of medullary cone formation and other methods of reducing the raised intracranial pressure should be tried, such as mannitol diuresis, dexamethasone or the use of hypothermia. As a last resort, surgical decompression may occasionally be required. Convulsions are controlled by diazepam or phenobarbitone. Antibiotics are required for secondary infection especially pneumonia. On recovery physiotherapy may be required for a long period. Emotional disturbances are common and require careful attention.

Poliomyelitis

Acute poliomyelitis is an acute viral illness, involving chiefly the lower motor neurones of the brain and spinal cord, caused by polioviruses (three serotypes). It is spread by human carriers and contact and is rare in countries with effective vaccination programmes against the disease. It may occur sporadically or epidemically.

Clinical features
The incubation period is 14 days. The infection tends to localise in the lower motor neurone of the brain and spinal cord, though the majority of infections are subclinical. The only symptoms may be of a 'flu-like illness with fever, nausea, vomiting, sore throat, headache and constipation. In these cases the virus may be cultured from the throat or stool.

Three to four days after the onset of the above symptoms the patient may develop a clinical illness similar to that due to aseptic meningitis (p. 177). Some days later a minority of patients develop lower motor neurone paralysis, (*paralytic polio*). The distribution of the paralysis is asymmetric and patchy and may affect the cranial motor nerves or the spinal nerves. In the *encephalitic* form there is drowsiness, disorientation, tremor and coma associated with some degree of motor paralysis.

Differential diagnosis
In the Guillain-Barré syndrome the paralysis is symmetrical and primarily affects the proximal muscles. *Peripheral neuritis* is distinguished by its symmetrical distribution and normal CSF findings. In *botulism* there is no neck stiffness and the CSF is normal. Encephalitis due to other viruses may cause difficulty, but patchy paralysis is characteristic only of acute polio.

Treatment
Patients with acute poliomyelitis should be isolated. Intensive care facilities should be available so that adequate ventilatory assistance can be given in cases with bulbar palsy. Bladder paralysis may respond to small doses of urecholine, local pressure, the effect of running water or, if all else fails, aseptic catheterisation and drainage. Physiotherapy is important to maintain joint mobility, to prevent deformities and to maintain pulmonary function. Spasm may be relieved by the skilful use of hot packs and muscle relaxants.

Prognosis
The majority of patients recover completely. Less than 2 % have permanent sequelae. Paralysis lasting six months is likely to be permanent.

Prevention
Oral live-attenuated poliomyelitis vaccine against the three serotypes of the virus should be given at the same time that the inoculation against diphtheria, tetanus and pertussis is carried out. Three doses are usually given at four to six week intervals. A booster dose should be given not later than school entry.

CEREBRAL PALSY

Cerebral palsy is a group of neurological disorders due to non-progressive brain injury occurring *in utero* or in early life. In all cases motor function is impaired because of an upper motor neurone lesion, or because of the occurrence of involuntary movements or ataxia. The condition may be complicated by mental handicap, blindness, deafness, epilepsy or orthopaedic deformities.

Classification

1 *Upper motor neuron lesions*:
   (a) Spastic diplegia (Little's disease).
   (b) Spastic hemiplegia.

(c) Spastic monoplegia.
(d) Hypotonic cerebral palsy.
2 *Extrapyramidal lesions*:
  (a) Athetoid type.
  (b) Choreo-athetoid type.
  (c) Ataxic type.

Upper motor neurone type of cerebral palsy

Lesions of the pyramidal tract may be unilateral or bilateral. The classical form was described by Little and consists of a spastic diplegia in which the legs are more severely affected than the arms. Marked adductor spasm produces 'scissoring' of the lower limbs. The deep reflexes are increased, ankle clonus is often marked and there is clasp-knife spasticity of the limbs. The superficial abdominal reflexes, however, are retained. During infancy the neck may be hypotonic and flops backwards when the infant is pulled off the couch by the arms, but later it may become spastic. Associated defects include mental handicap, speech difficulties, visual and auditory impairment and convulsions. The milestones of development are severely delayed. It is a matter of definition as to whether this group is to include microcephalics who also may have spastic quadriplegia. Many infants with spastic cerebral palsy are born pre-term or are light-for-dates. A proportion are associated with birth trauma, anoxia, or postnatal injury.

1 Spastic hemiplegia

Spastic hemiplegia is a disorder of the pyramidal tract in which the arm is usually more severely affected than the leg, and sometimes the one side of the face may be involved. It is a characteristic of the affected limbs that their growth is retarded. Usually there are no sensory changes.

The condition may be present from birth and is thought to be due to neonatal asphyxia or birth injury. It may develop after birth due to unilateral subdural effusion, or following meningitis. Neonatal polycythaemia may be a factor in some cases. In a proportion of cases, the infant is apparently normal and may have started walking when he suddenly develops a convulsion like a bolt out of the blue. He recovers from the attack with a permanent hemiplegia. The possibility that there is a congenital anomaly of the middle cerebral artery which suddenly occludes cannot be excluded.

Clinical features
A unilateral Moro response may be noted after birth or the parents may become aware that the patient only moves one arm when reaching or grasping. Some patients are brought to the doctor only when there is delay in sitting, standing or walking.

Examination reveals the typical features of spastic hemiplegia with hyper-reflexia and, in older children, an extensor plantar response on stroking the sole of the affected foot. Unlike the form of hemiplegia acquired in adulthood, the abdominal reflexes are usually present in children.

Treatment
Treatment is directed towards the family as a whole and this is usually best achieved by group discussions, so that parents can exchange experiences. For the child, physiotherapy is directed to preventing deformity and increasing his mobility. If the child has convulsions this must be treated. Speech problems and emotional problems require special attention.

2 Spastic monoplegia

This is a pyramidal lesion confined to one limb. If the one upper limb is affected little disturbance occurs as the opposite limb becomes the preferred limb. When the one lower limb is affected this will disturb gait considerably because the limb does not grow as rapidly as the healthy limb. Initially this is compensated for by walking on the toes of the affected limb and later by compensatory scoliosis of the spine. Physiotherapy and orthopaedic treatment can do much to minimise the damage. Prognosis depends on the mental ability of the child, as this may be normal or severely subnormal.

3 Hypotonic cerebral palsy

This is a curious phenomenon in that weakness predominates over spasticity. It is a common finding in cerebral palsy that the neck and spinal muscles may, in the early stages, be hypotonic, whereas the limbs may be spastic. In most cases the neck and back become hypertonic later, and the child may tend to lie in opisthotonos. This is specially liable to occur in severe microcephaly. However, there is a small group of children who remain persistently hypotonic and they may be difficult to distinguish from other types of 'floppy' baby. Careful examination usually reveals that the deep reflexes are increased despite the hypotonia.

Extrapyramidal cerebral palsy

The hallmark of extrapyramidal cerebral palsy is the presence of involuntary movements. These take the form of athetoid or choreo-athetoid movements and may be associated with varying degrees of lead-pipe rigidity. Kernicterus, associated with hyperbilirubinaemia due to Rh or ABO incompatibility, prematurity or other causes, is a common antecedent (see p. 48). Fetal distress and anoxia may be a factor.

Clinical features
Signs of kernicterus may have been present in the neonatal period. During the first year of life hypotonia may give way to hypertonia and attacks of opisthotonos. At about a year of age the characteristic athetosis appears. This consists of slow, writhing, involuntary movements which are aggravated by attempts at voluntary movements, and which disappear entirely during sleep. When jerky movements are superimposed on these athetotic movements we refer to them as choreoathetotic. These involuntary movements interfere with respiration and with speech which is painfully difficult for an outsider to understand. Persistence of the tonic neck reflex causes the arm and leg to extend when the neck is turned in the opposite direction. Voluntary movements are almost impossible due to the continual presence of involuntary ones. Deafness adds to the child's misery and should be suspected in every infant with a history of marked jaundice after birth. The constant salivation, due to inability to swallow properly, gives one the impression of gross mental handicap but this may not be the case. Every patient should be comprehensively assessed so that his handicaps can be defined and a plan of management formulated.

Treatment
Treatment will be multidisciplinary and demands the dedication of the paediatrician, physiotherapist, occupational therapist, speech therapist, psychologist, social worker, teacher and, above all, the parents.

Ataxic cerebral palsy

Ataxia takes the form of unsteady gait, tremor, titubation, nystagmus and scanning dysarthria. It is however a very rare form of cerebral palsy and most cases prove to have other diseases such as Friedreich's ataxia, cerebellar tumour or aqueduct stenosis. Each case therefore deserves full neurological investigation to exclude treatable causes.

MINIMAL BRAIN DYSFUNCTION (MBD)

Minimal brain dysfunction or *attention deficit disorder* refers to a wide spectrum of disorders in which specific disturbances of language, concentration, memory, spatial organisation, motor coordination and maturation occur. The child may have a normal IQ but has problems in learning to read, write or speak. He may confuse 'b' and 'd', 'b' and 'p' or other visual patterns. He may not be able to assemble objects, complete pictures or comprehend the concept of time or space. The teacher may complain that he does not concentrate, is easily distracted or is hyperactive.

Diagnosis and treatment
Many tests such as the Wechsler Intelligence Scale for Children (WISC),

Frostig's Developmental Test of Visual Perception and the Illinois Test of Psycholinguistic Abilities are able to detect many of the specific deficits in these children. Learning problems require special expertise by educationalists to correct though it should be emphasised that some of these children overcome their handicaps (or at least minimise them) by sheer hard work and determination. The practitioner may be consulted because the patient cannot concentrate or is hyperactive or has failed classes again. Solving these problems often requires the combined efforts of medical, paramedical and educationist teams. Medicines include central stimulants such as methylphenidate, tranquillisers, antidepressants and anticonvulsants. They should be used with discretion and as part of an overall plan in handling the child. Interested readers should consult larger works.

Other names for minimal brain dysfunction include hyperactive syndrome, learning disability, dyslexia, dysfluency, attentional disorder, and neurological immaturity. Recently the American Psychiatric Association has adopted the term *attention deficit disorder* (ADD).

EMOTIONAL PROBLEMS OF CHILDHOOD

The practitioner is often consulted for problems with a strong emotional element, such as temper tantrums, sleep disturbances, bad habits, enuresis, encopresis, thumb-sucking, nail-biting and tooth-grinding. Many of these are passing phases in the development of the child and quiet reassurance that they are temporary will often relieve the anxiety which is liable to build up around such situations. Sometimes there is an organic basis for some of these apparently 'psychological' disorders; for example the night cries of little girls which occur at 2 am and are due, not to nightmares, but to the movement of a threadworm across the child's hymen. (See p. 335).

It is not within the scope of this book to deal with these aberrations of development and the student is advised to read some excellent books that cover such common everyday problems. The first is Benjamin Spock's *Baby and Child Care* because a large percentage of intelligent mothers use this as their bible and it would be embarrassing for the practitioner not to know what Spock said—whether he agrees with his views or not. Two other sound books are R. S. Illingworth's *The Normal Child* (Churchill Livingstone), which is authoritative and provides sound advice, and Hugh Jolly's *Book of Child Care* (George Allen and Unwin).

Depression in children

Depression is being recognised increasingly in children. It may result from separation from the mother in early infancy, usually after a strong bond has already formed. It may occur as a result of divorce, death, imprisonment or other causes of deprivation. The infant becomes apathetic, cries silently, calls repetitively for his mother and stares into space. His emotional responses become flat.

In older children depression may also be precipitated by separation not only from parents as a result of death or divorce, but even separation from friends or pets. Movement from one location to another may result in a prolonged period of mourning for a child, a situation rarely recognised by parents until pointed out to them. The depressed child is sad, lonely and withdrawn with periods of aggressive behaviour. School work often suffers.

Management
The effects of separation in older children can be reduced if the child is allowed to 'talk it out'. Visiting in children's wards of hospitals should be unrestricted and the mother should be allowed to tuck her infant or child in before he goes to sleep. Where separation from the mother is not preventable, a substitute mother-figure (often Granny) should be provided at the earliest moment. Chronically depressed children, especially those that attempt suicide or risk their lives as though bent on self-destruction, should be referred to a child psychiatrist as a matter of urgency. Threats of suicide or suicidal attempts should always be taken seriously and should not be played down.

Infantile autism

Infantile autism is a rare disorder characterised by an inability of the patient to relate to people including his parents. As infants they are not cuddly, speech is markedly delayed and develops abnormally. Sufferers refer to themselves in the third person. A constant feature is the manner in which they avoid eye-contact. Their play routine is ritualistic and if these are interrupted they are liable to temper tantrums. The cause is unknown and therapy in specialised units offers these children their best chance of improvement.

HEADACHES

Headaches in the young child may cause irritability, quietness, pallor or head rolling. The significance of these symptoms may not be recognised if the child is unable to say his head is hurting. The older child and his parents, however, are usually more helpful and can give a detailed account of the headache. The two most common causes of chronic recurrent headache are migraine and functional or tension headaches.

Migraine

Migraine in the young child may present with episodes of pallor and vomiting apparently relieved by sleeping. There is usually a positive family history of the illness. Attacks may be precipitated by certain foodstuffs such as chocolate, or by fasting. Sometimes the headache is preceded by a visual aura which takes the form of flashing lights, stars, halos or scotomata which the child may find easier to draw than to describe. The headaches are usually unilateral but may be bifrontal, they last several hours and are relieved by darkness or sleep. During the attack the child may vomit and become pale. Occasionally migraine is complicated by ophthalmoplegia, dysphasia or hemiplegia.

Treatment
Precipitating factors should be avoided. The nature of the illness should be explained. Most children feel better after a sleep. A simple analgesic such as asprin or paracetamol often relieves the headache. Vomiting can be helped by using prochlorperazine suppositories. Ergotamine preparations are usually reserved for the older child who does not respond to other therapy.

Functional headaches

Functional headaches or tension headaches are usually due to underlying stress. The cause of the stress may not be obvious and one should look for an underlying emotional, social or educational problem. Functional headaches may be a sign of depression. The headache is usually generalised and may be described as pressing. It may come on suddenly and is constant, lasting days or weeks. There are no abnormal physical signs, though tension of the neck muscles may be noticed in some cases.

Treatment
The child and his parents should be reassured that there is no *serious* underlying cause. The underlying cause or causes should be identified and the child helped with his problem. Psychiatric help may be necessary.

Other types of headache may be due to local lesions in the head such as sinusitis or otitis media. Headache can be a feature of *any* febrile illness. Whenever neck stiffness is present meningitis, encephalitis, subarachnoid haemorrhage or an intracranial mass should be suspected. The headache of an intracranial mass is worse first thing in the morning and is eased by vomiting. Headaches may also be caused by hydrocephalus and hypertension. In all these cases physical signs are invariably present.

BRAIN TUMOURS IN INFANCY AND CHILDHOOD

At least half of all brain tumours in children lie under the tentorium, and the rest above. About three-quarters of all brain tumours lie in the midline. About three-quarters are gliomas.

Clinical features

Brain tumours may cause signs of sudden or insidious increase of intracranial pressure. In acute cases there may be severe headache, effortless vomiting, double vision, unsteady gait, dizziness, weakness, drowsiness and coma. If the increase in intracranial pressure develops slowly, the brain structures have time to adjust and the development of symptoms or signs may be delayed.

Ataxia and nystagmus with slowly developing increased intracranial pressure suggests an infratentorial tumour. Lesions above the tentorium are more likely to cause hemiparesis and varying cranial nerve palsies depending on the site of the lesion. Sensory defects may be very difficult to detect in children and the help of an ophthalmologist or audiologist may be required to establish an exact diagnosis. Weight loss is a common phenomenon but obesity is rare and suggests the presence of a hypothalamic tumour. Head tilting may compensate for ocular muscle paresis or may be due to a cerebellar tumour. Percussion of the skull may produce a 'cracked pot' sound (Macewen's sign). Papilloedema is usually present but may be a late sign.

Pathological notes

The term *glioma* is a blanket term covering *all* tumours of the supporting tissue of the brain. In children the most important are *astrocytomas.* Their variety is endless but fortunately they are rare in children.

Medulloblastoma means a tumour in the medulla, and does not refer to a cell type. They occur only in children, and are always in the mid-line of the medulla or cerebellar vermis.

Ependymomas arise from the lining cells of the ventricular system. They may be classified into four grades according to their degree of malignancy. At operation or autopsy they may resemble medulloblastomas on inspection, but histologically they differ markedly.

Other tumours such as oligodendroglias and neuroastrocytomas are uncommon. Vascular tumours are mentioned elsewhere (p. 166). Craniopharyngiomas are epithelial tumours related to the pituitary region.

Localisation of brain tumours

Suprasellar tumours

The most important in children are craniopharyngiomas and optic nerve gliomas (astrocytoma).

Craniopharyngioma

Craniopharyngioma is an ectodermal cystic tumour thought to derive from Rathke's Pouch. It is slow-growing and symptoms usually appear between 6 and 12 years of age. The cardinal features are:

1 Increased intracranial pressure due to obstruction to one or both foramina of Monro, and dilatation of one or both lateral ventricles.
2 Visual defects due to pressure on the optic chiasma. The classical finding is bitemporal hemianopia (blindness in the temporal fields).
3 Diabetes insipidus due to pressure on the hypothalamus or posterior pituitary gland. It may also appear for the first time *after* surgical removal of the tumour.
4 Growth retardation and sexual infantilism. Sometimes obesity with female distribution of fat may be present (Fröhlich's syndrome).
5 X-ray of the skull reveals enlargement of the sella turcica, flecks of calcification in or above it, and springing of the sutures.

Treatment
Surgical removal of the tumour is recommended. The neurosurgeon may prefer to aspirate the fluid from the tumour as this may provide immediate relief of symptoms and prevent blindness. Radiotherapy to the tumour may be of benefit. Hormonal replacement therapy is required during the operative period and postoperatively. The tumour may regrow slowly and require further aspirations or excisions.

Optic nerve glioma

Optic nerve glioma is a disease of early childhood and causes exophthalmos, visual impairment and optic atrophy. Squints and nystagmus sometimes occur. Large tumours may obstruct the foramen of Monro and cause hydrocephalus. Endocrine disturbances are rare.

Treatment
If the lesion is confined to a single optic nerve, excision is possible. If the optic chiasma is involved then radiotherapy is recommended. A ventricular shunt may be required to relieve hydrocephalus.

Diencephalic tumours

Glioma in the hypothalamus may produce a rare but striking symptom-complex, the *diencephalic syndrome*. Marked emaciation and hyperactivity in a baby of five or six months of age is associated with a striking alertness and euphoria. Vomiting is common but may not be severe enough to arouse comment. Peptic ulceration and intestinal haemorrhage may be a feature.

Brainstem gliomas

Gliomas of the brainstem, mostly astrocytomas but occasionally glioblastomas, occur in children between five and ten years of age. They produce cranial nerve palsies, pyramidal tract lesions and cerebellar tract disorders. The commonest cranial nerve lesion is facial palsy of the lower motor neuron type, but the V, VI, IX and X cranial nerves may also be affected. These may be bilateral. Pyramidal tract involvement is manifested by increased reflexes and extensor plantar response, but these may be masked by cerebellar ataxia. Nystagmus may be vertical or horizontal.

The cerebrospinal fluid is normal and *there is no increased pressure*. Air encephalography may be done therefore and the aqueduct of Sylvius and the fourth ventricle are displaced posteriorly and upwards on the lateral views. The pontine cistern is reduced in size because of the size of the tumour.

Treatment

Radiotherapy produces temporary improvement but relapse may be expected within a few months.

Cerebellar tumours

About a quarter of all brain tumours occur in the cerebellum. They can occur at any age. The commonest are astrocytomas, with medulloblastomas a close second. Ependymomas and choroid plexus tumours are rare.

Signs and symptoms may be non-specific. There is likely to be increased intracranial pressure causing effortless vomiting (i.e. without nausea), headache, double or blurred vision, squint, papilloedema and personality changes. Meningismus may be due to herniation of the cerebellar tonsil through the foramen magnum.

Unsteadiness of gait may be due to the cerebellar lesion or to the accompanying vertigo. Nystagmus with large amplitude on gaze to the side of the lesion may be present. There may be progressive involvement of cranial nerves V, VII and VIII causing facial numbness, facial weakness and deafness. Bulbar palsy may develop. Spasticity of the limbs is an indication of a pyramidal lesion. The head may tilt to the side of the lesion. Stupor, convulsions and coma may occur, usually shortly before the patient dies. Mid-line cerebellar tumours may cause none of the above focal symptoms except for ataxic gait. Raised intracranial pressure occurs early. There may be hydrocephalus with dilatation of the third ventricle which leads to obesity and polyuria. Papilloedema and secondary optic atrophy may occur.

Diagnosis

X-ray of the skull shows non-specific increase of intracranial pressure. Ventriculography and CAT scan may reveal hydrocephalus and the site and size of the tumour. Brachial or carotid angiograms may be of value in some cases to demonstrate distorted vascular patterns and herniation.

Treatment

Astrocytomas are slow-growing and successful removal is possible if diagnosed early. X-ray therapy should follow surgery. Medulloblastomas are very rapid-growing and seed along the CSF pathway or in the subarachnoid space. Nevertheless surgical decompression of the posterior fossa and deep X-ray therapy is advisable. Chemotherapy may be of value in some cases. Hydrocephalus may be relieved by an appropriate shunting operation.

Tumours of the cerebral hemispheres

These produce focal signs which may easily be confused with those of cerebellar tumours. There is usually obstructive hydrocephalus and signs of increased intracerebral pressure, unless the fontanelles and sutures are still open and the head is able to expand. In small children it is almost impossible to test for cortical functions such as hemianopia, aphasia or apraxia but sometimes gross pyramidal signs such as hemiplegia may be found. Focal convulsions of the Jackson type may occur. Occasionally cortical neoplasm may erode through the skull.

Diagnosis may be confirmed by full radiological studies including ventriculography and arteriogram to show local displacement of ventricle or blood vessels. Brain scans may be helpful in localising the tumour.

Treatment
The tumour should be eradicated if possible. This is followed by irradiation and/or chemotherapy. A high percentage of these tumours are malignant therefore the prognosis is poor.

CHAPTER 13

THE ENDOCRINE SYSTEM

Although the pituitary gland was once referred to as the 'conductor of the endocrine orchestra', it is now realised that the conductor is subservient to the 'director' in the hypothalamic nuclei, and to feedback from the very endocrine glands that it stimulates. The 'director' controls the secretion of the anterior pituitary by means of releasing factors formed in the hypothalamus by the supra-optic and para-ventricular nuclei. These are transmitted via the pituitary portal blood system to the anterior pituitary lobe. There is a finely balanced negative feedback system which exists between the hypothalamus and peripheral endocrine glands and which maintains the blood level of various hormones at their optimum level. It should be emphasised that, in children, not only are the metabolic effects of the endocrine system of prime importance but also the ability to stimulate physical growth and sexual maturation. There also seems to be a close association with centres for the regulation of sleep, temperature, blood pressure and appetite and with the pineal gland which seems to be concerned with circadian rhythms and melatonin formation (see Fig. 13.1).

DISEASES OF THE ANTERIOR PITUITARY GLAND

Idiopathic hypopituitarism

In the majority of patients with hypopituitarism the chief complaint is shortness of stature due to failure of somatotrophic (growth) hormone (GH). It should be suspected in any child growing less than 5 cm (2 inches) per year in whom no other organic cause for the retarded growth, including hypothyroidism, can be found. If there is failure of the pituitary gonadotrophic hormones the penis and scrotum are often poorly developed. Sexual infantilism becomes obvious after the expected age of puberty because the secondary sexual characteristics fail to appear. Occasional patients in whom there is isolated deficiency of thyroid stimulating hormone (TSH) or adrenocorticotrophic hormone (ACTH) have been described.

In *pure* GH deficiency the child is below the third percentile for his age, looks younger than his years and is often plump with a 'baby' distribution of fat. Skeletal and dental maturation are delayed. In many centres it is now possible to measure serum GH after stimulation with L-dopa, insulin or other means. The oral glucose test may suggest the

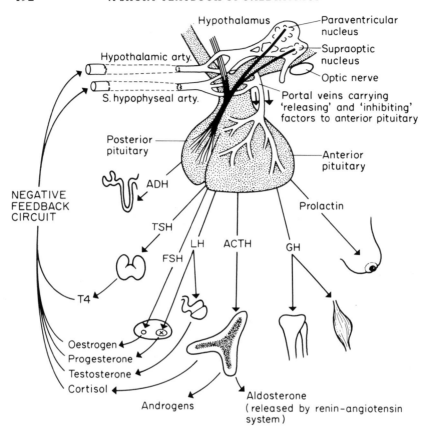

Fig. 13.1 The endocrine orchestra. The nerve cells in the hypothalamus secrete both releasing and inhibiting factors which reach the pituitary gland via the pituitary portal circulation. The cells of the pituitary gland release their appropriate hormones into the general circulation to stimulate their target organs. The serum levels of these hormones control the release of the hypothalamic and pituitary hormones by means of a negative feedback circuit

diagnosis of diabetes mellitus and there is often a reactive hypoglycaemia two to five hours later.

It is important to exclude organic causes of dwarfism before embarking on therapy. If the growth velocity measured over a year is less than 5 cm and the growth hormone responses to at least two provactive tests, such as L-dopa and insulin hypoglycaemia, are inadequate, the injections of human growth hormone (HGH) may be considered.

Treatment
This consists of injecting human growth hormone two or three times weekly. The hormone is very expensive as yet and should only be used for proved cases of GH deficiency. Associated ACTH or TSH deficiency can be treated with the appropriate hormones. Hydrocortisone and thyroxine in small doses are satisfactory. Sex hormones are used for sexual infantilism in order to stimulate the menstrual cycle in girls and to masculinise boys. Premature closure of the epiphyses may occur, however, if sex hormones are used too soon or in too big a dose. Psychological support is required for the patient and his family.

Organic hypopituitarism

Organic hypopituitarism is nearly always due to a craniopharyngioma or other tumours at the base of the brain. Rarely, it follows fracture of the base of the skull, tuberose sclerosis, or encephalitis. The primary symptoms usually relate to visual disturbances and increasing intra-cranial pressure. Pressure or invasion of the hypothalamus may cause an associated diabetes insipidus, obesity, drowsiness and seizures. X-ray reveals erosion of the clinoid processes of the sella turcica, or calcification in the suprasellar region due to craniopharyngioma. A CAT scan may help to delineate space-occupying lesions.

Treatment
Treatment involves radiotherapy and surgical excision. Postoperatively the appropriate hormone deficiencies due to excision of the pituitary gland should be treated.

Hyperpituitarism

GH-secreting adenomas produce an excess of somatotrophic hormone resulting in *gigantism*, a very rare disorder in children. After puberty it presents with *acromegaly*.

ACTH-secreting adenomas overstimulate the adrenal glands resulting in Cushing' syndrome (p. 196). In 80% of cases the tumours are very small and X-ray of the pituitary fossa may show no sign of enlargement.

Treatment
Radiation therapy may be used for hyperpituitarism to reduce the activity of the gland. When the tumour is large enough to press on the optic nerve, surgical excision or cryotherapy is required. Subsequently cortisol replacement is advised to maintain the activity of the suprarenal gland. Metyrapone and aminoglutethamide have been used as palliative therapy while awaiting response to radiotherapy in Cushings' disease. Many cases of Cushings' syndrome are due to tumours of the adrenal gland, thymus or ovary and these may require excision.

DISEASES OF THE POSTERIOR PITUITARY GLAND

Diabetes insipidus

Diabetes insipidus is a chronic disorder characterised by polyuria, polydipsia and an inability to concentrate urine. There are two forms now recognised.

1 Cranial diabetes insipidus
This is due to a lesion involving the posterior pituitary gland or its connections with the hypothalamus. It may follow trauma, encephalitis or neoplasms. Most cases are idiopathic and associated with a deficiency of antidiuretic hormone (arginine vasopressin).

2 Nephrogenic diabetes insipidus
This is due to an inherited disorder of the renal tubule in which there is diminished reabsorption of water. It is a sex-linked disorder occurring only in males. It is resistant to vasopressin injection.

The chief symptoms are polydipsia (excess thirst) and polyuria, in which the specific gravity of the urine is persistently below 1006 and the osmolality 50–200 mOsmol/kg H_2O. There is usually bed-wetting present and the child is often small for his age. Diagnosis is made by withholding water for 4–6 hours. The specific gravity of the urine does not exceed 1010 and the osmolality 300. The plasma osmolality also rises due to dehydration. If arginine vasopressin is administered, usually intranasally, the clinical picture improves dramatically and the urine output returns to normal. The dose of arginine vasopressin will be determined by trial. Failure of response suggests the possibility of nephrogenic diabetes insipidus or compulsive water drinking.

A number of drugs have been found effective in partial cranial diabetes insipidus, for example carbamazepine (Tegretol) and clofibrate (Atromid), but side-effects may limit their use. A low solute diet may be helpful. For nephrogenic diabetes insipidus chlorothiazide is used.

Excess antidiuretic hormone secretion

The syndrome of inappropriate ADH secretion may occur in a number of diseases such as bronchopneumonia, asthma or emphysema and in patients receiving positive pressure respiration. In such patients there is increased resistance to pulmonary flow which, for reasons uncertain, causes an 'inappropriate' secretion of ADH. It also occurs in hypothyroidism and diseases of the central nervous system such as meningitis, encephalitis, Guillain-Barré syndrome, head injuries and brain tumours. An increase in serum ADH also occurs in all hypovolaemic states. As a result the patient passes a *hypertonic* urine associated with a persistent *hyponatraemia*. The diagnosis is made by simultaneous measurements of serum and urine osmolality. The treatment is not to give extra salt, as seems logical to correct the hyponatraemia, but to reduce the water intake until the underlying causes have been corrected. In the case of lesions of the central nervous system many respond to the simple procedure of raising the foot of the bed. Postoperatively, water should be moderately restricted for a few days.

THE ADRENAL GLAND

Hyperadrenocorticalism

The clinical picture in hyperadrenocorticalism depends on which of the adrenal cortical steroids is produced in excess.

1 *Androgen-producing lesions* lead to adrenogenital syndrome with masculinisation of the female and the occurrence of ambiguous genitalia. In males virilisation may cause an 'infant Hercules', or may present as a hypoadrenal state.
2 *Cortisol-secreting lesions* produce Cushing's syndrome.
3 *Hyperaldosteronism* produces Conn's syndrome, in which hypertension, hypernatraemia, hypokalaemia and metabolic alkalosis occur.

Adrenogenital syndrome

The adrenogenital syndrome is due to the inherited inability of the adrenal cortex to synthesise cortisol. A number of different enzyme deficiencies have been described. The pituitary gland produces an excess of ACTH (due to lack of cortisol feedback) and this in turn stimulates the formation of an excess of adrenal androgens. In girls this results in virilisation of the external genitalia. The urogenital sinus may persist with a common opening of the vagina and urethra into the perineum. At birth the female baby may resemble a cryptorchid male with hypospadias. In the male the sex organs may look normal but precocious pseudopuberty may occur before four years of age. Tremendous muscular development may occur ('infant Hercules'). The testes, however, remain small due to the suppression of pituitary gonadotrophic hormone by the excess androgens. Cushing's syndrome does not occur because cortisol is not formed.

In one-third of infants evidence of acute adrenocortical insufficiency develops in the second week of life and the infant is likely to die unless he is treated promptly ('salt-losing' type of adrenogenital syndrome). In these patients both cortisol and aldosterone are deficient, resulting in hyponatraemia and hyperkalaemia. Occasionally some patients develop hypertension due to the accumulation of a cortisol precursor, desoxycorticosterone. Diagnosis is made by steroid assays of the urine or blood. Pregnanetriol, 17–ketosteroids in the urine, 17–hydroxy-progesterone in the serum and various other metabolites are increased.

These should return towards normal when cortisol therapy is given. The serum electrolytes should always be measured.

Treatment

Hydrocortisone (Cortisol) is urgently indicated; a suppressive dose of $20-25$ mg/m^2 per day is given in two divided doses orally or by injection, the dose being gradually increased according to the age and needs of the patient. It must be continued for life. In the salt-losing form intravenous saline is given initially, together with a salt-retaining hormone such as aldosterone or fludrocortisone orally. Extra salt, $3-5$ g daily, should be administered orally every day. Corrective surgery may be required at a later stage in girls. Problems in relation to correct sexing should be referred to the appropriate team.

Cushing's syndrome

Cushing's syndrome is characterised by obesity and protein wasting. Polycythaemia, hirsutes, moon-face, hypertension, hyperglycaemia with glycosuria, and decalcification of the skeleton occur. Pathological fractures may be found. Purple striae are seen on the skin of the chest, buttocks and thighs. The excess fat tends to accumulate on the cheeks, shoulder girdle ('buffalo hump') and hips. Potassium wastage, salt retention and growth retardation is usual.

The commonest cause of Cushing's syndrome in children is iatrogenic, i.e. it is due to the prolonged use of pharmacological doses of corticosteroids for diseases such as rheumatoid arthritis, nephrosis or leukaemia. Other causes include pituitary-dependent Cushing's syndrome or cortisol-producing tumours of the adrenal cortex, thymus or ovary (see Fig. 13.2).

Diagnosis

Diagnosis is clinical but can be confirmed by finding an abnormal excretion of both 17-ketosteroids and 11-oxysteroid in the urine. The dexamethasone suppression test may be helpful in distinguishing hyperplasia from malignancy of the adrenal, though the validity of this test has been questioned. Blood ACTH levels can be measured in some centres.

Treatment

In children requiring long-term corticosteroid therapy it has been found that if the dose is given on alternative days there is a considerable reduction in 'Cushingoid' side-effects without reduction of clinical efficacy. Reduction of dosage or complete stoppage of the hormone nearly always reverses the iatrogenic disorder.

Patients with neoplasms of the adrenal gland, ovary or thymus require surgical excision of the tumour. Temporary replacement therapy with corticosteroids is usually necessary because prolonged excess of cortisol production due to the neoplasm suppresses ACTH production.

CUSHING'S SYNDROME – Characteristics

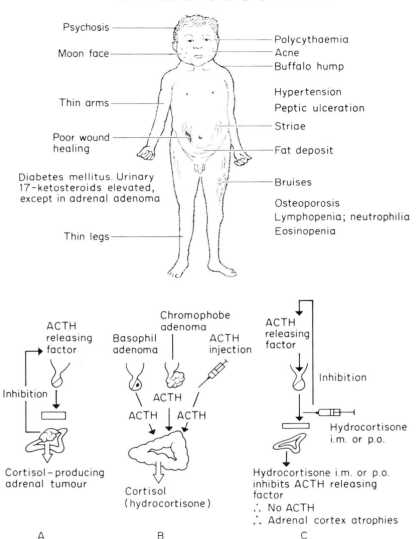

Fig. 13.2 Effect on adrenal gland of: **A** adrenal tumour; **B** pituitary tumour or ACTH therapy; **C** other corticosteroid therapy

On removing the cortisol-producing neoplasm the patient has none of his own. This may cause unexpected collapse during anaesthesia or in any stress situation requiring circulating cortisol.

When Cushing's syndrome is due to a pituitary tumour (rare)

microsurgical excision should be contemplated, or the diseased gland irradiated.

ACTH and corticosteroids in therapy

Corticotrophin (ACTH; adrenocorticotrophin) is used to stimulate the patient's own adrenal cortex to produce cortisol and androgens. It does not stimulate aldosterone secretion. Short- and long-acting preparations are available for injection only.

The normal adult produces about 20 mg (10–15 mg/m^2) of *cortisol* (hydrocortisone) per day. A large number of analogues of hydrocortisone have been produced which are more powerful but have a reduced salt-retaining effect. Table 13.1 shows the approximate equivalent doses of these analogues.

Table 13.1 Equivalent doses of corticosteroids

Name of corticosteroid	Dose equivalent mg
Hydrocortisone	20
Prednisone and prednisolone	5
Methylprednisolone	4
Dexamethasone	0.75
Betamethasone	0.7

Pharmacological doses of corticosteroids are five to ten times the physiological dose and, if used for any length of time, produce Cushing's syndrome. Side effects can be reduced by prescribing the minimum therapeutic dose and by giving the drug on alternate days.

Prolonged corticosteroid therapy suppresses endogenous corticosteroid secretion, therefore therapy should always be tailed off slowly to avoid an Addisonian crisis, (see below). Any patient who has received prolonged corticosteroid therapy may respond poorly to stress situations such as infection or anaesthetic for at least six months after stopping treatment. These patients should be 'covered' by reinstituting a short course of treatment.

Topical corticosteroids

Many skin infections, notably infantile eczema, respond remarkably well to corticosteroids topically. The most useful are fluocinolone (Synalar) and betamethasone (Betnovate) both of which can be diluted in aqueous cream B.P. up to ten times for the sake of economy and to permit the mother to spread the ointment over large areas if necessary. If used with care, systemic absorption is rarely a problem.

Adrenal insufficiency

The commonest cause of adrenal insufficiency is prolonged suppression of the adrenal glands with pharmacological doses of corticosteroids in diseases such as nephrosis, rheumatoid arthritis or rheumatic fever. Insidious failure of the adrenal gland (Addison's disease) in children may occur as an auto-immune phenomenon, or rarely it may be due to tuberculosis of the gland. Weakness, loss of appetite and bouts of vomiting occur. The blood sugar is often low causing dizziness, trembling and gnawing epigastric pains. Any stress may precipitate cardiovascular collapse (adrenal crisis). Pigmentation is due to increased secretion of ACTH by the pituitary. It gives the skin a dirty brown colour, any freckles present are darkened and there is usually pigmentation of the gum margin and inside the cheeks.

Diagnosis
This may be confirmed by the ACTH stimulation test. In Addison's disease there is no increase of plasma cortisol or urinary corticoids. There is usually a low serum sodium, raised potassium level, metabolic acidosis and hypoglycaemia. The disease is not always as clear-cut as in adults.

Treatment
The use of oral glucocorticoids in physiological doses is usually sufficient to maintain the patient in good health. Extra salt should be added to their food. Some patients may require fluorocortisone (a mineralocorticoid) to maintain salt balance. The dose of this should be increased in anticipation of stress situations such as dental extraction or major surgery. Infections should always be treated vigorously.

Waterhouse-Friderichsen syndrome
See meningococcal infections (p. 175).

ADRENAL MEDULLA AND SYMPATHETIC NERVOUS TISSUE

Phaeochromocytoma

Phaeochromocytoma is a very rare noradrenaline- and/or adrenaline-secreting tumour arising from the adrenal medulla, commonly the right, or from chromaffin tissue anywhere else in the body. It is usually benign. Symptoms may begin at any age but most cases are diagnosed after six years of age. In children sustained hypertension is much more common than the paroxysmal type seen in adults. Headache, tachycardia, excessive sweating, abdominal pain, vomiting and visual disturbances occur.

Diagnosis

This depends on finding excess catecholamines and their metabolites in the urine. Tests such as the phentolamine test, glucagon or intravenous histamine test may be dangerous in children and are seldom used nowadays.

Treatment

The tumour must be localised first by means of X-rays of the chest to reveal mediastinal or paravertebral masses, or IVP to show displacement of the kidney by an adrenal mass. In many cases ultrasound or CAT scan may be useful. Serial collection of plasma for catecholamines from the inferior vena cava and its tributaries may be helpful. When the diagnosis is certain but the tumour cannot be localised, extensive surgical exploration may be necessary.

Pre-operatively hypertension is controlled by phenoxybenzamine, an alpha-adrenergic blocking agent. It is sometimes advisable to use beta-blockers to prevent cardiac arrhythmias. Fluid and electrolytes should be carefully monitored. The blood pressure should be carefully checked as there may be a sudden drop after removal of the tumour. This may be controlled by a noradrenaline infusion. It should be remembered that phaeochromocytomas may be bilateral. The urinary catecholamines should be measured five or six days after operation to be sure that all functional tissue has been removed.

Neuroblastoma

A neuroblastomata is a malignant tumour of one of the ganglia of the sympathetic chain or of the adrenal medulla. Its peak incidence is three years of age and it is rarely seen after the age of six years. It commonly occurs in the retroperitoneal tissue of the chest or abdomen. It metastasizes early to the skeleton, brain, lymph nodes or liver. A retro-orbital deposit may be the first evidence of the tumour. In infants it may present with massive infiltration of the liver.

Fever, bone pain, weight loss and progressive anaemia occur. Paraplegia occurs if the spinal canal is invaded. Sometimes paroxysmal hypertension occurs due to the secretion of excess noradrenaline (see also phaeochromocytoma above).

Diagnosis

Diagnosis depends on finding excess catecholamines and/or their metabolites VMA or HVA in the urine. An IVP may reveal displacement of one kidney by a suprarenal mass. X-ray of the chest may reveal paravertebral shadows or a tumour in the posterior mediastinum. Ultrasound or CAT scan may help to localise the tumour. Bone-marrow puncture may reveal secondary deposits.

Differential diagnosis

Phaeochromocytoma is distinguished by its clinical features and the fact that it is not an invasive tumour. Wilm's tumour, Ewing's sarcoma and lymphomas do not produce abnormal catecholamines or their metabolites in the urine.

Treatment
As much of the tumour as is feasible should be excised and this is followed by radiotherapy and/or chemotherapy. The tumour is very sensitive to this attack which should be undertaken even in advanced cases. Cyclophosphamide may be combined with vincristine sulphate intravenously.

Prognosis
The younger the patient the better the prognosis. Over the age of five years the prognosis is hopeless. Infants with massive infiltration of the liver may respond surprisingly well to therapy. Occasionally spontaneous cures have been documented. Response to therapy can be judged by the return of catecholamines and their metabolites in the urine to normal levels.

Ganglioneuroma

A ganglioneuroma is a benign tumour containing mature ganglion cells. It is thought that some neuroblastomas mature into ganglioneuromas. The condition is not associated with increased excretion of catecholamine or its metabolites. It is usually found during palpation of the abdomen. The tumour should be excised.

Occasionally ganglioneuroma and other neural crest tumours may be associated with a syndrome in which chronic watery diarrhoea, failure to thrive, abdominal distension, cough, malar flush and hypokalaemia occur. The symptoms clear when the tumour is removed.

THE THYROID GLAND

The physiologically active hormones secreted by the thyroid gland are the organic iodine compounds tri-iodothyronine (T3) and thyroxine (T4). Their release into the circulation is governed by thyroid releasing hormone (TRH) and thyroid stimulating hormone (TSH).

Hypothyroidism

The term 'cretin' is commonly used as a synonym for hypothyroidism occurring in infants. It is characterised by myxoedema, mental deficiency and dwarfism. The commonest causes are congenital absence of thyroid tissue and inborn errors of thyroid hormone synthesis. Hypothyroidism due to iodine deficiency in the diet still occurs in some parts of the world and can be prevented by using iodinised salt. Goitrogens given to a mother with thyrotoxicosis may cross the placenta and depress the fetal thyroid hormone production.

Clinical features

Neonatal screening has shown that the incidence of congenital hypothyroidism is 1 in 4000. Hypothyroidism should be suspected in neonates who feed sluggishly and in whom 'physiological' jaundice persists for more than ten days. The bowels, like the baby, may also be sluggish, the temperature is low and some harshness of the voice may be noted. Skeletal retardation may be present at an early age.

The full-blown cretin is hypothermic with a pig-like face due to the accumulation of myxoedema in the subcutaneous tissues and tongue (Fig. 13.3). There is a harsh cry and generalised hypotonia. An umbilical hernia and pot-belly is constant. The heart rate is slow and the pulse pressure is small. The ECG shows low voltage leads and a prolonged

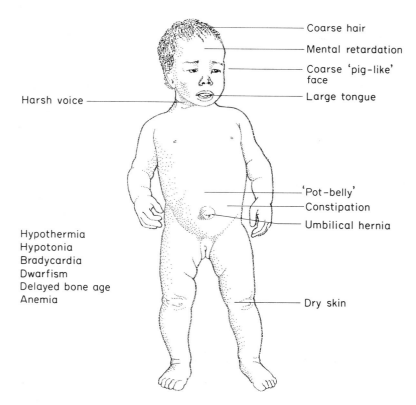

Fig. 13.3 Signs of advanced hypothyroidism (*early* hypothyroidism should be suspected in neonates whose jaundice is *prolonged*)

conduction time. X-ray reveals retarded skeletal maturation and stippling of the epiphyses. Laboratory findings include a normochromic anaemia and a raised TSH. The T4 is usually low. Neonatal screening for hypothyroidism has been introduced in centres in the United Kingdom, the USA, Japan and Australia.

Treatment
The hypothermic child should be warmed up gradually. Cretins are highly sensitive to sedative drugs, vitamin D and other substances such as bilirubin, due to impaired conjugation and excretion. Thyroid replacement may be made with thyroxine (T4) or tri-iodothyronine (T3) according to the needs of the patient. With thyroxine one usually starts with 50 μg once daily and increases by 25 μg every 10–14 days until the pulse, growth, general activity and bowels are normal. The dose at one year is usually 75–100 μg daily, and at 7 years 150–200 μg daily. The starting dose of tri-iodothyronine is 25 μg daily. Response to therapy may be determined by TSH, T3 and T4 levels in the serum. The bone age may be assessed at six-monthly intervals. Overdose produces tachycardia, nervousness and loose bowels. Initially, if not used with care, it may precipitate sudden death.

Prognosis
The prognosis depends on the degree of prenatal and postnatal hypothyroidism. Neonatal screening is recommended to diagnose cases early. If treatment is begun before three months of age the chances for normal or near normal intellectual development are good in cases developing after birth but less good in those developing prenatally.

Goitre

A goitre is an enlarged thyroid gland. It may be present in the newborn of mothers who have taken goitrogens during pregnancy. The commonest cause has been iodine-containing cough mixtures or antithyroid drugs such as carbimazole or thiouracils. Sulphonamides, para-aminosalicylic acid (PAS) and cobalt-containing haematinics have been implicated. It may occur in cretinism due to inborn errors of metabolism but obviously not in athyrotic cretinism. It may be due to the over-production of thyroid-stimulating hormone (TSH) or thyroid stimulating immunoglobulin (TSI). Functionally, a goitre may be associated with hyper-, hypo- or euthyroidism.

Hashimoto's struma (auto-immune thyroiditis)

This is an enlargement of the thyroid gland most commonly occurring in girls. It may progress to hypothyroidism. Circulating antithyroid antibodies are found. The patient has an unusual sensitivity to iodides, and iodine should never be used for therapy. Thyroxine is given if there is definite evidence of hypothyroidism or as a means of reducing TSH and thus reducing the size of the goitre.

Hashimoto's struma is probably the commonest cause for thyroid enlargement in children. Fifty per cent of patients with so-called 'simple goitre' have this as the cause.

Lingual goitre and thyroglossal cysts

A swelling at the base of the tongue or along the course of the thyroglossal duct may be due to ectopic thyroid tissue. It may be the sole thyroid tissue that the patient has. Enlargement may cause pressure symptoms and dysphagia. Before removing midline masses from the neck of children radioisotopic scans should firstly be performed. If the mass is indeed the only available thyroid tissue, treatment with full doses of thyroxine will cause shrinkage and avoid the need for surgery. However, it must be given for life.

Hyperthyroidism

Overactivity of the thyroid is rare in childhood, occurring chiefly in girls after the age of puberty. It is mediated by an immunoglobulin derived from lymphocytes, called thyroid stimulating immunoglobulin (TSI). This may also be found in the serum of babies born to thyrotoxic mothers.

The clinical picture is similar to that in adults. Initially sleeplessness, nervousness, jumpiness and falling-off in school performance occur. The usual signs of exophthalmos, tachycardia and fine tremor of the outstretched hands occur. The skin is warm and moist and there is an increase in pulse pressure. A bruit may be heard over the enlarged thyroid gland. A voracious appetite may compensate for the increased metabolism but weight loss usually occurs.

Diagnosis
An absent TSH response to intravenous TRF usually indicates hyperthyroidism. The T3 and T4 are elevated. Agglutinating antibodies to thyroglobulins may be found. TSH is usually present in the plasma. X-rays may reveal accelerated skeletal maturation.

Treatment
Drugs such as carbimazole or thiouracils are used to block thyroid synthesis. In selected cases subtotal thyroidectomy may be used.

Thyroid nodules in children

A solitary thyroid nodule is malignant in 50% of children. It never causes thyrotoxicosis, therefore lack of symptoms should not prevent one from referring the child for surgical opinion and excision-biopsy of the affected lobe.

DISEASE OF THE PARATHYROID GLANDS

Parathyroid hormone has three actions:

1 It mobilises calcium and phosphorus from bone.
2 It inhibits renal tubular reabsorption of phosphate thus causing a reduction in serum phosphate.
3 It increases reabsorption of calcium by the renal tubules.

Hypoparathyroidism

Transient hypoparathyroidism may occur in the neonate, particularly those who are fed from the start on milk with a high phosphate-calcium ratio. It may also occur in babies of low birth-weight and in babies of diabetic mothers. The serum calcium is lowered, and the serum phosphate increased. Latent or overt tetany may occur, or the infant may have a convulsion.

Di George's syndrome is the rare association of congenital absence of parathyroids, aplasia of the thymus with defects of the eye, heart and brain.

Chronic hypoparathyroidism due to parathyroid antibodies may be associated with persistent moniliasis, anaemia, Addison's disease and steatorrhoea.

Clinical features
Parathyroid deficiency causes hypocalcaemia, convulsions and tetany. In prolonged cases blepharospasm, conjunctivitis, cataracts, diarrhoea, alopecia, skin rashes, thickened irregular nails, moniliasis, dental hypoplasia and occasionally symmetrical calcification of the basal ganglia may occur.

The convulsions may be focal or mimic grand mal epilepsy. There may be a typical EEG pattern of grand mal. Therefore all children with seizures should have a serum calcium done to exclude hypoparathyroidism as a treatable cause.

The classical findings of tetany are a positive Chvostek's sign, carpopedal spasm (Trousseau's sign) and laryngospasm, but are not often present.

Diagnosis
Hypocalcaemia plus raised serum phosphate plus normal renal function. In hypoparathyroidism parathyroid hormone (PTH) levels are low. In such cases an intravenous injection of PTH causes an increase in serum calcium, an increase in urinary cyclic AMP, and a reduction in tubular reabsorption of phosphate. In *pseudohypoparathyroidism* the intravenous PTH test does not increase urinary cyclic AMP, and changes in calcium and phosphate are small.

Treatment

Acute hypocalcaemia is best treated by intravenous calcium gluconate, 5% or 10%. Prolonged hypocalcaemia requires the addition of large oral doses of calcium and the use of vitamin D to increase the serum calcium and reduce the serum phosphate. Alfacalcidol (One-Alpha) has a similar effect but is more rapid in action and more potent. The serum calcium should be monitored and not be allowed to rise above 2.7 mmol/l lest calcium be precipitated in the kidneys and other organs.

Pseudohypoparathyroidism

The parathyroid secretion is normal but the end organs fail to respond in this congenital disorder. There are associated disturbances of bone growth with short fingers and toes. Mental retardation may be present. The biochemistry is the same as for hypoparathyroidism except for the failure to respond to the hormone. As if this is not complicated enough, pseudo-pseudohypoparathyroidism has also been described!

Hyperparathyroidism

1 Primary hyperparathyroidism

This is even more rare than hypoparathyroidism. It causes hypercalcaemia, hypophosphataemia, demineralisation of bone and hypercalciuria. In infants it is one of the many causes of failure to thrive. It may also cause constipation. Prolonged hypercalcaemia leads to precipitation of calcium in soft tissues, including kidneys and blood vessels. X-rays of the long bones reveal diffuse or patchy demineralisation. Subperiosteal erosion of the phalanges occur, and loss of the lamina dura surrounding the tooth buds is characteristic. Sometimes the X-ray picture closely resembles that of rickets, sometimes of osteitis fibrosa cystica. The serum calcium and parathyroid hormone levels are increased.

Treatment

Treatment consists of surgical exploration for a parathyroid adenoma provided that all other causes for hypercalcaemia have been excluded.

2 Secondary hyperparathyroidism

This may be associated with lowering the serum calcium and raising of the serum phosphate level due to phosphate retention in the kidney. This occurs in renal failure and leads to demineralisation of bone, rickets or osteitis fibrosa cystica in an attempt to raise the serum calcium. The term *renal osteodystrophy* is sometimes used. The common renal lesions associated with this disease are hypoplasia of the kidneys, chronic pyelonephritis, chronic nephritis or hydronephrosis. Progressive deformity of the bones ('renal rickets') occurs (p. 76). This must be distinguished from the hypophosphataemic rickets associated with renal tubular defects (vitamin D resistant rickets), a rare familial disorder.

Treatment
Treatment is that of the underlying renal failure. In selected cases parathyroidectomy may be considered.

GONADAL DEFICIENCY

Testicular deficiency may be due to failure of luteinising hormone (LH) of the anterior pituitary, testicular atrophy or intra-uterine hormonal influences. Of infections, syphilis, tuberculosis and mumps are important causes of testicular disease. Testicular tumours and surgical removal also cause hypogonadism. An important genetic cause is *Klinefelter's syndrome* (see below). A rare cause is the *testicular feminisation syndrome* in which the male end organs fail to respond to testosterone and the patient resembles and is brought up as a girl.

In the female, ovarian hypofunction may be due to failure of pituitary gonadotrophins (luteinising hormone) or disease or surgical removal of the ovaries. An important genetic cause is *Turner's syndrome.*

Turner's syndrome

This syndrome of gonadal dysgenesis (streak ovaries) is associated with 45 XO sex chromosomes and negative sex chromatin. A few are XO/XX with positive sex chromatin. These patients are girls who do not develop secondary sexual characteristics at puberty. Their growth is stunted, they have amenorrhoea, there may be webbing of the neck, cubitus valgus and coarctation of the aorta, an anomaly which usually occurs in boys. Mental retardation may occur and other congenital anomalies may be found. At birth oedema of the extremities and loose neck folds are recognisable.

Treatment
Oestrogens may be given between 13 and 15 years to stimulate sexual maturation. Thereafter sequential oestrogen/progesterone therapy may be given to simulate the normal menstrual cycle as closely as possible. These patients remain infertile. Recently small doses of androgens have been used to stimulate skeletal growth.

Klinefelter's syndrome

This is a syndrome of seminiferous tubule dysgenesis (tubular fibrosis) associated with 47 XXY chromosomes and positive (female) sex chromatin. The patient looks like a boy, is usually tall with long legs, but the testes are very small. After puberty there is usually aspermia, gynaecomastia and eunuchoidism. Urinary gonadotrophin is increased.

Treatment consists of androgen replacement. This does not, however, reverse the gynaecomastia or the testicular lesion and these patients are all infertile.

Numerous other disturbances of the sex chromosomes have been described such as XXYY, XXX and various mosaics such as XY/XXX. These are fortunately all very rare, and are sometimes associated with other congenital anomalies.

Cryptorchidism (undescended testes)

Normally during descent the testes reach the inguinal canal by the 32nd week of pregnancy and enter the scrotum by the 39th week. The scrotum is initially small but becomes pendulous with extensive rugae at the time that the testes enter it. During cold weather or by stimulating the thigh, the testes retract into the inguinal canal and can be induced to return to the scrotum by manipulation (*retractile testes*). Failure to descend is called *cryptorchidism*. A testis which loses its way *en route* to the scrotum is called an *ectopic testis*.

Treatment

When it is certain that the testes will not descend, especially after a hot bath or by manipulation, then orchidopexy is advised between two and three years of age. If only one testis is undescended the results of operation are good, but if both testes are intra-abdominal, sterility or subfertility are extremely common. Nevertheless they should be brought down as torsion is not uncommon in undescended testes. There is also the possibility of malignancy to be considered. The use of chorionic gonadotrophin is no longer recommended as it may stimulate the early onset of puberty, premature closure of epiphyses and does not bring the retained testes into the scrotum.

Infants with intra-abdominal testes and a small phallus should be investigated for pseudohermaphroditism (p. 211).

Precocious puberty

Precocious puberty means the development of secondary sexual characteristics before the expected age. The age at which puberty normally develops varies with race, sex, and socio-economic conditions. It may be between 9 and 16 years, average 12 years. In the majority of children the cause of precocious puberty is unknown but it is thought to be due to the early triggering of the gonadotrophic hormones or their releasing factor in the hypothalamus. The serum FSH and LH may be increased above the normal pubertal level in most female patients. In boys there may be an increase in testosterone production, and most boys with precocious puberty have a CNS lesion such as an hamartoma of the tuber cinereum, tuberculous meningitis, or measles encephalitis injuring the hypothalamus. Adrenal hyperplasia, adrenal tumours and ovarian tumours should be excluded as causes of pseudopuberty.

Treatment

The main problems of precocious puberty are psychological and wise counselling is needed. Affected girls should wear clothes that minimise the size of their breasts and should be encouraged to behave appropriately for their chronological age, not their sexual age. Pregnancy is possible at a very early age, even before seven years. Menopause on the other hand occurs late. The development of secondary sexual characteristics can be retarded by the use of progestational agents such as medroxyprogesterone acetate or cyproterone acetate which is an anti-androgenic which suppresses gonadotrophins in both sexes. These substances cause cessation of menstruation and regression of breast development in girls and depress testosterone levels in boys. Linear growth and skeletal maturation may remain accelerated. As these drugs cause pituitary-adrenal axis suppression this should be carefully monitored on cessation of therapy.

Pseudoprecocious puberty

This refers to a condition in which the secondary sexual characteristics are initiated outside the normal hypothalamic-pituitary mechanism. The gonads do not mature and the patient is sterile. It may be associated with adrenogenital syndrome (p. 195), granulosa cell tumour of the ovary (which is nearly always palpable by the time the patient presents with symptoms), or interstitial cell tumour of the testis. Occasionally chorionepithelioma or teratomas may secrete gonadotrophins. In some cases it is iatrogenic as a result of gonadotrophic hormone treatment for cryptorchidism or the prolonged use of oxymetholone, an anabolic steroid for aplastic anaemia. Treatment depends on the cause.

Menstrual disorders

In temperate climates menstruation normally begins at about 9–12 years of age, but not later than 17 years. In the tropics the range is 9–14 years. Vaginal bleeding in the newborn is due to oestrogen withdrawal following transplacental passage of maternal oestrogen, and is of no consequence. In pre-pubertal girls bleeding is more likely to be due to a foreign body in the vagina than to menstrual disorders.

Delayed onset of menstruation may be due to an imperforate hymen, hypoplasia of the uterus, ovarian dysgenesis (see Turner's syndrome, p. 207), endocrine deficiency (especially thyroid or pituitary) or it may be constitutional or familial. Psychological factors are often implicated.

At puberty the first few periods are likely to be irregular, of variable flow and of the oestrogen breakthrough type. Occasionally they may be dangerously excessive. Pain before or during the flow may or may not be present.

Ambiguous sexual differentiation

Any infant with ambiguous sex organs should be investigated to determine their correct sex (see Figs. 13.4 and 13.5). Features which should arouse suspicion are:

1 Males with bilateral undescended testes, especially if the phallus is small (is it a large clitoris?).
2 Girls with an oval mass in the groin or labium majora (is it a testis?).
3 Newborns with oedema of the extremities and loose neck folds (is it Turner's syndrome?).
4 The occurrence of siblings with similar problems of sex identification.

It should be remembered that in genetic *gonadal disorders* such as Turner's or Klinefelter's syndromes the external genitalia are not ambiguous. Other features, however, are diagnostic (p. 207).

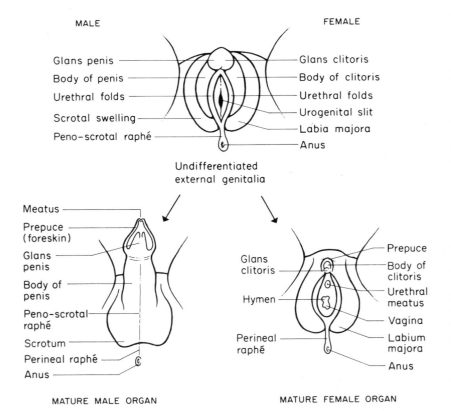

Fig. 13.4 Differentiation of sex organs

VIRILISATION OF THE FEMALE

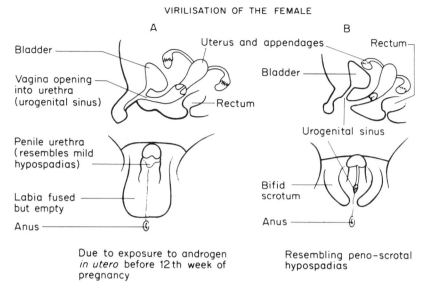

Fig. 13.5 Ambiguous sex organs

A true hermaphrodite
A hermaphrodite is a case of intersex in which the individual has both a functioning ovary and testis or ovotestis. It is extremely rare.

A male pseudohermaphrodite
This is a male phenotype with testes but ambiguous sexual structures resembling severe hypospadias. The labioscrotal folds are usually fused. Rarely the external genitalia are female (feminising testis syndrome).

A female pseudohermaphrodite
This is a female with ovaries but ambiguous sexual structures such as an enlarged clitoris resembling a penis. This may occur when the female fetus is exposed to excess androgens *in utero* (see adrenogenital syndrome p. 195).

Investigation of intersex

The history should include a family history of problems of sexual identification. The occurrence of 'cryptorchidism' may be significant. The use of androgens or progestogens for threatened abortion has caused virilisation of the female fetus and one should watch for the possibility of salt-losing crises in the first weeks of life. Physical examination should include palpation of the groin and labium-scrotum. Investigation should include culture for karyotype (chromosome type). Urinary excretion of

17-ketosteroids and pregnanetriol may indicate the presence of excess androgen formation.

Laboratory diagnosis

In female pseudohermaphroditism the genotype is XX whether induced by androgens or not. In these patients the urinary 17-ketosteroids and pregnanetriol should be investigated as they are increased only in the androgen-induced type of pseudohermaphrodite. The serum electrolytes should be tested to exclude the 'salt-losing' type. If the urinary hormones are normal a laparotomy and gonadal biopsy is required to distinguish non-androgen-induced pseudohermaphroditism from true intersex. An IVP is required to detect anomalies of the urinary tract in the former. A 'vaginogram' delineates the urogenital organs.

An XY genotype associated with abnormal external genitals is due to male pseudohermaphroditism or to true intersex. They are distinguished by bilateral gonadal biopsy.

Management

It is important to diagnose intersex problems early in order to prevent or minimise the development of serious social and psychological problems for both parent and child. Such problems should be tackled by an appropriately trained team which includes the general practitioner, paediatrician, gynaecologist, psychiatrist, geneticist, psychologist, social workers and other interested parties.

In adrenogenital syndrome virilisation can be suppressed by the administration of corticosteroids, and the external organs corrected surgically in the first year of life.

In other forms of intersex the gonadal and chromosomal sex are the most important guide to the child's sex. However if plastic surgery is unable to correct a deficiency, for instance to create a functioning penis in a male pseudohermaphrodite, then it may be necessary to bring the child up as the opposite sex, in this example as a girl. Once the sex has been assigned the parents should adhere firmly to the decision.

THE PANCREATIC ISLANDS

Diabetes mellitus

Diabetes mellitus in children is a metabolic disease characterised by polydipsia (excess thirst), polyuria (excess urination), hyperglycaemia, glycosuria and keto-acidosis, and is usually due to an absolute deficiency of insulin. It can occur at any age. Two types of *juvenile onset diabetes* (JOD) are recognised by the British Diabetic Association (1978):

Type IA—JOD with antibodies to exogenous insulin (90% of cases).
Type IB—JOD with auto-antibodies to own thyroid, adrenal or islet cells (10% of cases).

Transient diabetes of the newborn occurs and responds to insulin therapy. It tends to disappear in a month or two and the insulin can be stopped.

Clinical features

In children the onset of overt illness is relatively acute. Premonitory symptoms are thirst, polyuria, enuresis in a patient who was previously dry, loss of weight, hunger, tiredness and abdominal or limb pains. Vulvitis and cystopyelitis are common. Early in the disease attacks of spontaneous hypoglycaemia may occur. Stupor due to diabetic keto-acidosis may be the presenting feature of the illness.

Diagnosis

This is confirmed by the finding of glucose and acetone in the urine. The smell of acetone in the breath is noteworthy. Blood sugar values of over 14 mmol/l are common. A blood sugar, 1–2 hours after a meal of 9 mmol/l or more, or a fasting blood sugar of 6 mmol/l or more is diagnostic.

Therapy and management

Dehydration should be corrected urgently. If the patient is stuporose one can assume that 10–15% dehydration is present. Thus a child weighing 20 kg will require 2–3 litres of fluid in the first 4–6 hours. This should be corrected initially with intravenous normal saline followed by a maintenance fluid containing 0.45% normal saline to which 2 g potassium chloride is added per litre. When the blood glucose falls to 14 mmol/l, 5% dextrose may be added. It is not necessary to correct acidosis unless the blood pH is less than 7.1, in which cases sodium bicarbonate may be given.

Insulin should be given in all cases. For stupor or coma a short acting insulin (Actrapid MC) may be given by intravenous infusion using a constant infusion pump. The usual dose is 0.1 units/kg stat, followed by 0.1 units/kg/h until the blood glucose level falls to 14 mmol/l. A change is then made using insulin subcutaneously on a sliding scale.

Intragastric suction to prevent vomiting and catheterisation of the bladder should be done at the onset of therapy so that the urine volume and glucose loss can be estimated. As soon as the patient recovers consciousness he should be placed on a suitable diabetic diet. His insulin can be given subcutaneously on a sliding scale half-an-hour before meals and before retiring, as follows:

Blood glucose (mmol/l)	*Actrapid SC (units/kg)*
> 20	0.5
16–20	0.4
13–16	0.3
10–13	0.2
10	0.1

Once the daily insulin requirements are stabilised the total dose for the day may be given as a twice daily injection. We have found the combination of monocomponent insulins, Actrapid and Monotard cover most cases. About two-thirds of the dose is given subcutaneously in the morning half an hour before breakfast and one-third half an hour before supper. A selection of monocomponent insulins is listed in Fig. 13.6. Until recently the only available insulins were prepared from the ox or pig, so had an animal amino acid sequence. Insulins with a human amino acid sequence are now marketed but they have not yet been shown to be less immunogenic than highly purified ox or pig insulins.

In 1983 single strength insulins containing 100 units of insulin per ml (U100) were introduced into the UK to replace all the other strengths within eighteen months. U100 insulins can be used only with U100 syringes and are safer and easier to give than the old strengths of insulin. *Never use U_{40} or U_{80} insulins with U_{100} syringes. Never use U_{100} insulins with U_{40} or U_{80} syringes.*

What is good control?
We believe that *good control* of diabetes means a blood sugar of under 10 mmol/l throughout the 24 hours and a glycosylated haemoglobin within normal limits when estimated every three months— the better the control the less the likelihood of late cardiovascular, renal and ocular complications.

It should be remembered that on discharge from hospital the dose of insulin may become reduced and many patients may require none at all for many months. This is known as the *honeymoon period of juvenile onset diabetes.* However this should not be taken as a sign of cure because the vast majority will again relapse and then require their insulin for life. The usual dose is 0.8 units/kg/day. During and after puberty the dose may increase to 1 unit/kg/day or more in many cases.

Home monitoring
The corner stone of diabetic 'control' has been routine urine testing for glucose and ketones. Unfortunately the amount of glucose in the urine may not accurately reflect the blood glucose. Many children find routine urine testing irksome and are reluctant to do it. We have found routine blood glucose estimation at home more acceptable and are increasingly recommending it. Capillary blood can be drawn virtually painlessly by using a spring-loaded gadget called an Autolet (Ames), shown in Fig. 13.7. The blood glucose can be estimated by using Dextrostix with a suitable electronic meter, for instance Ames Glucometer or Gluco-Chek. Blood is tested half an hour before breakfast and two hours after lunch. A third test half an hour before supper is useful. If early morning hypoglycaemia is suspected the parents should do a test at 4 am! If a high blood glucose is found the urine should be tested for ketones. The aim is to keep the blood glucose between 3 and 10 mmol/l. Levels below

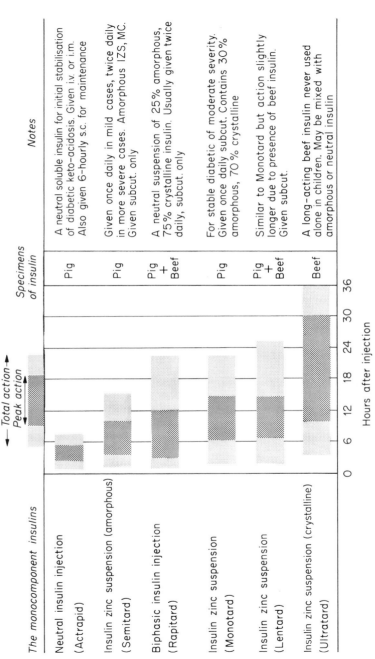

Fig. 13.6 The action of monocomponent insulins
(Courtesy of Novo Industries (Pharmaceuticals) (Pty) Ltd, South Africa)

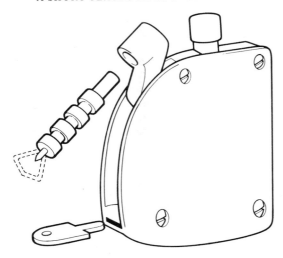

Fig. 13.7 The Autolet—a capillary blood letting device
(Courtesy of Owen Mumford Ltd, Medical Division)

2.5 mmol/l are likely to be associated with symptoms of hypoglycaemia and should be avoided.

Diet
There are two schools of thought with regard to diet—the free dieters and the strict dieters. The *free dieters* allow a normal diet but restrict concentrated carbohydrates such as sweets, sugar, cakes and biscuits. They allow small amounts of brown bread and bran porridges. Protein and fats are limited only by the patient's appetite, though many would substitute vegetable fats for animal fats. The *strict dieters* believe that children do better if the daily diet is carefully worked out. The child requires a basic 4200 kJ (1000 Calories) plus 420 kJ per year of age. Thus a five year old child requires:

$$4200 + (5 \times 420) \text{ kJ}$$
$$\text{i.e.} \quad 4200 + 2100 = 6300 \text{ kJ}$$

About 60 % of this is given as carbohydrates, preferably in the form of unrefined starches and high fibre foods, 8–10 % as proteins and the rest as fats, mainly polyunsaturated. The details should be worked out with a dietician. It is important that the patient's kilojoules are equally distributed over the three main meals and that he have a mid-morning, mid-afternoon and a late night snack.

Parents require continuous guidance and psychological support, and should join a Diabetic Association. *Your child has Diabetes* and *Living with Diabetes: the problem for the younger patient under 18* are two books suitable for children, available from the British Diabetic Association (10 Queen Anne Street, London WIM 0BD).

Initially, the parents have to give injections (an automatic spring-loaded syringe is a god-send). In the future it is likely that portable continuous infusion insulin pumps will become a practical method of delivering insulin to some children.

Parents should be taught the symptoms of hypoglycaemia and the child should always carry a few lumps of sugar in his pocket for just such an emergency. For hypoglycaemic coma an injection of glucagon should be given. The patient usually regains consciousness rapidly and should be given food on awakening.

Intercurrent infections such as sore throats or upper respiratory infections may precipitate the child into diabetic keto-acidosis unless he is given *additional* doses of insulin. Before operations the child should be given half his normal dose of insulin because he misses breakfast. Half-strength saline or half-strength Darrow's solution in 5 % dextrose-in-water is given to ensure an open venous line for the anaesthetist, who can give supplementary insulin during the operation as required. The blood sugar should be carefully monitored both during and after the operation.

Exercise reduces the need for insulin and one should advise regular and relatively constant daily exercise.

Hypoglycaemia due to overdose of insulin causes shakiness, dizziness and an uncomfortable sensation of hunger. Sweating, abdominal pain and headache may occur. Immediate oral glucose (4 lumps of sugar or 4 ounces of 25 % sugar) usually reverses it. In severe cases the patient may become comatose or have a seizure indistinguishable from grand mal epilepsy. An intravenous infusion of 20 % glucose should be given by a deeply placed intravenous catheter. This produces a prompt return to consciousness. Glucagon 1 mg may also be given by injection, intravenously, intramuscularly or subcutaneously.

Patients on long-acting insulin such as Monotard may not get the usual warning symptoms of hypoglycaemia, as these attacks tend to occur after midnight. If the child has difficulty in waking in the morning or complains of headache, it may be assumed that he is hypoglycaemic. A snack at bed-time or a slight reduction in the dose of Monotard may prevent this.

Long-term complications

Patients with badly controlled diabetes are liable to staphylococcal infections (boils, styes and abscesses) and thrush. Tuberculin negative patients should be given BCG. Vascular complications occur 10–20 years after the onset of diabetes leading to retinopathy and nephropathy (Kimmelstiel-Wilson disease). These are due to changes in the small vessels. They may lead to blindness, hypertension and nephrotic syndrome. These complications can probably be postponed by keeping the blood sugar consistently under 10 mmol/l (180 mg/dl).

Hypoglycaemia

Hypoglycaemia may be defined according to the blood sugar level during an attack. Thus in a low birth-weight baby less than 1.1 mmol/l in a full-term infant less than 1.6 mmol/l and over the age of one month less than 2.2 mmol/l may be regarded as a hypoglycaemic blood glucose level. In such cases there is the danger of convulsions. In the newborn, hypoglycaemia may present with apnoeic attacks, cyanosis, refusal to feed, jitteriness, sweating and subnormal temperature. In older children weakness, tremor, sensations of hunger, pallor, ataxia, squinting and confused behaviour occur. Sympathetic discharge causes sweating and tachycardia. Convulsions and coma may occur leading to mental retardation. The diagnosis is confirmed by finding a low blood glucose during the attack and by rapid response of the patient to the administration of sugar and glucagon.

The treatment of hypoglycaemia is that of the underlying cause though this is sometimes easier said than done. Dietary management is often possible. A high protein diet containing unrefined sugar and starch usually helps, but may aggravate leucine-sensitive hypoglycaemia which requires leucine restriction. Adrenaline and glucagon injection increase the serum glucose temporarily and are useful in emergency prior to setting up an intravenous glucose drip. Cortisone and ACTH have a more prolonged effect which may be useful in some patients. In severe recurrent cases for which other causes cannot be found, the possibility of partial or total pancreatectomy should be considered carefully if the serum insulin is raised.

Hypoglycaemic attacks occurring during puberty ('black-outs') tend to be self-limiting and usually respond to a couple of lumps of sugar.

Diazoxide inhibits insulin release and is used for severe cases of hypoglycaemia due to hyperinsulinism. However, side-effects are troublesome including hypertrichosis, oedema, neutropenia and hyperuricaemia.

In general refined sugars should be avoided in the long-term management of hypoglycaemia as one may be caught in a 'hyper-hypoglycaemia see-saw'. Unrefined carbohydrates which are broken down slowly to sugars are preferable and may be given frequently during the day.

Infants with cold injury are liable to develop severe hypoglycaemia.

Hypoglycaemia—a check list

1 Metabolic:
  (a) Neonatal due to immature regulatory mechanisms.
  (b) Ketotic hypoglycaemia.
  (c) Protein-calorie malnutrition and starvation.
  (d) Inborn errors of metabolism, e.g. galactosaemia, glycogen storage disease of the liver, fructose intolerance.
  (e) Leucine-sensitive hypoglycaemia.
2 Massive liver necrosis (including Reye's disease).
3 Poisoning by alcohol, salicylates, oral hypoglycaemic agents, beta-adrenergic blockers and plant alkaloids.
4 Endocrines:
  (a) Insulin overdose
  (b) Islet cell tumour or hyperplasia
  (c) Hypopituitarism
  (d) Thyroid deficiency
  (e) Cortisol deficiency
  (f) Infant of diabetic mother.
5 Hypothermia, especially in small babies.
6 Idiopathic:
  (a) Familial.
  (b) Non-familial.

CHAPTER 14

INHERITED METABOLIC DISEASES

Garrod's list of four inborn errors of metabolism described in 1905 has now been expanded to hundreds of these inherited metabolic diseases. The majority are inherited as autosomal recessive characters, and appear to be due to the absence of a single enzyme which disrupts that particular metabolic pathway. Inborn errors of metabolism are all relatively rare, nevertheless they are of great intrinsic interest.

Many inheritable errors of metabolism are totally or partially treatable. In some cases delay in treatment can lead to irrepairable damage, as in phenylketonuria, which causes mental retardation. In such cases it is essential that the diagnosis is made as soon as possible. Screening programmes have been introduced to diagnose the more common (and treatable) inborn errors of metabolism in the neonatal period. However, screening is not possible in the majority of first affected children who are usually diagnosed after signs and symptoms have appeared. As many of these disorders are so rare the detailed investigation and management of affected patients is often carried out in regional centres. Once an inborn error of metabolism has been diagnosed in a child other members of the family should be screened to unearth unrecognised cases. The family should be given expert genetic advice. They should be told the risks for further affected children, the expected clinical course of the disorder and the current treatment available. A rapidly increasing number of errors of metabolism can be diagnosed prenatally. Where appropriate this can be offered to women who might have children with a serious progressive disease for which no treatment is available, such as neurolipidoses, or in cases where effective treatment should be given as soon as possible, such as galactosaemia.

An account of some of the more common inborn errors of metabolism is given below.

DISORDERS OF AMINO ACID METABOLISM

Phenylketonuria (PKU)

The metabolic pathway of phenylalanine and the points at which blocks can occur are shown in Fig. 14.1. The frequency of the disorder is about 1 in 10 000. Phenylketonuria was the first inherited disorder of amino acid metabolism for which widespread screening tests were introduced in various countries. In Britain the most widely used test is the Guthrie

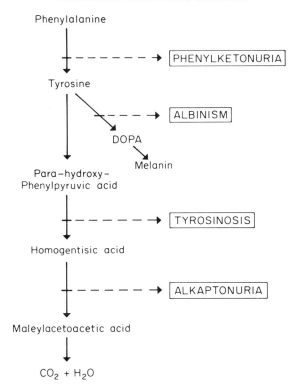

Phenylalanine

→ PHENYLKETONURIA

Tyrosine

→ ALBINISM

DOPA

Melanin

Para-hydroxy-
Phenylpyruvic acid

→ TYROSINOSIS

Homogentisic acid

→ ALKAPTONURIA

Maleylacetoacetic acid

$CO_2 + H_2O$

Fig. 14.1 Disorders of phenylalanine metabolism

test. One drop of blood is taken by heel prick on the sixth day of life for phenylalanine estimation by the bacterial inhibition assay method. In babies in whom the introduction of milk feeds have been delayed, the Gurthrie test should also be delayed until the child is on a normal protein intake. In PKU the plasma level of phenylalanine exceeds 1.2 mmol/l. Without treatment patients may develop neonatal jaundice or have seizures. Mental retardation nearly always occurs.

Treatment
A low phenylanaline diet, such as Albumaid XP or Lofenalac, should be introduced as soon as possible. The diet should contain adequate amounts of tyrosine. Expert dietary supervision is essential. In infancy one should keep the plasma phenylanaline level below 0.3 mmol/l but the diet may gradually be relaxed in later childhood.

Prognosis
With adequate treatment most patients have normal intelligence. Adult women with PKU stand a very high risk of bearing children with major

congenital malformations such as microcephaly or congenital heart disease. There is now some evidence to suggest that these complications can be avoided if a low phenylalanine diet is started *before* conception.

Albinism

An inherited disorder of tyrosinase activity in which the melanocyte is unable to form melanin. It occurs in all races and also in mammals, fish and birds. The skin is milk- or pink-white, the hair often yellowish or white. The iris is pink or light blue in colour. The pupils are red in children, often becoming darker in adults. Photophobia, lacrimation and nystagmus are present. The skin is very sensitive to light. Partial albinism may occur, limited to an area of skin, to a white forelock or to the retina only.

Treatment
The skin should be protected from sunlight by suitable creams. Refraction errors should be corrected and tinted glasses worn.

Alkaptonuria

A genetic metabolic error due to absence of the enzyme homogentisic acid oxidase. The child seems perfectly normal but the urine that he passes turns dark brown or black on standing. Urinalysis reveals a positive Clinitest tablet test for reducing substances but negative enzyme tests for glucose. The ferric chloride test is positive. A strip of exposed undeveloped photographic film dipped in the urine turns black, due to the presence of homogentisic acid. As this metabolite is fully excreted in the urine it does not accumulate in the blood. During childhood there are no symptoms but one can predict that by 30 years of age *ochronosis*, the deposition of dark brown or blue pigment in the fibrous tissue and cartilage of the body, will occur. Arthritis and degeneration of the intervertebral discs are likely to develop.

Maple syrup urine disease

This is a genetic disorder of the branched-chain amino acids leucine, isoleucine and valine. The excretion of the branched-chain keto acids gives the urine, the skin and the hair its characteristic caramel-like odour. It is rare but important because symptoms start within 2 or 3 days of starting milk feeds and, untreated, leads to convulsions, opisthotonos, generalised muscular rigidity or flaccidity and death within 2–3 weeks. Milder forms may occur.

Treatment
Treatment demands early diagnosis and the use of synthetic amino acid mixtures containing reduced amounts of branched-chain amino acids. Despite this mental handicap may occur.

Cystinuria

Cystinuria is an inherited defect of renal tubular function in which there is impairment of reabsorption of cystine, lysine, arginine and ornithine. The symptoms can be explained by the formation of cystine stones in the urinary tract. The stones vary in size from gravel to staghorn calculi. This leads to recurrent urinary infection, renal colic and obstructive lesions. Uraemia is a common terminal event. Diagnosis is confirmed by finding cystine in the urine.

Treatment
Treatment aims at preventing cystine stones forming in the urinary tract. The urine should be alkalised to at least pH 7.6 or more. Fluid intake should be increased. Oral penicillamine forms soluble cystine disulphide. The cystine excretion and concentration in the urine must be carefully assessed and the dose adjusted accordingly.

Cystinosis (Cystine storage disease; Lignac-de Toni-Fanconi-Debré syndrome)

Cystinosis differs from cystinuria in that cystine is deposited in the tissues of the kidney, cornea and bone-marrow. There is no excess of cystine in the urine. Glycosuria, generalised amino-aciduria, and phosphaturia (which cause low phosphate 'renal' rickets or osteodystrophy) occurs. Polyuria, hypokalaemia and metabolic acidosis may be features. The infant fails to thrive, attacks of vomiting occur and there is stunting of growth. Diagnosis is confirmed by finding cystine crystals in the cornea by slit lamp, or in lymph nodes or bone marrow by phase microscopy. It can be diagnosed *in utero* by amniocentesis and cell culture.

Treatment
Acidosis may be corrected with sodium citrate, hypokalaemia with potassium chloride, and rickets, which is usually resistant to normal doses of vitamin D, with large doses of calciferol or alfacalcidol.

DISORDERS OF CARBOHYDRATE METABOLISM

Galactosaemia

Galactose is derived from the disaccharide lactose (milk sugar) which splits in the bowel to form glucose and galactose. In the liver it is converted to glucose-1-phosphate by means of the enzyme galactose-1-phosphate transferase (G-1-PUT). If this enzyme is deficient (as in galactosaemia) then the intermediate product galactose-1-phosphate accumulates in the blood and tissues.

Clinical features
Galactosaemia occurs soon after the baby starts his first milk feeds. Vomiting and poor weight-gain may be the initial symptoms. Hepatomegaly, jaundice, hypoglycaemia and convulsions may lead to death. If the patient is less severely affected, cataracts, renal damage and severe mental retardation occur.

Diagnosis
Diagnosis is confirmed by finding galactose, as well as protein and amino acids, in the urine. Defective G-1-PUT enzyme activity in the red cells is diagnostic. Several variants have been described, the Duarte variant being the commonest.

Treatment
A galactose-free diet is life-saving and may be brain-saving if started early enough. Nutramigen with added dextri-maltose or glucose contains no galactose. Mothers of known cases should take a galactose-free diet during subsequent pregnancies.

THE GLYCOGENOSES

Glycogen storage disease

There are at least a dozen known types of glycogen storage disease, each due to a specific enzyme deficiency in the synthesis or breakdown of glycogen. They are almost all inherited as autosomal recessive conditions and are very rare. The commonest is *von Gierke's disease (type I)* with an incidence of 1 in 400 000 live births. It is due to glucose-6-phosphatase deficiency. It results in the accumulation of glycogen in the liver, kidney and intestines. The affected infant is usually seen in his first year with massive enlargement of the liver, and he may or may not have hypoglycaemic convulsions. Ketonuria (otherwise unusual in infants) may be found. Growth is retarded and respiratory infections are common, causing ketoacidosis. Hyperuricaemia occurs. There may be a haemorrhagic tendency which makes any operative intervention dangerous.

Laboratory diagnosis
Overnight fasting causes hypoglycaemia, ketosis, increased lactic acid and lipids in the blood. These return to normal when glucose is given. Subcutaneous adrenalin or glucagon does not cause an increase in the blood glucose. Liver biopsy reveals increased fat and glycogen, the glucose-6-phosphatase activity being absent.

Treatment
In order to prevent hypoglycaemic convulsions frequent carbohydrate feeds day and night may be required. Adequate protein should be

supplied. Infections should be treated urgently and sodium bicarbonate should be given during the infection to prevent metabolic acidosis. After puberty gout may be a problem.

INHERITED DISORDERS OF LIPID METABOLISM

Hyperlipoproteinaemia

The plasma lipoproteins contain protein, phospholipid, triglyceride and cholesterol. They can be separated electrophoretically and by ultra-centrifugation into very low density lipoprotein (VLDL; pre-β-lipoprotein), low density lipoprotein (LDL; β-lipoprotein) and high density lipoprotein (HDL; α-lipoprotein). Chylomicrons, which are predominantly dietary triglycerides, do not migrate on electrophoresis. Most types of hyperlipoproteinaemia can be classified by the naked eye appearance of the plasma after being kept at 4°C for 18 hours, by fasting plasma cholesterol and triglyceride levels and by electrophoretic mobility of the lipoproteins. High levels of low density and very low density lipoprotein are atherogenic but high density lipoprotein is thought to be protective.

Familial hypercholesterolaemia (familial hyperbetalipo-proteinaemia; type II hyperlipoproteinaemia)

Heterozygous familial hypercholesterolaemia (FH) is the most important disorder of this group occurring in 1 in 500 of the population. As young children with this disorder appear normal, the only hope of making an early diagnosis lies in screening the children of parents who have had a myocardial infarction in early middle age. When this has occurred before 40 years of age there is a 1 in 8 chance of the child being affected. Affected patients have raised levels of plasma cholesterol, mostly of the low density lipoprotein (LDL) fraction (about twice normal for age). Xanthomata, manifestations of coronary artery disease and a premature corneal arcus may appear in the second or third decade. Treatment with a low fat diet (using polyunsaturated fat), or with drugs such as cholestyramine or probucol should be started as early as possible.

Homozygous FH is the most devastating form of the disease and is fortunately rare. Xanthomata around the large joints may occur in early childhood while plasma cholesterol levels, even in infancy, may be very high. Symptoms of coronary artery disease may occur before puberty, and fatal myocardial infarction in the early teens. Treatment includes the use of low cholesterol diet and medication as above. Portocaval shunts and plasmaphoresis have been tried in order to reduce the serum cholesterol levels with variable results.

Secondary hyperlipoproteinaemia

Hyperlipoproteinaemia occurs in many forms of liver disease, diabetes, the nephrotic syndrome and hypothyroidism. These disorders must be excluded before entertaining a diagnosis of *primary hyperlipidaemia.*

Hypolipoproteinaemia (familial high density lipoprotein (HDL) deficiency; Tangier disease)

In the *homozygous* form of HDL deficiency there is absent α-lipoprotein in the plasma due to deficiency of apoprotein A. The plasma cholesterol is low and the plasma triglyceride is high. Patients have corneal opacities, enlarged lymph glands, hepatosplenomegaly, bright orange coloured tonsils and a peripheral neuropathy. Histological examinations show an accumulation of cholesterol esters in the tissue macrophages. *Heterozygotes* also have low levels of HDL.

A-β-Lipoproteinaemia

A-β-lipoproteinaemia is a recessively inherited disorder in which there is absent plasma VLDL, LDL, chylomicrons and hypocholesterolaemia due to deficiency of apoprotein B. It causes steatorrhoea, acanthocytosis, ataxia and a retinopathy. A low fat diet and fat soluble vitamin supplements (A, D and K) should be given. Treatment with vitamin E may slow the development of neurological complications.

The neurolipidoses

There are a number of neurolipidoses inherited as recessive autosomal characters most of which are fatal and are associated with progressive mental deterioration. Those mentioned below can be diagnosed prenatally.

Tay Sachs' disease

Tay Sachs' Disease is the commonest of the lipidoses, being especially common amongst Ashkenazi Jews. It is due to deficiency of the enzyme hexosaminidase A.

The affected patient is normal until six months of age and undergoes progressive mental deterioration. Blindness is associated with a characteristic cherry red macula on ophthalmoscopy. The head is usually bigger than normal due to accumulation of Tay Sachs' ganglioside in neurones. The liver and spleen do not enlarge. Hexosaminidase levels can be estimated from cultured leukocytes or fibroblasts.

Gaucher's disease

This is a disorder in which glucocerebroside accumulates in brain and reticulo-endothelial tissue. It is due to glucocerebrosidase deficiency. Several forms are recognised. The *infantile form* is rapidly progressive with dementia and organ enlargement. In the *juvenile and adult forms* the

CNS is usually spared. Juveniles develop hepatosplenomegaly whereas adults have a slowly progressive disease and have anaemia and thrombocytopenia, due to involvement of the long bones. The diagnosis can be made by finding typical foam cells (Gaucher cells) on bone-marrow puncture and an increase in serum acid phosphatase.

Metachromatic leukodystrophy

This demyelinating disorder is caused by the accumulation of sulphated cerebrosides due to a deficiency of aryl sulphatase. Infantile, juvenile and adults forms occur, depending on the age of onset. A previously normal patient develops ataxia, spasticity and peripheral neuropathy associated with speech loss and dementia. The course is rapidly downhill. The diagnosis is made by finding decreased levels of aryl sulphatase A in white blood corpuscles. Macrophages containing blue staining material (with toluidine blue) may be found in the urine or on rectal or brain biopsy.

INHERITED DISORDERS OF PROTEIN METABOLISM

These include a wide variety of disorders:

1 Absent clotting factors (p. 105).
2 Immunoglobulin deficiency (p. 119).
3 Serum complement deficiency (p. 121).
4 Metal-binding protein deficiency (Wilson's disease).
5 Alpha-1-antitrypsin deficiency.
6 The porphyrias.

Metal-binding protein disorders

Hepatolenticular degeneration (Wilson's disease) is an autosomal recessive metal-binding protein disorder characterised by excess copper deposition in the basal ganglia, cirrhosis of the liver and a deficiency of serum ceruloplasmin. The total body copper is increased due to increased absorption. The onset of the illness is usually about eight years of age, but it can start in late middle age. In early childhood the patient manifests signs of liver involvement with jaundice, hepatosplenomegaly and the development of cirrhosis. Neurological signs due to basal ganglia involvement occur later.

Diagnosis

Diagnosis may be confirmed by slit lamp examination of the eye which reveals a deposit of yellow-brown copper salts in the corneal limbus (Kayser-Fleisher ring). There is an increased concentration of copper in the plasma, urine and liver.

Treatment

The damage caused by excess copper deposition is partially reversible.

The drug of choice is penicillamine 10 mg/kg/day twice daily (*adult dose*: 500 mg twice daily), together with 20 mg pyridoxine daily for life.

Alpha-1-antitrypsin deficiency

The protein alpha-1-antitrypsin is manufactured in the liver. About 10 % of homozygotes are liable to develop neonatal hepatitis of varying severity. Affected neonates may have a fatal hepatitis or recover completely. A proportion go on to develop hepatic cirrhosis. The majority of patients with alpha-1-antitrypsin deficiency develop basal panlobular emphysema in middle age. Patients at risk should be advised not to smoke.

The Porphyrias

The porphyrias form a group of disorders caused by abnormalities of haem synthesis. Symptoms are due to excess production of porphyrin and its precursors. They may be acute or non-acute.

Acute hepatic porphyrias
Acute hepatic porphyrias are all inherited as autosomal dominants. Symptoms are unusual before puberty. Attacks may be precipitated by drugs such as barbiturates, phenytoin, and sulphonamides, by acute infections or by fasting. Patients develop acute abdominal pain, vomiting and constipation. Some of the acute porphyrias are associated with photosensitivity of the skin. Cranial nerve palsies, respiratory paralysis or seizures may occur. Sometimes patients develop acute psychiatric disturbances. The diagnosis is made by finding excess porphobilinogen (Hoesch Test) and delta-amino-laevulinic acid in the urine. A Burgundy red urine is due to uroporphyrins. Enzyme studies on blood, leucocytes and skin may be helpful.

Treatment
Drugs known to induce porphyrias are contra-indicated. Precipitating factors should be avoided. The patient may be given antiemetics, such as metoclopremide, and should be kept well fed, intravenously if necessary. Assisted ventilation is required for respiratory paralysis.

Non-acute porphyrias
These cause photosensitive skin eruptions. They may be precipitated by drugs and sunlight.

Erythropoietic porphyria may occur in infancy and causes a burning sensation in the skin. Affected children may be afraid to go out in the sunlight. The commonest non-acute porphyria is *cutaneous hepatic porphyria* which is not inheritable.

The severest and rarest form is *congenital porphyria* which is inherited as an autosomal recessive disorder. Photosensitive skin eruptions cause scarring. The spleen is often enlarged.

Treatment
Children should avoid direct sunlight. Barrier creams or sunscreen lotions may be used over exposed parts. Splenectomy may help congenital porphyria. Regular venesection to remove iron is used for cutaneous hepatic porphyria.

MUCOPOLYSACCHARIDOSES

Mucopolysaccharidoses are a group of inherited disorders of the extracellular matrix synthesised by connective tissue cells. As a result these patients are dwarfed, with restriction of joint movement, skeletal deformities, hepatosplenomegaly and cardiac abnormalities.

Hurler's syndrome is perhaps the best known of the mucopolysaccharidoses. It is characterised by extremely coarse facial features, hence the term 'gargoylism'. Excess hair on face and body, low set ears, hydrocephalus and lumbar gibbus are present in addition to the features mentioned above. Mental retardation is present and there is clouding of the cornea. The diagnosis is confirmed by finding a deficiency of α-L-iduronidase in cultured fibroblasts.

The mucopolysaccharidoses are autosomal recessive disorders, except for *Hunter's syndrome* which is an X-linked recessive condition, and can be diagnosed antenatally. Treatment by bone marrow transplantation has been successful. The severer mucopolysaccharidoses cause death in early childhood.

CYSTIC FIBROSIS OF THE PANCREAS
(cystic fibrosis; CF)

Cystic fibrosis is a Mendelian recessive disorder with an incidence of about 1 in 2500 births, characterised by excessive sodium chloride excretion of the sweat glands, and increased viscidity of the mucus secretions of the pancreas, lungs and elsewhere.

Clinical features
Cystic fibrosis may present in three ways:

1 Meconium ileus
This is a form of intestinal obstruction in the newborn due to the presence of viscid meconium plugs in the small bowel. It is due to the absence of trypsin which fails to digest and soften the meconium. Sometimes perforation occurs *in utero* (meconium peritonitis, p. 247).

2 Steatorrhoea
Ninety per cent of patients with cystic fibrosis have a malabsorption syndrome. The viscid mucus plugs in the pancreatic ducts cause atrophy

of the acini and secondary fibrosis of the pancreas. This results in failure of pancreatic secretion, which causes steatorrhoea. This is characterised by the passage of large, pale, greasy foul-smelling stools several times daily. It may be accompanied by a voracious appetite ('each meal is like a Christmas dinner'), and progressive wasting. Prolapse of the rectum is common.

3 Respiratory disease
Recurrent respiratory infection may occur in early infancy but is sometimes postponed until two or three years of age. Here again problems arise because of the presence of viscid sputum which is difficult to cough up. This leads to patchy areas of bronchial obstruction with areas of absorption collapse, obstructive emphysema and secondary infection. The anterior-posterior diameter of the chest is usually increased due to the widespread emphysema, air entry is diminished, expiration prolonged and crepitations are frequently heard. Sometimes there is bronchospasm with musical rhonchi and expiratory wheezing. Small areas of consolidation due to bronchopneumonia may be found. Diffuse bronchiectasis eventually leads to *cor pulmonale*.

The affected child coughs frequently and this may sometimes be mistaken for whooping cough. The patient becomes progressively disabled by respiratory insufficiency. Clubbing of the fingers with cyanosis and dyspnoea may occur fairly early but in very mild cases may be postponed to later childhood and occasionally to adolescence. Adults with minimal disease have been detected, usually in the families of known patients.

Other features
Retarded growth and delayed puberty are invariable. Partial intestinal obstruction may occur due to collections of tenacious faecal material in the small bowel, so called 'meconium ileus equivalent'. Biliary cirrhosis and portal hypertension may result from the plugging of bile ducts with viscid secretions. Diabetes mellitus is an occasional late complication of pancreatic fibrosis.

Family history
There is often a history of another affected child in the family. Death due to intestinal obstruction shortly after birth (meconium ileus) or severe recurrent respiratory infection or 'coeliac disease' is highly suggestive. Attempts to distinguish homozygotes and heterozygotes by estimations of sodium chloride levels in the sweat have not been satisfactory.

Diagnosis
Diagnosis may be confirmed by finding a sodium concentration of more than 60 mmol/l in the sweat. Strict attention to detail in performing the test is important and it should be repeated two or three times if there is any doubt about the diagnosis. Duodenal intubation will show reduced or absent pancreatic enzyme concentrations.

Prognosis

Prognosis has improved considerably with treatment. Previously death in infancy was the rule, whereas patients are surviving now into their twenties. Very mild cases may be discovered in adulthood. Various methods of screening neonates and young children for cystic fibrosis have been introduced in the belief that early diagnosis and treatment improves the prognosis. None of the screening methods is entirely satisfactory. Antenatal diagnosis is not yet possible.

Treatment

Respiratory infections should be treated promptly and energetically. *Staphylococcus aureus* and *H. influenzae* are the two most common organisms found in the sputum. Treatment is usually started with an isoxazolyl penicillin such as flucloxacillin. In infancy this is given until the child's symptoms have abated. Some centres give continuous antibiotics during the first year of life. After prolonged antibiotic therapy *Pseudomonas aeroginosa* is invariably found. Aerosols containing suitable antibiotics and mucolytics may be helpful. Oxygen, which should be humidified, is often required. Physiotherapy to help drain viscid material from the lungs is helpful. The parents should be taught how to give this regularly at home.

Steatorrhoea can be controlled by the use of Pancreatin B.P., which is available in powder form to sprinkle over food, and as tablets and capsules. Gelatine capsules may not be digested in cystic fibrosis, therefore the capsule should be opened and the contents spread over the food. The dose is adjusted according to the needs of the patient. Reduction in appetite is often a sign of improved digestion. A normal diet is often possible though it may be necessary to reduce the fat in individual cases or to use medium-chain fatty acids. It is advisable to supply vitamins in soluble form, for example Vi-Daylin or Abidec multivitamin drops 0.6 ml two or three times daily.

The family should be given long-term emotional support and many parents find membership of the local Cystic Fibrosis Association helpful. As far as possible patients should be encouraged to lead a 'normal' life.

CHAPTER 15

THE GASTRO-INTESTINAL TRACT

THE MOUTH

The oral cavity may be too small because of the presence of a large tongue (macroglossia) such as occurs in cretinism, or the presence of a small jaw (Pierre-Robin syndrome and Treacher-Collins syndrome). In Down's syndrome the mouth seems to be too small for the tongue. The tongue may be displaced by a large cyst (ranula), by a tumour such as an ossifying fibroma, or malignancies such as Burkitt's lymphoma or osteogenic sarcoma. Most of these conditions are discussed elsewhere.

Teething

The deciduous teeth appear between 6 and 24 months of age (p. 54). Teething is a physiological process and may cause excessive salivation and discomfort. Other symptoms should not be attributed to teething. *Delayed teething* occurs in rickets and hypothyroidism. *Premature teething* is occasionally noticed at birth. Usually the lower two incisors (natal teeth) are present. Their presence rarely interferes with breast feeding, as the teeth are usually loose. The danger of inhalation of loose teeth has probably been exaggerated.

Anodontia means absence of teeth. If no teeth have appeared by one year of age it is justifiable to have an X-ray of the jaws to determine whether the tooth-buds are present or not. Anodontia may be complete, as occurs in ectodermal dysplasia, or it may be incomplete, involving perhaps only the second or third molars or the lateral incisors.

Disturbances in the calcification of the teeth include:

1 *Amelogenesis imperfecta*, in which the enamel is thin and easily abraded.
2 *Dentinogenesis imperfecta*, in which the dentine is poorly calcified. The overlying enamel tends to flake. The tooth has an opaque pearly appearance. It may be associated with *osteogenesis imperfecta* (p. 378).
3 *'Growth disturbance lines'*, occurring during periods of illness and analogous to similar lines seen in long bones.
4 *Mottled enamel*, which is an unsightly discoloration of the teeth due to dental fluorosis. Normally it is recommended that drinking water should contain one part of fluorine per million to reduce the incidence of dental caries. In many areas of the world the drinking water contains more than treble this amount and most children will show

mottled enamel. Despite their ugly appearance, these teeth are very resistant to caries. However, if the fluorine content exceeds six parts per million, hypoplasia of the enamel may occur.

Discoloration of the teeth has also been observed in *erythroblastosis fetalis* due to the deposition of pigment in the deciduous teeth. The colour may be dark green, blue or black. The *tetracyclines* form a coloured chelate in tooth and bone. The primary teeth of the fetus may be affected if the mother takes a tetracycline from the fourth or fifth month of pregnancy onwards, or the baby takes it in the first year of life. The permanent teeth can also be affected *in utero*, and during the first seven or eight years of postnatal life. After this only the cusps of the molars are affected and these teeth are not of cosmetic interest. The affected teeth fluoresce under ultra-violet light.

Dental caries
Tooth decay is one of the commonest problems of civilisation and children are its first victims. It may destroy both deciduous and permanent teeth.

A highly refined diet plays a major role, sweets, cakes and biscuits being perhaps the worst offenders. They impact between the teeth and along the gum line forming an ideal substrate for bacterial growth and the formation of *dental plaque*. An area of the underlying tooth decalcifies and the supporting matrix breaks down, leaving an area of caries. This extends until the whole tooth is destroyed. Pain may be severe. It is felt in the affected tooth but more often along the jaw or referred to the ear. Dental abscesses may form and cause swelling of the jaw.

Prevention and treatment of caries
This depends on the elimination of refined sugars and starches from the diet and the avoidance of sugars which stay in the mouth for a long time, i.e. sweets and sweetened dummies. Although the causes of dental caries are well known and documented, there is extraordinary resistance to applying the cure.

Fluoridation of water supplies may reduce the caries rate by 30–40 %. It should not be regarded as the answer to the problem. Topical fluorine and fluorine supplements should only be prescribed where the drinking water is known to be low in fluorine. Regular brushing and, failing that, a thorough mouth rinse immediately after meals may help reduce caries. Apart from brushing, dental floss should be used to eliminate debris between the teeth. When caries is detected the child should be referred for dental treatment.

The dentist should be honoured for what he is, a specialist in disorders of teeth. He should be consulted for any child with a malocclusion which causes overlapping of the bite; for periodontal disease, gum recession, overcrowding of the teeth or traumatic lesions of the teeth. The dentist can often make appliances which ease the management of cleft palate or even thumb-sucking.

Hare-lip

Hare-lip may vary from a small notch in the vermilion border of the lip to a deep cleft extending into the nose. The cleft is usually off-centre and may be unilateral or bilateral. It may involve the alveolar ridge and there may be abnormalities of the upper incisors when they cut. The ala nasi on the affected side is usually flattened and requires cosmetic attention. A median cleft is rare and may be associated with absent corpus callosum in the brain.

Treatment
Hare-lip is usually repaired when the baby weighs about 6.5 kg, but some surgeons prefer early closure. It is advisable therefore to notify the plastic surgeon immediately after the birth of the patient in case he should wish to undertake early repair. Repair facilitates both breast and bottle feeding.

Cleft palate

Cleft palate may involve the soft or the hard palate, or both. The soft palate lesion may be represented as a double uvula, or as a complete mid-line split. Involvement of the hard palate may be either in the mid-line or it may be lateral. Lateral clefts may be unilateral or bilateral and invariably involve the lip as well. In the severest forms there is persistence of the embryonic vomer.

Treatment
The optimum time for operation for repair of cleft palate remains a controversial issue. The majority of plastic surgeons operate between 15 and 18 months of age, but some believe that operation should be delayed until 7 years of age to allow full development of the facial bones.

Feeding may be a very difficult problem in these children because of the opening between the oral cavity and nose. Nevertheless breast feeding can be established in the majority of cases. Only when this is not possible should a large teat which partially blocks the palatal opening be used. Enlarging of the hole in the teat or cutting slits next to the central hole of the teat may help many patients. A great deal of experimentation may be required to establish proper feeding habits. Occasionally special cleft palate teats may be helpful. Sometimes the use of a pipette solves the problem. Tube feeding should be avoided as it discourages the use of the oropharyngeal muscles.

Operation should preferably be done by a surgeon with special experience in this work. Infection of the wound should be prevented by appropriate antibiotics. A speech therapist should be consulted in all cases and a plan worked out to ensure adequate speech development.

Dental consultation will be required in all cases involving the alveolar margin to ensure the proper alignment of the unaffected teeth. Orthodontic appliances may be required. Otitis media is a common complication and should be treated vigorously in order to prevent progressive deafness.

The parents of the child require support and many 'cleft palate units' keep a photo-album of 'before-and-after' pictures of successful cases to show the parents and reassure them that the baby will look fine after the operation.

Inflammation of the mouth

Stomatitis
Stomatitis may be due to *metabolic disturbances* such as uraemia, *deficiency diseases* such as pellagra or ariboflavinosis, *blood dyscrasias* such as agranulocytosis or leukaemia, or various *infections* which are described below.

Thrush
Oral thrush is the most common infection in infancy and is due to the fungus *Candida albicans*. It forms white raised patches on the tongue and mucous membrane of the mouth resembling milk curds. On attempting to remove them with a cotton bud the underlying mucous membrane is found to be red and may bleed. This is not the case with milk curds. Diagnosis may be confirmed by adding a drop of 10% potassium hydroxide solution to a smear from the lesions applied to a slide. Rounded and oval spores may be seen.

The condition is favoured by abrasions to the mouth, lack of oral hygiene, superinfection following antibiotic therapy, malnutrition, immunological defects and hypoparathyroidism. Severe infection may spread down the oesophagus. Lesions may also occur at mucocutaneous junctions or systemically. *Candida* often causes a napkin rash.

The condition should be prevented by ensuring that feeding bottles are properly sterilised, and the hands of attendants are free of the fungus. Underlying conditions should be treated. An effective topical treatment in infants is nystatin suspension, 50 000–100 000 units dropped on the tongue three times daily for a few days. Alternatively, miconazole gel can be applied to the lesions after feeds. Systemic moniliasis responds to amphotericin B, a comparatively toxic relative of nystatin, or to oral ketoconazole.

Herpetiform stomatitis
See page 303.

Herpangina
Herpangina is a viral disease due to group A coxsackie virus. It forms vesicular lesions on the fauces, soft palate and tonsillar pillars. The floor

of the ulcer is greyish-white with a red areola. The condition is self-limiting.

Frenular ulcer

An ulcer on the frenulum of the tongue is associated with whooping cough and is due to abrasion of the frenulum against the teeth during coughing spasms. Treatment is not usually required but the lesion may be touched with a silver nitrate stick to hasten healing.

Hyperplasia of the gums

Prolonged use of phenytoin in epilepsy may cause hyperplasia of the gums. The swelling is nodular and pink and may cover most of the teeth. It is said to occur only when dental hygiene is poor. Treatment consists of excision of the excess tissue by a dental surgeon. The phenytoin may be continued if this is thought necessary for the adequate control of the seizures. The patient should be taught to brush his teeth after meals.

Haemorrhage into the gums

Gum haemorrhages suggest investigation of the child for thrombocytopenia, leukaemia and scurvy.

Bullous stomatitis

Bullous stomatitis may be associated with generalised skin disease such as Stevens-Johnson syndrome and the treatment is that of the underlying condition.

The tongue

Tongue-tie

Tongue-tie is a congenital lesion in which the frenulum of the tongue is abnormally short. In severe cases the patient cannot push his tongue beyond the gum margin, and the tip of the tongue puckers with the attempt. In such cases there may be feeding problems and speech problems may develop later. In severe cases the frenum should be cut at 2–3 years, under generalised anaesthesia.

Geographic tongue

This is a very common and benign lesion in which one or more irregular smooth red patches appear on the dorsum of the tongue, each patch being surrounded by a greyish-white raised serpiginous edge. The patches may have a map-like shape, hence the term 'geographic tongue'. The shapes change from day to day. They usually last a few days but may undergo repeated and frequent recurrences. The mother should be reassured that it is not an illness and treatment is unlikely to have any effect.

Black hairy tongue

This refers to a dark patch which occurs in the V-shaped line of circumvallate papillae. It is due to hypertrophy of the filiform papillae.

It may occur after antibiotic therapy or following a persistent bleed subsequent to tooth extraction. The mouth may have a foul smell. The condition tends to clear spontaneously.

White tongue
This is a coating on the tongue due to the accumulation of food debris and bacterial products. Filiform papillae may be hypertrophied. The condition is usually self-limiting. It may be aggravated by fever, dehydration, lack of tongue movement or simply poor oral hygiene. When seen in the early stages of scarlet fever it is known as a *white strawberry tongue* (p. 313) and when it sheds it leaves a *red strawberry tongue*.

Atrophy of the papillae of the tongue
This produces a smooth glazed tongue which may be seen in *pellagra*. A pale salmon colour is seen in *atrophic glossitis* due to severe anaemia or steatorrhoea. A magenta coloured tongue is noted in *riboflavin* or other *nutritional deficiency*. It is associated with photophobia and lacrymation.

Oedema
Oedema of the tongue is often seen in anaemias and malnutrition and is recognised by the indentation of the teeth on the edge of the tongue. The underlying causes should be attended to.

Salivary glands

Mumps (epidemic parotitis) is the commonest salivary gland disease of childhood (p. 306). Bilateral enlargement of the submaxillary glands may be due to chronic malnutrition and to cystic fibrosis.

Unilateral submaxillary swelling occurring during eating is usually due to a calculus in the submaxillary duct. The duct should be gently milked or the stone should be removed surgically.

Excess drooling may be associated with enlarged adenoids, mental deficiency or cerebral palsy. In normal infants it usually disappears by three years of age. In older children poor dental hygiene and caries may be a factor.

Recurrent parotitis
This is a swelling of unknown cause occurring in the parotid glands of otherwise healthy children. These glands are involved either singly or together and several recurrences may occur. It is usually painless and subsides after 2–3 weeks. In some patients pressure on the glands causes the discharge of pus from the opening of Stenson's duct, and *Staphylococcus aureus* can sometimes be cultured. A sialogram may reveal dilated salivary ducts (sialectasis). In such patients specific antibiotic therapy should be given. Non-infective parotitis does not require therapy.

Ranula

A ranula is a large cyst of the sublingual salivary glands, occurring in the floor of the mouth. It pushes the tongue upwards and backwards and may cause feeding problems. It should be excised or marsupialised.

THE OESOPHAGUS

Tracheo-oesophageal fistula

In its commonest form, tracheo-oesophageal fistula consists of a short upper oesophagus which ends in a blind pouch above the level of the bifurcation of the trachea. A short fistula connects the trachea to the lower portion of the oesophagus (Fig. 15.1 A). In this form the baby chokes on its very first feed and becomes cyanosed. Aspiration may occur into the lung. For this reason in many infant nurseries it is the rule to give only sterile water with the first feed, so that if aspiration occurs no harm will come of it. Regurgitation of stomach contents into the trachea frequently occurs via the fistula.

Diagnosis

As the fetus with oesophageal obstruction cannot swallow amniotic fluid the mother usually suffers from hydramnios. This should be a warning to anticipate trouble! If the baby salivates excessively after birth, even after repeated suction of the throat, suspicion should turn to

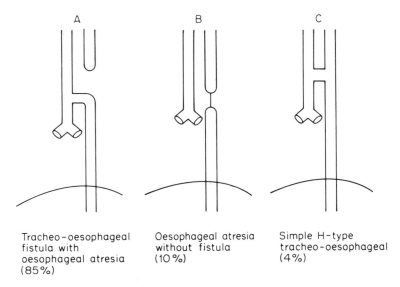

Tracheo-oesophageal
fistula with
oesophageal atresia
(85%)

Oesophageal atresia
without fistula
(10%)

Simple H-type
tracheo-oesophageal
(4%)

Fig. 15.1 Congenital anomalies of the oesophagus and trachea

certainty. Choking, cyanosis and regurgitation after the first swallow or two of feed is practically diagnostic. An attempt should be made to pass a radio-opaque catheter into the stomach. It usually curls up in the oesophageal pouch or comes back via the mouth or nose. This can be demonstrated on screening or X-ray. A diagnosis can usually be made without the use of contrast media which may aggravate the aspiration pneumonia. X-ray of the abdomen in the vertical position reveals gas in the stomach. This gas comes direct through the tracheo-oesophageal fistula.

Treatment
Surgery may be life-saving. Early diagnosis and proper pre-operative preparation are essential to success. Primary end-to-end anastomosis is usually attempted with excision of the fistula. If anastomosis is not possible then gastrostomy is done and the blind pouch is exteriorised so that swallowed saliva does not enter the lungs.

Postoperative treatment consists of parenteral feeds for 48 hours. Gastrostomy feeds are then begun with half-strength saline, followed by 5 % dextrose-in-water for two to three feeds, then gradually increasing milk feeds. The tube can usually be eliminated by the tenth day and the feeds given orally. A barium swallow should be done if there is dyspepsia in order to determine whether or not stenosis has developed.

Oesophageal atresia may occur without a fistula (Fig. 15.1 B). It is distinguished by absence of air in the stomach on percussion and by straight X-ray of the abdomen. Ten per cent of cases are of this type.

Occasionally a fistula may occur between an intact oesophagus and trachea (Fig. 15.1 C). Symptoms may occur at any age. The infant or child characteristically chokes and coughs after fluids but not after solids. It is one of the causes of recurrent pneumonia. The fistula may be quite difficult to detect even with cine-radiography.

Dysphagia

Difficulty in swallowing in the neonate may be due to incoordination of the pharyngeal muscles such as occurs in cerebral palsy or other forms of bulbar palsy. There is a distinct danger of recurrent aspiration pneumonia. In severe cases tube feeding may be required. In older children infection of the throat is the commonest cause of dysphagia, and resolves with resolution of the infection.

Hiatus hernia

Hiatus hernia is a congenital defect in which a variable portion of the stomach slips through the enlarged oesophageal hiatus. As a result, the baby vomits, especially when it is laid down after a feed, and fails to thrive. There may be specks of altered blood present due to oesophagitis. Eventually scarring leads to a 'congenital short oesophagus'. In older children curious writhing movements of the neck may be required to facilitate swallowing. These may be referred to by the mother as 'fits' but their relationship to swallowing should make the diagnosis clear. Occasionally oesophageal stenosis may occur.

Diagnosis
Diagnosis may be confirmed by barium swallow which should be done in the head-down position in order to demonstrate the presence of part of the stomach in the chest. There is free reflux of barium from the stomach into the oesophagus.

Treatment
If diagnosed early, the baby may be treated medically. A special chair is made with suitable straps so that the baby sits propped up day and night. Recent work suggests that if a baby lies prone regurgitation is less likely. Feeds may be thickened with Nestargel or cereals, and water should be given between feeds to prevent hyperosmolar dehydration. Metoclopramide and domperidone have been suggested to reduce vomiting. A large number of infants may be cured in this way before one year of age. Surgery may be indicated if oesophageal stenosis is present, or in older infants with symptoms not responding to conservative therapy.

Chalasia cardia (gastro-oesophageal incompetence)

Chalasia cardia is due to persistent relaxation or incompetence of the lower end of the oesophagus (cardia). It may be very difficult to distinguish from hiatus hernia clinically but on barium swallow reflux of the gastric contents up the lower end of the oesophagus is detected without evidence of an anatomical hernia. The medical treatment of chalasia cardia is the same as for hiatus hernia.

Achalasia cardia (cardiospasm)

This is a disorder in which failure of the lower oesophageal sphincter to relax leads to progressive dilatation and hypertrophy of the oesophagus. Symptoms usually take several years to develop and rarely occur in infancy. The patient has difficulty in swallowing and regurgitates undigested food. Cough on lying down at night is associated with aspiration pneumonia. Failure to thrive and lack of appetite is usual.

Diagnosis
Diagnosis is confirmed by barium swallow which reveals the grossly dilated oesophagus.

Therapy
Therapy consists of dilating the lower oesophagus at regular intervals. In advanced cases, a Heller oesophagocardial myotomy (analogous to a Rammstedt operation) may be considered.

Foreign bodies in the oesophagus

Children are liable to swallow almost anything big enough to get into the mouth. The objects may lodge in the upper oesophagus, at the level of the cricoid cartilage, at the level of the bifurcation of the trachea or in the lower oesophagus. Sometimes respiratory distress induced by pressure on the larynx may require a preliminary tracheostomy. In all cases of suspected ingestion or inhalation of foreign bodies an X-ray of the neck, chest and abdomen should be taken, as many foreign bodies are radio-opaque. If a radiotranslucent foreign body is suspected, oesophagoscopy may be warranted. Repeat X-rays may be required to follow the progress of the object. Once it has passed the pylorus it is unlikely to get stuck lower down. It is surprising how often pointed objects such as pins and nails pass through the bowel without harming the patient. However, if they stick for more than 72 hours in one place, surgical exploration may become necessary. Similarly pain, vomiting, fever or local tenderness may force one to explore the abdomen.

THE STOMACH

Congenital diaphragmatic hernia

See page 40.

Congenital hypertrophic pyloric stenosis

The cardinal features of a 'Py' are *projectile vomiting*, visible *gastric peristalsis* and a *palpable pyloric tumour*. The condition is five times more common in boys than in girls and may occur in one or both of identical twins. Symptoms rarely begin before the tenth day after birth, whether the baby is born prematurely or not. Initially there may be small vomits which become increasingly more frequent and more forceful. Within a few days baby vomits after every feed and the food is ejected with such force that it may spurt over the edge of the cot (projectile vomiting). It is never bile-stained because the obstruction is proximal to the duodenum. Constipation is usual but baby may sometimes have 'hunger stools' which are small, loose and tinged with green.

At first the baby is ravenously hungry but neglected cases develop dehydration and alkalosis which leads to lethargy. There is a progressive loss of weight. Gastric peristalsis is visible in the left hypochondrium, the waves passing towards the umbilicus. Given sufficient patience and experience the pyloric tumour is palpable in the right hypochondrium in all cases. The examiner should sit to the left of the baby and palpate the baby's right hypochondrium with the index and third finger of the left hand. The best time to feel the tumour is during a feed when baby is relaxed, or just after a vomit. The tumour feels very much like the tip of a nose except that it tends to come and go. Its presence is virtually pathognomonic of the disease and one should not be satisfied with the diagnosis until the pyloric tumour has been palpated.

Barium meal is sometimes used to confirm the diagnosis in difficult cases.

Treatment

Intravenous correction of dehydration and hypochloraemic alkalosis should first be carried out. The stomach should be washed out repeatedly with normal saline until the return is clear. The intragastric tube is left in place to ensure gastric deflation.

The subsequent treatment is the Rammstedt operation. This should only be carried out when the patient has been made fit for operation. It may be done under local or general anaesthetic and consists of longitudinal incision across the hypertrophied circular muscle. If the muscle is not completely cut through, symptoms will recur. Care must be taken not to cut the mucous membrane.

Oral feeds are begun about four hours postoperatively. Initially 15 ml of 5% dextrose-in-water is given followed by 30 ml three hours later. If this is retained then 30 ml of a suitable milk feed is given. The quantities are then rapidly increased until the baby is able to take a full feed. If the baby continues to vomit persistently after operation, it is likely that the pyloromyotomy was incomplete and may have to be repeated.

Haematemesis neonatorum

In the newborn period, blood in the vomitus may be maternal, the baby having swallowed it during birth, or it may come from the baby as a result of pharyngeal trauma, from gastric erosion or haemorrhagic disease of the newborn. The blood may be tested spectroscopically or by means of alkali denaturation to determine whether it contains fetal or adult haemoglobin. If it is mother's blood the stomach should be washed out with normal saline. If it is fetal blood, the baby's haemoglobin level should be closely watched and he should be given a blood transfusion if necessary.

THE INTESTINES

Small-bowel obstruction

Complete obstruction may be due to congenital atresia of a portion of the bowel, to the presence of abnormal bands compressing the bowel or to volvulus. If the site of obstruction is in the duodenum above the ampulla of Vater the vomitus contains no bile. If the lesion is below this level bile will always be present. Duodenal atresia is the commonest form of intestinal obstruction in Down's syndrome.

Vomiting is an early sign of obstruction. The lower the obstruction, the longer it takes for vomiting to occur but rarely longer than 24 hours after birth. There is usually progressive abdominal distension, but in high obstruction the abdomen may be flat. Visible peristalsis may become prominent around the umbilical region and dehydration sets in. Constipation may be absolute, but small amounts of lightish coloured meconium formed distal to the obstruction may be passed. X-rays of the abdomen should be taken in the upright position. The distribution of air may give an indication of the site of the obstruction. Fluid levels are usually present. If the obstruction is complete there will be no air beyond the site of obstruction. Free air under the diaphragm indicates perforation of the bowel. The presence of a mottled appearance at the site of the terminal ileum may be due to tiny bubbles of gas in meconium, such as occurs in meconium ileus (p. 247). Barium or gastrografin enema should be done to exclude meconium ileus, intussusception and volvulus, all of which may cause small-bowel obstruction.

Treatment
Surgery is usually required to relieve the obstruction. The patient should be made safe for surgery by intestinal decompression. Salt and water deficits should be replaced intravenously before surgery and the patient sent to theatre on maintenance infusion using one-third strength Darrow's solution in 5 % dextrose-in-water. Blood loss should be replaced during surgery. After surgery renal flow should be monitored so that oliguria can be spotted quickly. If renal flow is satisfactory the above infusion may be continued for 48 hours, thereafter half-strength Darrow's solution may be more satisfactory. Oral feeds may be started cautiously as soon as they are tolerated.

Stenosis of the small bowel

As the bowel is narrowed but not completely obstructed, symptoms may take much longer to manifest themselves. Vomiting may be intermittent rather than progressive and there may be intermittent abdominal pain and distension. Diagnosis may be delayed for months or even years and is usually made when an X-ray of the abdomen is taken during an episode of acute abdominal distension. Treatment is surgical.

Meckel's diverticulum and vitelline remnants

The vitelline duct usually disappears before the 12th week of fetal life. However it may remain patent causing a faecal fistula at the umbilicus. A small mucosal polyp may persist at the umbilicus, closely resembling an umbilical granuloma. A persistent vitelline artery joining the umbilicus to the small bowel may act as a pivot for volvulus. Lastly a diverticulum of the small bowel occurring about 25–50 cm (10–20 inches) from the ileocaecal junction in children, known as Meckel's diverticulum, may occur. It may be long and thin and produce a symptom-complex identical to acute appendicitis. The treatment is the same, and it is usual to remove both the diverticulum and appendix at the same time. Meckel's diverticulum may be broad and short and often contains ectopic gastric mucosa. This may ulcerate and bleed and, despite the distance from the anus, the blood may appear to be fresh on being passed. Characteristically the passage of an unexpectedly large quantity of red blood may be entirely painless. It results from ulceration secondary to ectopic gastric mucosa. If it perforates it may cause a dangerous peritonitis. Five per cent of volvuli are said to be due to rotation of a Meckel's diverticulum.

The diagnosis of Meckel's diverticulum is made difficult by the fact that it is rarely visualised on X-ray even when specially looked for. It is commonly found during the course of a laparotomy and should be actively searched for in every patient with a 'surgical abdomen'.

Intussusception

Intussusception is the telescoping of one part of the bowel (the intussusceptum) into a more distal part (the intussuscipiens). The commonest age for this to occur is from 4–14 months, and the commonest site for an intussusception to begin is at the ileocaecal valve (ileocaecal type). In 8–10 % of cases the head point is a polyp or a Meckel's diverticulum. The cause is unknown but sometimes enlarged Peyer's patches and mesenteric lymph nodes have been found at operation. The baby is usually healthy and chubby at the onset of the illness, which begins with recurrent attacks of sharp abdominal pain. With each attack the baby screams, sweats and pulls up his legs to relieve the pain. Between paroxysms he is apparently well and cheerful. However, vomiting usually develops and the baby rapidly becomes alkalotic and dehydrated. If neglected shock may develop.

On examination a sausage-shaped mass may be palpated along the course of the colon, usually in the right hypochondrium. The right iliac fossa is said to feel empty but this is not a very convincing sign unless other evidence of intussusception is found. Rectal examination usually results in blood and mucus appearing on the examining finger (red currant jelly). If one feels the point of the intussusceptum it means that it has already reached the rectum (see Fig. 15.2). Sometimes the mass is expelled through the anus and should not be confused with a prolapsed anus. The main danger of an intussusception is that the blood supply to the affected part is cut off and gangrene of the bowel may occur. As with any strangulating obstruction there is a considerable fluid deficit at the time of presentation.

Treatment

In *early* cases reduction may occur during the course of a diagnostic barium enema. The barium should be run in from a height of one metre above the baby, and if it enters the terminal ileum then the intussusception is fully reduced. Close observation for 24 hours after reduction is essential as recurrences are possible.

If the enema is not successful, or in advanced cases, surgical reduction is mandatory. Fluid and electrolytes should be corrected prior to operation. Whole blood should be given as the manual reduction may be very shocking to the patient. Gentleness is of the essence as the congested bowel may easily perforate. It is a wise precaution to give all cases prophylactic broad-spectrum antibiotics and metronidazole.

Postoperatively parenteral feeding should continue for at least 2–3 days as paralytic ileus is a common sequel to manual reduction. Feeding should begin cautiously after bowel sounds return.

Prognosis
Prognosis depends on the viability of the bowel after reduction. The earlier the diagnosis the better the prognosis. The occurrence of peritonitis indicates that the course will be stormy though not necessarily fatal.

Intestinal polyps

Intestinal polyps are spheroidal structures growing on a broad base from the mucosa, or attached to a stalk of varying length. They may be single or multiple.

Juvenile polyps are the commonest in children from 1–10 years. They are usually single and found in the rectum, or a little higher in the sigmoid colon. They tend to ulcerate and cause small bleeds during defaecation. Abdominal colic may occur and iron-deficiency anaemia may develop. They never become malignant and usually disappear without treatment. Rarely they initiate an intussusception. Troublesome polyps may be fulgurated. Juvenile polyposis should be differentiated from:

1 *Peutz-Jeghers syndrome*, in which polyps occur throughout the intestine and there are pigmented deposits on the lips, fingers and toes.
2 *Multiple familial polyposis*, in which innumerable polyps crowd the rectum and colon.
3 *Gardner's syndrome*, in which colonic polyps are associated with multiple osteomas and multiple epidermoid cysts.

Malignant change is a definite danger in the latter two conditions.

Hirschprung's disease

Hirschprung's disease is a rare functional obstruction of the rectum or colon due to a congenital absence of the myenteric nerve plexus. The affected area is known as the *aganglionic segment*. The lesion is limited to the rectosigmoid area in 80 % of patients or it may involve large areas of the colon and even the small bowel (long segment type). Skip areas of unaffected bowel may occur on rare occasions.

Symptoms are due to absence of peristalsis across the affected area. In the neonatal period there may be signs of rectal obstruction with progressive abdominal distension and vomiting. Sometimes bloody diarrhoea may occur. There is hyperperistalsis in the colon proximal to the obstruction, and pressure necrosis may lead to perforation and peritonitis. Rectal examination characteristically reveals a small empty rectum. On removing the finger there may be partial relief of the obstruction due to the explosive discharge of liquid meconium mixed with faeces. In infants failure to thrive and chronic diarrhoea may be a problem, while in older children there is a long history of persistent constipation, slowly progressive abdominal distension and failure to gain weight adequately. Attempts to dislodge the faecal masses by enemas are only partially successful. Large volumes of fluid are required and patients have died as a result of water intoxication. Care must therefore be exercised during this procedure to limit the amount of water used.

Diagnosis
Diagnosis may be suggested by barium enema. The grossly dilated colon contrasts with the small rectum. Rectal biopsy (full thickness) reveals absent ganglion cells of the myenteric plexus in the affected area.

Treatment
Treatment may be conservative in mild cases. Repeated saline enemas may be used to assist emptying of the colon. Tap water should not be used because of the danger of water intoxication. Liquid paraffin, wetting agents like Dioctyl-Medo and *mild* laxatives like cream of magnesia may be given orally. Unfortunately conservative therapy may lead to faecal impaction, therefore a proximal colostomy may be necessary to relieve the obstruction. Surgical therapy is aimed at the removal of the aganglionic segment at about one year of age. A small percentage of patients may be expected to have anal leakage and diarrhoea but this should improve with time. Staphylococcal enterocolitis may cause a very toxic diarrhoea or, as a result of muscular damage, cause an apparent recurrence of constipation. Anal or even colonic decompression may be required.

Imperforate anus

Congenital malformations of the rectum and anus include:

1 *Rectal agenesis*, in which both rectum and anus are absent.
2 *Anal agenesis*, in which only the anus is absent.
3 *Imperforate anal membrane*, in which the anal opening is sealed by a membrane of varying thickness. The anal opening may be represented by a dimple.

Diagnosis

Diagnosis should be made by inspection after birth, but sometimes the first warning is the nurse's complaint that she cannot get a thermometer into the anus. Radiological examination may reveal a fistulous opening between the blind pouch of the anus or rectum and the bladder, vagina or perineum. The urine should be examined microscopically for meconium and the vagina should be inspected carefully. X-ray of the abdomino-perineal area may be helpful in assessing the extent of the defect. This is important because 'high anomalies' (i.e. those which terminate above the puborectal sling) have a worse prognosis and poorer functional result than 'low anomalies' in which the rectum ends below this sling. If the lower spine reveals any bony abnormality, an intravenous pyelogram is often abnormal.

Treatment

Surgery is required to reconstruct a proper passage. An imperforate anal membrane is the easiest to treat, but unfortunately is the rarest of these anomalies. The bulging transparent membrane is incised and the anus dilated daily. Other low lesions can also be treated surgically with good results. In high lesions a colostomy should be performed as an emergency procedure and a correction done at about one year of age.

Anal stenosis

Narrowing of the anus at birth is usually diagnosed by the ribbon-like appearance of the stool. It is confirmed on rectal examination. Dilatation with bougies is carried out initially and thereafter the mother should be taught to carefully dilate the anus daily with her well-lubricated and gloved little finger for 3–4 months. A good result is likely.

Meconium plug

Occasionally an infant may present with all the signs of a low intestinal obstruction but passes a plug of inspissated white meconium after a rectal examination. This relieves the symptoms. Sometimes an enema is required to unblock the obstruction. Thereafter there is no further trouble except in the rare case which develops signs of cystic fibrosis.

Meconium ileus

Meconium ileus is an obstruction of the small gut due to extremely viscid clay-like meconium. It is caused by the lack of digestive enzymes which occurs in cystic fibrosis of the pancreas. The diagnosis may be suspected if there is a family history of this disease. It may be confirmed by plain X-ray of the abdomen in which a granular appearance of the terminal ileum reveals a microcolon, i.e. a colon that has never been expanded by meconium. Calcification in an area devoid of gas is diagnostic of

meconium   peritonitis   due   to   perforation   of   the   ileum
in utero.

Treatment

Treatment is surgical. A Mikulicz ileostomy relieves the obstruction and permits irrigation of the distal bowel with digestive enzyme-containing solutions. Hypertonic contrast medium Gastrografin has been given rectally to draw water into the bowel and loosen up the inspissated meconium. It cannot of course relieve the atresia, perforation or peritonitis. The patients that recover from meconium ileus develop the full-blown picture of cystic fibrosis (p. 229).

Prolapse of the rectum

Rectal prolapse (Fig. 15.2) is a rare condition and usually occurs in wasting conditions in which perirectal fat and supporting tissue is diminished. It is most common before five years of age. Usually there is an accompanying diarrhoea or steatorrhoea. It may be the presenting sign in cystic fibrosis. Polyps and parasites may be present. Whooping cough may precipitate the prolapse. The underlying cause should be treated and the prolapse returned manually by pressing it back with a piece of toilet paper. Recurrent uncontrolled prolapse may require surgery.

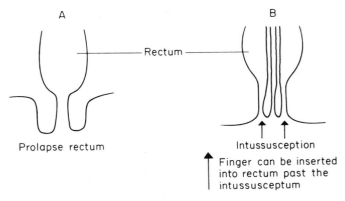

Fig. 15.2 Comparison of the appearance of a prolapsed rectum and intussusception

INFECTIONS OF THE BOWEL

Infantile gastroenteritis

Diarrhoea and vomiting in infants may be due to bacteria such as *Shigella, Salmonella, Staphylococcus, Yersinia enterocolitica, Campylo-*

THE GASTRO-INTESTINAL TRACT 249

bacter species or enteropathogenic *E. coli*, or it may be due to enteroviral infections such as rotavirus or parvo-like particles. In many epidemics the cause remains obscure. Disturbances in the diet such as over-feeding, excess sugars or other imbalance may be precipitating factors. Sometimes it may be associated with infection outside the bowel such as tonsillitis, otitis media, pneumonia or pyelonephritis (parenteral infections). It is a common complication of kwashiorkor.

Clinical features

The infection may be mild, moderate or severe. Mild gastroenteritis is characterised by the onset of fever, irritability, diarrhoea and vomiting. The stools are usually loose, green, slimy and foul smelling. They may vary in number from two or ten or more per day. The volume of stool may be small or large. The attack may be over in 12–24 hours without the patient becoming seriously ill or dehydrated.

Moderate gastroenteritis is characterised by 5 % dehydration while in severe cases 10 % of body-weight may be lost as a result of an explosive diarrhoea and repeated vomiting. In severe cases of gastroenteritis the eyes and fontanelle are sunken, the tongue dry and the skin inelastic. If pinched between the fingers it does not spring back into position as occurs with normal skin. In fat babies these signs may be less obvious because the fat masks the signs of inelasticity of the skin. Also fat babies are especially prone to develop metabolic acidosis, the respiration being fast and deep. This may be mistaken for pneumonia but the lungs are clear to percussion and auscultation. Hypovolaemic shock may set in very rapidly and is characterised by grey cyanosis or pallor, dry skin, thin rapid pulse and staring half-open eyes. Potassium depletion causes apathy, marked hypotonia, ileus and ECG changes. Oliguria is invariable.

Laboratory findings

These depend on the severity of the illness. In most cases the dehydration is isotonic but in severe cases there may be hypertonic dehydration, i.e. the serum sodium is above 145 mmol/l and the serum osmolality increased above 300 mOsmol/kg. The serum chloride may be very low (say 85 mmol/l) but sometimes high values above 110 mmol/l associated with blood urea values of 10 mmol/l or more reflect dehydration and haemoconcentration. This increase in blood viscosity may lead to cerebral thrombosis. The total body potassium is usually low though this is not always reflected in the serum potassium values, which may be normal. Hypernatraemia may cause swelling and permanent damage to the brain cells during rapid rehydration.

Clinically it may be very difficult or even impossible to distinguish hypertonic from hypotonic dehydration. In the latter the serum sodium is below 135 mmol/l and the osmolality less than 270 mOsmol/kg.

Stool culture may reveal the guilty bacteria or enteroviruses, but in many epidemics of gastroenteritis the yield of pathogenic organisms is surprisingly low.

Differential diagnosis

Shigella infection affects most members of the family. Vomiting may be a prominent feature and fever and convulsions are common. The stools are watery, odourless, yellow-green, and often contain mucus and blood. *Salmonella* presents abruptly with diarrhoea and vomiting. Fever is variable and may be high in severe infection. Abdominal pain is usually present. The stools are green, contain mucus and blood and smell of rotten eggs. *Campylobacter* infection is similar but affects mainly infants and produces a profuse watery diarrhoea. *Enteropathogenic E. coli* is limited to infants and does not cause vomiting, fever or convulsions. The stools are loose, green and slimy, and no blood is present. *Rotavirus* is nearly always associated with a previous upper respiratory tract infection. The diarrhoea is profuse and may lead to dehydration. Vomiting is often present at the onset or precedes the diarrhoea. It is most likely to occur in infants six months to two years of age and is thought to be the commonest cause of winter diarrhoea. In all cases of infantile gastroenteritis parenteral causes should be sought for and treated. Cholera should be considered in explosive epidemics.

Prevention

Breast feeding reduces the chances of gastroenteritis by providing appropriate immunoglobulin A which protects mucous membranes. Bottle-fed babies are more likely to be infected in over-crowded, fly-infested, unhygienic conditions. Hospital staff in nurseries and paediatric wards should have regular throat and rectal swabs taken during periods at risk.

Treatment

In mild cases of gastroenteritis it is usually enough to stop solids for 12 hours and to give fluids by mouth. Kaolin and pectin mixtures and anti-emetics are not recommended. Recent studies have shown the efficacy of oral rehydration, even in moderately dehydrated children. A glucose-electrolyte solution such as Dioralyte can be used. If vomiting is a problem small amounts should be given frequently. Aliquots of 5–10 ml can be administered every five minutes if necessary and in this way 100 ml or more fluid can be taken in every hour.

Severe cases of gastroenteritis always require parenteral fluids (see Table 15.1). If shock is present an isotonic fluid should be given initially to expand the blood volume and ensure urinary flow. As a rough rule 10 % of the body-weight in kilogrammes may be given as litres of fluid in the first 4–6 hours (e.g. a baby weighing 5 kg who is dehydrated and shocked requires 10% of 5 kg = 0.5 litres of fluid). Normal saline, Ringer's lactate or other isotonic solutions may be given.

Table 15.1 Approximate dose of intravenous fluids in gastroenteritis

Severity of illness	First 24 hours ml/m²	Maintenance/24 hours
Mild	2000	After acute phase is over the
Moderate	2250	patient may be given 1500–
Severe	2500	1800 ml/m² plus estimated
plus shock	2750	continuing losses by diarrhoea

Subsequently a potassium-containing *hypotonic* fluid should be used. We have found half-strength Darrow's solution in 2.5% or 5% dextrose-in-water ideal in that it contains an excess of water over electrolyte. This permits the body to use those electrolytes that it requires for repair, and to excrete the balance. If metabolic acidosis is severe it may be wise to counteract this with 1.2% sodium bicarbonate solution intravenously. Each 7 ml of this solution provides 1 mmol sodium ions. The dose in millimoles is:

$$\text{Weight in kg} \times 0.3 \times \text{base deficit}$$

where the base deficit is estimated by blood gas analysis.

Usually when an intravenous drip is set up (often in a scalp vein or on the dorsum of the hand) and oral feeds are stopped, vomiting ceases. Recovery from shock is rapid once intravenous fluids are given. It is customary to give oxygen in the acutely ill baby, but this should be stopped on recovery from shock.

Antibiotics should be given in severe cases of bacterial infection showing evidence of toxaemia, septicaemia or meningitis. However, most cases of *Salmonella*, *Campylobacter* and enteropathogenic *E. coli* infections do not require antibiotics as they tend to prolong the diarrhoea. Nowadays many cases of gastroenteritis are due to enteroviruses for which antibiotics have no effect whatsoever and may even be deleterious. Salicylates are contra-indicated in gastroenteritis— they do no good and may precipitate severe metabolic acidosis.

As soon as improvement sets in, usually in 24 hours, oral glucose-electrolyte solution may be started cautiously. If fluids are taken well the diet may be enlarged to include the infant's usual foods. Sometimes there is a temporary lactase deficiency and milk is not well tolerated. Substitutes such as Nutramigen may be used temporarily. However, in most infants suffering from gastroenteritis, milk feeds may be given soon after vomiting has ceased and the patient is rehydrated. Temporary flare up of the diarrhoea is usually of no consequence.

Patients with infective diarrhoea who are admitted to hospital should be isolated and barrier-nursed in order to prevent cross infection. After recovery from the acute illness some children continue to excrete pathogens in their stools. Patients with *Shigella*, *Salmonella* or pathogenic *E. coli* should not mix with infants (for example in nurseries) until three negative stool cultures have been obtained.

Other causes of diarrhoea

Acute, chronic or recurrent diarrhoea may be due to:

1 Irritable colon syndrome.
2 Antibiotic-induced colitis.
3 Crohn's disease, ulcerative colitis.
4 Typhoid fever, amoebiasis, giardiasis.
5 Any other cause of intestinal malabsorption.

The irritable colon syndrome (Toddler diarrhoea)

The irritable colon syndrome (mucous colitis) is characterised by diarrhoea which varies from day to day and from stool to stool. The stool frequently contains mucus and undigested vegetable matter, especially carrots and peas. Despite this the infant thrives and seems perfectly happy and active. The diarrhoea may commence at six months or earlier and usually clears by four years of age. A few may go on to intermittent abdominal pain with or without loose muculent stools. Stool cultures are negative and there is no evidence of malabsorption.

Management
The mother should be reassured and a normal diet given. Loperamide 2–4 mg a day helps some patients.

Antibiotic-induced colitis

Antibiotic-induced colitis is an acute severe form of diarrhoea occurring in patients who have been on antibiotics, notably clindamycin, lincomycin, tetracyclines, chloramphenicol and ampicillin. It is caused by destruction of the normal bowel flora and overgrowth with *Clostridium difficile*, resulting in pseudomembranous colitis. There are white plaques of mucin, fibrin and necrotic material attached to the mucosa.

Treatment
The antibiotic should be stopped, fluid and electrolyte balance corrected and vancomycin administered orally (adult dose 125–500 mg 6-hourly for 5 days). If relapse occurs the therapy should be repeated with added cholestyramine.

Crohn's disease

Crohn's disease is rare in childhood. Any segment of the intestinal tract can be affected leading to anorexia, abdominal pain and diarrhoea. Systemic features are fever, anaemia, arthritis, iritis and hepatitis. The child may fail to thrive. A mass may be palpable on abdominal examination. When symptoms are non-specific there may be a long delay in making the correct diagnosis.

Treatment
Corticosteroid therapy is the most effective form of medical treatment. Sulphasalazine may also be of value. Deficiency states due to malabsorption should be corrected. Complications such as intestinal fistula and stricture are treated surgically.

Ulcerative colitis

Ulcerative colitis may occasionally occur in children and cases have been reported in infancy. The onset may be acute or insidious. Diarrhoea with tenesmus and blood in the stool may suggest the diagnosis of dysentery. A particularly unpleasant symptom is uncontrollable soiling. The initial symptoms may be those of abdominal pain, anorexia and weight loss. Fever and hepatosplenomegaly may complicate the picture while iron-deficiency anaemia, responding poorly to oral iron, may be present. Wasting, hypoproteinaemia and oedema may develop. Tenderness over the colon may be found.

Diagnosis
Diagnosis is made on sigmoidoscopy in which the rectum and colon are found to be hyperaemic and friable and bleed to the touch. Ulcers and pseudopolyps may be seen. Barium enema in the early stages reveals colonic irritability. Later shaggy barium-filled ulcers may be noted. Eventually the typical 'pipestem colon' develops in which the colon is rigid and haustral markings are lost.

Treatment
The disease is characterised by remissions and exacerbations. Of medicines, corticosteroids have proved the most effective, the dose being adjusted to the needs of the patient. Some do well on long-term sulphonamides of which sulphasalazine (Salazopyrin) is recommended by some. Corticosteroid enemas may be helpful in some patients and reduce the need for oral corticosteroid medication.

Symptomatic therapy includes dicyclomine for colic and loperamide for diarrhoea. Water-soluble vitamins and iron should be given in all cases. A low residue diet is usually recommended.

In view of the long-term danger of malignant change, colectomy is recommended for patients who do not respond to medical therapy, in whom high doses of corticosteroids are required to control the disease, and in patients with fulminant attacks. Acute dilatation of the colon calls for emergency colectomy.

Typhoid fever (enteric fever)

The classical description of typhoid fever may be found in William Osler's *Textbook of Medicine* published at the turn of the century. In the

United Kingdom most cases occur in the families of travellers, particularly in immigrants who have returned from visiting their families abroad. The infecting organism is *Salmonella typhi*. In children the disease is rarely classical. In infants the illness may resemble infantile gastroenteritis but often the child is constipated. The occurrence of fever and splenomegaly should arouse one's suspicion of typhoid. Rose spots occur in 50 % of patients but are easily missed. The patient may present with a prolonged fever and the diagnosis is made unexpectedly by finding a positive culture or positive Widal test.

Older children are usually more ill and may develop abdominal distension, anaemia and leucopenia.

Diagnosis
Salmonella typhi may be grown from the blood (first week), urine or stools.

Treatment
In patients with diarrhoea and vomiting, or with anorexia, fluid and electrolyte losses should be replaced and adequate nutrition maintained. Isolation should be strict. Co-trimoxazole, chloramphenicol or high dose amoxicillin should be given.

Amoebiasis

Amoebic dysentery is due to infection with *Entamoeba histolytica*, a parasite which occurs in both vegetative or cystic forms. Its distribution is world-wide and it tends to be endemic in hot humid climes. It is carried by infected faeces, contaminated food and water. It occurs commonly in the tropics and has been diagnosed in neonates.

The clinical manifestations are very variable. Some patients may pass cysts yet be entirely without symptoms. Others may have an explosive dysentery-like picture due to extensive inflammation of the colon. Abdominal pain and tenesmus may be associated with blood and mucus in the stools, which are passed frequently. Severe infection may be associated with the perforation of the colon and peritonitis. Spread of the infection to the liver leads to fever, rigors and hepatic tenderness. An amoebic hepatic abscess may form. Diagnosis is confirmed by detecting the amoeba in a fresh, warm stool. A rapid amoebic latex agglutination test has been developed, a negative result excluding the disease.

Treatment
The drug of choice for both intestinal and hepatic amoebiasis is metronidazole (Flagyl) the dose being 220–440 mg/m² three times daily for 5 days. For amoebic hepatitis the smaller dose is satisfactory and is usually followed by chloroquine phosphate 280 mg/m² once daily for 14 days. If an hepatic abscess forms, penicillin should be given systemically and the advice of a surgeon sought.

Giardiasis

Giardia lamblia is a protozoon parasite which lives in the duodenum and upper jejunum (see p. 333). Heavy infestation may cause abdominal discomfort, steatorrhoea, malabsorption, diarrhoea and other more non-specific complaints. Treatment is with metronidazole.

Malabsorption syndromes

Malabsorption from the bowel causes steatorrhoea, abdominal distension, weight loss and stunting of growth. It may be due to:

1 Cows milk protein intolerance.
2 Cystic fibrosis (p. 229).
3 Gluten-induced enteropathy (coeliac disease).
4 Disaccharidase deficiency.
5 Short-bowel syndrome: bowel resection, fistulas or short-circuiting operation involving the small bowel.
6 Lymphatic (lacteal) obstruction due to tuberculosis, Hodgkin's disease or lymphomas.
7 Acrodermatitis enteropathica.

Cows milk protein intolerance

Intolerance to cows milk protein is often diagnosed but is probably uncommon. It usually presents with diarrhoea, vomiting and failure to thrive. Hypoproteinaemia and iron-deficiency anaemia may occur. As there is no *reliable* laboratory test to confirm the diagnosis, the practitioner must depend on the response to withdrawal of milk protein from the diet, and the exacerbation of symptoms on re-introducing milk. It is thought that the beta-lactoglobulin in milk is the offending agent.

Treatment
Cows milk protein should be replaced by milk in which the protein has been hydrolysed (such as Nutramigen) or with a soya bean formula. The condition is usually temporary and cows milk protein can be re-introduced into the diet by two years of age without problems.

Gluten-induced enteropathy

Coeliac disease is a disturbance of the small bowel which is precipitated by ingestion of gluten in susceptible patients. The term *coeliac syndrome* is sometimes used synonymously with *malabsorption syndrome*.

The illness begins shortly after the introduction into the diet of wheat or rye cereals, which contain the protein *gluten*. The patient develops steatorrhoea, the stools being large, pale and greasy, but not nearly as foul smelling as in cystic fibrosis. Anorexia is a feature, unlike the ravenous appetite of the child with cystic fibrosis. Progressive wasting and growth retardation is usual. Watery diarrhoea may occur at times and cause acute dehydration. Chronic malabsorption of vitamin D may cause rickets (*coeliac rickets*) while folate deficiency is commonly found. Diagnosis may be confirmed by peroral intestinal biopsy with a child-size Crosby-type capsule. The intestinal villi are flat but return to normal with treatment.

Treatment
Treatment consists of permanent withdrawal of gluten-containing foods from the diet. This includes all wheat, oats, barley and rye products including certain 'hidden' sources such as commercial ice-cream and many types of confectionery. Fried fish and chicken in which the batter contains wheat, is taboo. Vitamin supplements including folic acid and vitamin K should be given initially during recovery.

Disaccharidase deficiencies

Disaccharidase deficiency is a disorder characterised by watery diarrhoea, flatulence, abdominal pain and bloating after the ingestion of milk. It is most commonly due to lactase deficiency in the intestinal mucosa, but in rare cases enzymes such as maltase, iso-maltase and invertase may be involved. It may be congenital or acquired. The acquired form is commonly associated with infantile gastroenteritis and protein-energy malnutrition. It is due to the temporary reduction or absence of lactase in the small bowel and, in severe cases, sucrase may be absent as well.

Diagnosis
Diagnosis is suggested by the presence of watery stools of low pH, containing an excess of lactic acid. The Clinitest tablet test for reducing substances is positive.

Treatment
The offending sugar should be eliminated by using a lactose-free milk. It has been found that in protein-energy malnutrition, despite the persistence of diarrhoea, milk protein and fat are adequately absorbed and retained. Milk therefore should *not* be stopped unless the diarrhoea is severe or a milk substitute is easily available.

Short-bowel syndrome

Malabsorption may occur in any condition which reduces the absorptive area of the small bowel, such as after extensive bowel resection, short-circuiting due to surgical intervention or fistulous tracts. A similar syndrome may be due to obstruction of the lacteals by Hodgkin's disease or tuberculosis. Treatment consists of surgical correction where possible. Medical treatment consists of careful dietary control, the use of medium chain triglycerides and the parenteral injection of vitamins A, B, C, D and K including vitamin B_{12} and folic acid. Underlying causes such as tuberculosis and Hodgkin's disease must be treated.

Lymphatic obstruction

Obstruction of the lacteal vessels of the bowel by tuberculosis, Hodgkin's disease or lymphoma prevents the absorption of long-chain fats, whether saturated or unsaturated. This causes steatorrhoea, which can be minimised by replacing long-chain fats with medium- and short-chain fats in the diet.

Acrodermatitis enteropathica

This is a rare, recessively inherited, often fatal disease characterised by symmetrical bullous lesions, loss of hair and chronic diarrhoea. The skin lesions commonly occur around the mouth and anus. Some patches resemble eczema, others psoriasis. This rarity is mentioned here because many respond dramatically to zinc sulphate 50–100 mg three times daily.

CONSTIPATION

Constipation means the passage of hard stools at infrequent intervals. It may be due to lack of fluid intake, excess loss of fluid in hot weather, or from increased resorption of fluid from the colon. There may be reduced food intake, especially insufficient fibre. Lack of exercise predisposes to colonic stasis after surgery and may be an important cause for constipation during other illnesses. Often it may be due to the child ignoring the call to stool. The toilet may be unsuitable for a child—too high, too low or too noisy. Bed pans are badly designed aids to elimination.

One of the commonest causes for constipation in babies is the change-over from breast milk, which tends to cause frequent stools, to cows' milk, which tends to form hard dry stools. The effort to pass such a stool may cause an anal tear which is exquisitely painful and inhibits further bowel movements. If not treated adequately this could lead to chronic constipation and, in some cases, to 'false diarrhoea'. Rectal examination in these cases reveals a large hard stool partially blocking the rectum with the escape of liquid, foul smelling faecal matter around the mass (encopresis).

Constipation almost always accompanies hypothyroidism, hypercalcaemia and neurological disorders such as mental deficiency and meningomyelocele. A rare but important cause is Hirschprung's disease (see p. 245). Chronic lead poisoning is usually associated with constipation.

Iatrogenic causes of constipation include abuse of purgatives which result in the bowel being emptied completely. It takes about 36 hours before the bowel is filled again and many parents get upset if the bowel does not act every day. They therefore give another dose of purgative which maintains the vicious circle. Cough suppressants such as codeine are constipating, as are the related antidiarrhoeal preparations paregoric (Tincture of camphorated opium) and its more modern counterpart diphenoxylate. The barium sulphate used in radiological studies of the gastro-intestinal tract (the Barium meal) can cause impaction of the rectum if suitable precautions are not taken. Certain antacids especially calcium salts and anticholinergic drugs can also inhibit peristalsis and cause constipation.

There may be a strong psychological element in some cases of constipation and there is often abnormal tension between parent and child. Many constipated children appear to have parents who are obsessively concerned about their own bowels.

Management

The underlying cause should be eliminated wherever possible. Before drugs are used an attempt should be made to eliminate family tensions. An increase of dietary fibre seems to help, particularly bran fibre and a breakfast which includes 1–2 tablespoonsful of Kellogg's Hi-Bulk Bran seems to be particularly helpful. Many children however refuse bran in any form however well disguised and one must then turn to artificial aids.

Bulk laxatives such as Agiolax or Normacol may be found useful. They should be swallowed with plenty of water. Hard stools can be softened with liquid paraffin but prolonged use may lead to malabsorption and sufficient may be absorbed into the lacteals to cause lipoid granulomas. Dioctyl sodium sulphosuccinate is a wetting agent for softening stools and is available in many forms. To stimulate peristalsis either senna glycosides or bisacodyl may be used.

To remove impacted faeces from the rectum an olive oil enema or a phosphate enema may be used. In extreme cases it may be necessary to remove the faecal mass manually under anaesthesia.

THE CHILD WITH ABDOMINAL PAIN

Any practitioner who is troubled with little 'belly-achers', is referred to John Apley's classic monograph *The Child with Abdominal Pains* (Blackwell Scientific Publications, 1975). Recurrent abdominal pain is a very common symptom in childhood and it is rare to make a satisfying pathological diagnosis. Some children have been subjected to extensive investigations, including laparotomy, appendectomy and even tonsillectomy, without anything being established. There is frequently a certain degree of anxiety in the parent-child relationship and the assurance that the pain is *real* but *not organic* is often helpful. The use of anticholinergic drugs such as Belladonna Mixture for Infants or dicyclomine syrup may be of actual or placebo value. Extensive investigations are not advised unless other symptoms point to a definite pathology such as peptic ulcer, urinary tract problems or malabsorption. Sometimes lactose intolerance may be the underlying cause and the use of a lactose-free milk may help.

Appendicitis

Acute appendicitis is perhaps the commonest cause of an 'acute abdomen' in childhood. It may be preceded by a respiratory infection or may be due to impaction by a faecolith or worm in the appendix. In most cases no cause is found.

Clinical features

The illness usually starts with acute pain around the umbilicus. After 2–4 hours the pain may become localised in the right iliac fossa. Often by the time the doctor sees the patient he has had a single vomit. If the appendix lies retrocaecally there may be diarrhoea, but often there is constipation. If the inflamed appendix crosses the ureter, ureteric pain and frequency of micturition may mislead one from the diagnosis.

There is usually a fever of 38°C and a pulse of 130–140 beats per minute, both of which increase in the presence of perforation and peritonitis. The patient is often anxious and may double up with pain. The right psoas muscle may go into spasm causing flexion of the right hip. Examination confirms tenderness over McBurney's point. Rebound tenderness indicates involvement of the peritoneum. Rectal examination may reveal tenderness on the right side and even a mass due to omentum covering the inflamed appendix. In girls the vagina should be inspected for pus as gonococcal peritonitis can mimic appendicitis.

Laboratory diagnosis

The white blood count is usually about 18 000/mm^3 with over 70 % neutrophils. A single white blood count may be misleading but repeated tests at 4-hourly intervals may reveal a rising white count with a left shift. The urine is usually clear but a few blood cells may be found if the appendix irritates the ureter. Purulent urine is probably due to pyelonephritis which should be treated conservatively. An X-ray of the chest should be taken to exclude basal pneumonia and pleurisy as a cause for the abdominal pain. Abdominal plates may be negative but a soft tissue mass may be found in the right iliac fossa due to abscess formation. Free gas and fluid indicates perforation. Occasionally a faecolith or abnormal gas pattern may be found. A barium enema may show pressure deformity of the caecum or incomplete filling of the appendix.

Differential diagnosis

Intussusception may mimic appendicitis but the presence of blood and mucus in the stool on rectal examination clarifies the diagnosis. *Mesenteric adenitis* is due to swelling of the mesenteric lymph nodes. It is often associated with a preceding upper respiratory infection; there may be high fever but vomiting is unusual. *Pyelonephritis* has been mentioned and thorough examination of the urine will help clarify the diagnosis. *Peritonitis* causes generalised abdominal pain. Pneumococcal peritonitis is usually associated with nephrosis while gonococcal peritonitis occurs in girls with vulvovaginitis. *Threadworms* may, on rare occasions, cause obstructive appendicitis. Diabetes mellitus, infections, hepatitis and sickle-cell disease may all present with acute abdominal pain but should not require laparotomy to exclude them.

Treatment

The patient should be prepared for surgery. Oral feeds are stopped and adequate fluids and electrolytes are given intravenously. Antibiotic therapy should be started immediately with a large dose of ampicillin. Kanamycin or metronidazole may be given at the same time. Gastric suction prevents further vomiting and deflates the stomach.

At the operation the appendix is removed and some surgeons take the opportunity of exploring the last two or three feet of small bowel for Meckel's diverticulum.

If the appendix has already ruptured a drain is inserted in the right iliac fossa and the patient nursed in Fowler's position, preferably in an oxygen tent. Blood or plasma may be given. Gastric suction and parenteral feeding are continued postoperatively until bowel sounds reappear. Pain may be controlled by the more powerful analgesics such as morphine, pethidine or dipipanone. Cultures from the appendix will determine subsequent antibiotic therapy.

A late complication may be intestinal obstruction due to the formation of adhesions. This will require a repeat laparotomy.

Vomiting—a check list

Common causes which should be excluded are:

1 Gastro-intestinal obstruction at any level from oesophagus to anus.
2 Acute appendicitis.
3 Acute intussusception.
4 Congenital hypertrophic pyloric stenosis.
5 Enteral infections such as food poisoning, infantile gastroenteritis and the dysenteries.
6 Parenteral infections such as acute otitis media, tonsillitis, pneumonia or pyelonephritis.
7 Intracranial diseases including meningitis, encephalitis, subdural haemorrhage or expanding tumours.
8 Vestibular disease and motion sickness.
9 Regurgitation and rumination in babies.
10 Heart failure and digitalis poisoning.
11 Hiatus hernia and achalasia cardia.
12 Psychic vomiting due to excitement.

13 Over-eating.
14 Drug-induced vomiting.
15 Poisoning.

Most of these are discussed elsewhere. This is merely intended as a quick check list in case of diagnostic difficulties. No case of vomiting should be treated with powerful anti-emetics until 'surgical' conditions have been excluded, lest the symptoms be masked.

Diarrhoea—a check list

1 Physiological 'diarrhoea' of breast-fed babies.
2 Feeding disorders:
   (a) Excess carbohydrate and sugar intolerance
   (b) Excess fat and fat intolerance
3 Enteral infections:
   (a) Bacterial—*Staphylococcus, Shigella, Salmonella* and entero-pathogenic *E. coli*
   (b) Enteroviral
   (c) Amoebic dysentery
   (d) Giardiasis or worm load
   (e) Antibiotic induced colitis
4 Infantile gastroenteritis.
5 Parenteral infections such as otitis media, tonsillitis, pneumonia, pyelonephritis and others.
6 Toxins, e.g. food poisoning.
7 Allergy, especially foods.
8 Ulcerative colitis and irritable colon syndrome.
9 Purgatives.
10 Poisoning.

Rectal bleeding—a check list

Infants
1 Swallowed maternal blood.
2 Haemorrhagic disease of the newborn.
3 Allergy (?).
4 Anal fissure.

Children
1 Dysentery:
   (a) Bacterial
   (b) Amoebic
2 Intussusception and volvulus.
3 Peptic ulcer.
4 Meckel's diverticulum.
5 Duplication of the bowel.
6 Blood diseases.

7 Iatrogenic, e.g. antileukaemic agents.
8 Portal cirrhosis with varices.
9 Rectal polyps.
10 Trauma from foreign body.

LIVER DISEASE IN CHILDREN

Hepatomegaly in children

In healthy babies and young children the edge of the liver may often be felt 1–2 cm below the costal margin in the mid-clavicular line. The edge is sharp, smooth and fairly soft. Undue enlargement, especially when associated with hardness or irregularity should be regarded as abnormal and the following are the main causes to be considered for the hepatomegaly.

Hepatomegaly—a check list

Neonatal hepatomegaly
1 Haemolytic disease, especially Rh and ABO incompatibility, acholuric jaundice or thalassaemia.
2 Congestive heart failure.
3 Hepatitis due to viruses (hepatitis A or B virus, rubella, herpesvirus and cytomegalovirus), bacteria (umbilical sepsis and septicaemia) and spirochaetes (syphilis).
4 Congenital absence of bile ducts.
5 Metabolic diseases such as glycogen storage disease, lipoidoses or galactosaemia. Also infant of diabetic mother.

For neonatal jaundice see p. 45–48.

Hepatomegaly in infancy and childhood
1 Infections:
Viral
    (a) Viral hepatitis type A and type B
    (b) Non A, non B hepatitis
    (c) Infectious mononucleosis
    (d) Yellow fever
    (e) Herpesvirus and cytomegalovirus.
Bacterial
    (a) Pyogenic abscesses
    (b) Tuberculous hepatitis.
Spirochaetal
    (a) Syphilitic hepatitis.
    (b) Weil's disease.

Parasitic
  (a) Amoebic hepatitis
  (b) Bilharzial hepatitis
  (c) Echinococcus cyst
  (d) Tropical infections
  (e) Toxoplasmosis.
2 Cirrhosis of the liver:
  (a) Portal cirrhosis of Laennec
  (b) Biliary cirrhosis
  (c) Hepatic vein thrombosis (Chiari's syndrome)
  (d) Veno-occlusive disease of the liver.
3 Neoplasms such as leukaemia, lymphomata, Hodgkin's disease and sarcoma. Also secondary deposits from tumours elsewhere, e.g. Wilm's tumour of the kidney, osteogenic sarcoma or neuroblastoma.
4 Blood diseases such as thalassaemia or sickle-cell anaemia.
5 Congestive heart failure and constrictive pericarditis.
6 Drug toxicity, hypersensitivity reactions, or poisoning by carbon tetrachloride, chloroform or mushrooms.
7 Endocrine disorder especially diabetes mellitus.
8 Metabolic diseases (mostly very rare):
  (a) Glycogen storage disease
  (b) Lipoidoses (Gaucher's disease; Niemann-Pick)
  (c) Amyloidosis
  (d) Galactosaemia
  (e) Letterer-Siwe's disease
  (f) Xanthomatoses.

Viral hepatitis

Three types of viral hepatitis are known:

1 *Type A hepatitis* (HAV infectious hepatitis, short incubation hepatitis or epidemic jaundice).
2 *Type B hepatitis* (HBV homologous serum hepatitis, long incubation or syringe transmitted hepatitis).
3 *Non-A/Non-B hepatitis*

Type A hepatitis

This is due to the hepatitis A virus (HAV). It is spread by the faecal-oral route, but water- and food-borne epidemics occur. Rarely it has been syringe-transmitted.

The lower the living standard of the population the more common the infection. The virus is an acid stable particle 27 nm in diameter which is destroyed by heating at 100°C for 5 minutes. The incubation period is 30 days (range 15–45). The stool is infectious for one week before symptoms develop and for two weeks after.

Clinical features

The prodromal illness consists of fever, nausea, vomiting and upper abdominal pain. Sometimes pain in the joints occurs and the illness may resemble influenza or an 'acute abdomen'. The intensity of symptoms may vary from very mild to very severe. A few days later the urine becomes dark, the stools pale and the patient may become yellow. The jaundice may last a few days or persist for weeks. Most cases however are anicteric. The liver may be enlarged, firm and tender and the spleen is often palpable. The vast majority recover, but in a small percentage of children marked liver damage occurs which may lead to acute liver failure with metabolic acidosis, hyperammonaemia and encephalopathy.

As a rule the course of type A hepatitis in children is mild while type B tends to be severe. In pregnancy viral hepatitis tends to run a severe course and the incidence of abortion, stillbirth and prematurity is increased.

Laboratory findings

1 Urine contains bile giving it a dark, brown-yellow colour. If the urine is agitated the foam is a bright canary yellow.
2 The stools are often pale for a day or two due to temporary biliary obstruction.
3 Serum bilirubin, mainly conjugated, is increased.
4 Serum proteins are altered. The alpha-2-globulin and gammaglobulin increase in the second week. In massive hepatic necrosis both alpha- and betaglobulins *decrease*. Hypoalbuminaemia is often a bad prognostic sign.
5 AST and ALT increase early, the alkaline phosphatase a week later.
6 The blood sedimentation rate and the serum bilirubin may be useful for following the course of the disease.
7 The prothrombin time should be measured to anticipate hypo-prothrombinaemia in severe cases of hepatitis, and prior to doing a liver biopsy.
8 Virus is demonstrable in the stool in type A but not in the blood.

Differential diagnosis

Infectious mononucleosis may present with hepatitis but other signs like tonsillitis, generalised lymphadenopathy and splenomegaly are likely to be present. *Cytomegalovirus infection* usually has a positive complement fixation test. In *yellow fever* there are accompanying signs of renal damage. *Drugs* such as chlorpromazine and erythromycin may on rare occasions cause cholestatic jaundice.

Treatment

Bed rest is advisable until recovery. Toilet privileges and quiet play may be permitted as soon as the child's condition permits. In the early phase nausea and vomiting may lead to dehydration and electrolyte imbalance and this should be corrected. Once the patient becomes yellow, the appetite often improves dramatically and a normal palatable diet may be given. Fats are restricted only if the patient has nausea, a symptom of cholangitis. Severely ill patients may benefit by prednisone for a few days, the dose being tailed off as soon as possible. Blood transfusion should be given for any bleeding tendency. If hepatic coma develops protein intake should be reduced and neomycin $2-3$ g/m^2/day may be given orally to reduce ammonia-forming organisms. Intravenous dextrose 10% may be given but amino acids should be avoided. Exchange transfusion, repeated as necessary, has on occasion been helpful in these very severe cases. Perfusion of blood through a pig's liver has been attempted, as has liver transplantation.

Hygienic measures to prevent spread of type A virus within the family or closed communities are important. Frequent hand washing and the use of disposable plates, cups and eating utensils are advised.

Type B hepatitis

This is thought to be due to the Dane Particle, a viral nucleoid $40-42$ nm in diameter. It has a double shell and inner core. The Australia antigen, now called the hepatitis B surface antigen (HB$_s$Ag) is a smaller particle found in the serum of some patients and may represent viral coat antigen to which antibodies occur during convalescence. Hepatitis B core antigen (HB$_c$Ag) is the core of the Dane Particle which stimulates antibody during the acute attack of HBV infection. Many cases also have a soluble 'e' antigen (HB$_e$Ag) in their serum.

In children hepatitis B virus is most likely to be transmitted by blood transfusion, renal dialysis or during cardiac by-pass. In adolescent drug addicts it may be transmitted by syringe. It may be transmitted from mother to child during delivery. The virus may be reactivated in patients who are given immunosuppressive drugs.

Clinical features
The clinical picture of hepatitis B is very similar to hepatitis A except that the incubation period is three times longer, i.e. 90 days (range $40-180$ days). In the prodromal period urticaria and arthritis may occur. The illness tends to be more severe than in hepatitis A, yet 80% recover fully, 15% develop chronic persistent hepatitis (which tends to be benign) and 5% develop chronic active hepatitis. Of the latter one-half develop cirrhosis of the liver. Immunological sequelae may occur due to the deposition of antigen-antibody complexes on the glomerular basement membrane.

Diagnosis
Antihepatitis B core antibodies occur in the serum at the onset of the acute illness, while antibodies to the surface antigens (Anti-HB$_s$) occur during convalescence. Their presence indicates that the patient is not

suitable for use as a blood donor. Virus may be demonstrated in the blood, but not in the stools.

Laboratory findings and treatment
See type A hepatitis above.

Prognosis
Prognosis for type B hepatitis is worse than for type A. Even so the vast majority recover (80 %).

Chronic active hepatitis

Formerly called chronic aggressive hepatitis, chronic active hepatitis is a chronic inflammatory and fibrosing lesion of the liver which may complicate type B hepatitis. It may occur after apparent recovery or following a symptomless infection. The insidious onset of fatigue leads to cirrhosis with oedema, ascites, bleeding oesophageal varices and hepatic encephalopathy. To distinguish this disorder from the more benign chronic persistent hepatitis liver biopsy is essential. Liver function tests are not very helpful. Corticosteroids appear to be helpful in chronic active hepatitis.

Non-A non-B hepatitis

The discovery of the Australia antigen and the elucidation of hepatitis types A and B has led to the discovery that there are a large group of cases of post-transfusional hepatitis that are neither type A nor B. The incubation period is half way between A and B virus. The risk of developing chronic active hepatitis is similar to that for B virus. The diagnosis is made by exclusion.

Prevention of hepatitis, types A and B
Hepatitis A contacts may be given small doses (usually 0.4–2 ml depending on size) of human immunoglobulin. In the case of HBV exposure, for example by needle prick, hepatitis B hyperimmune serum 0.06 ml/kg should be given within 7 days of exposure and repeated 30 days later. Infants born to mothers with acute hepatitis B or with HB_sAg in the blood should be given 0.13 ml/kg intramuscularly. The serum has also been used to prevent outbreaks in haemodialysis units.

Cirrhosis of the liver

Cirrhosis is common in developing countries, uncommon in developed countries. In the latter biliary atresia is the commonest cause of cirrhosis whereas in the former syphilis, bilharzia and virus infections are probably the most important. Certain genetic diseases may be associated with cirrhosis, namely cystic fibrosis, Wilson's hepatolenticular degeneration, alpha-1-antitrypsin deficiency, glycogen storage disease and galactosaemia.

Postnecrotic cirrhosis may occur after a severe attack of viral hepatitis or after chronic active hepatitis. Some cases are due to neonatal hepatitis. Initial symptoms refer to the gastrointestinal tract, i.e. anorexia, flatulence, nausea and vomiting. There may be an insidious development of ascites and portal hypertension, in which case the spleen becomes enlarged. The liver may have shrunk so that it is not palpable, but it may be large and nodular. Spider angiomata and 'liver palms', which are red and warm, may be noted. Clubbing of the fingers may develop though jaundice is usually absent.

Laboratory findings
These usually include marked bromosulphonphthalein retention, the serum albumin is low and the gammaglobulins increased. Conjugated bilirubin may be increased in the serum. Barium swallow may reveal oesophageal varices. Liver biopsy will establish the type of cirrhosis. Blood count reveals reduction in formed elements if there is hypersplenism.

Treatment
Treatment is symptomatic. Hepatic coma is treated by withdrawing protein from the diet, and antibiotics such as neomycin are given orally to sterilise the bowel and prevent the absorption of ammonia. Corticosteroids may be tried for progressive disease. Severe hypersplenism may require splenectomy to control it. In the presence of bleeding oesophageal varices, surgical shunting procedures should be considered. Ascites tends to be resistant to treatment but a good response may be obtained by combining a thiazide diuretic with spironolactone (Aldactone). Frusemide (Lasix) and ethacrynic acid may be used but the serum electrolytes must be monitored carefully.

Portal hypertension

Portal hypertension may be due to intrahepatic or extrahepatic obstruction of the portal vein (Fig. 15.3).

1 Intrahepatic causes:
   (a) Cirrhosis of the liver
   (b) Veno-occlusive disease
   (c) Hepatic vein thrombosis (Budd-Chiari syndrome).
2 Extrahepatic causes:
   (a) Congenital anomalies of portal venous channels, stenosis and atresia
   (b) Compression of portal veins by bands or lymph nodes
   (c) Splenic or portal vein thrombosis.

Anastomotic channels between the portal and systemic circulations open up, being prominent at the lower end of the oesophagus. In children one does not see the caput medusae or varicose leg veins such as

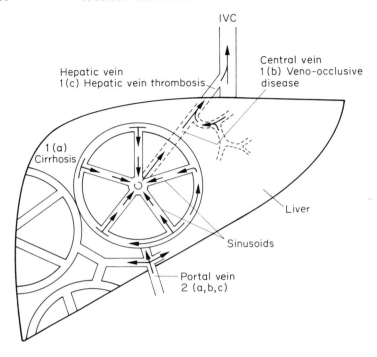

Fig. 15.3 Some causes of portal hypertension (the numbers refer to those in the text)

occurs in adults, despite high intraportal vein pressures of 300 or 400 mmH$_2$O (3 or 4 kPa). The spleen is enlarged and becomes firm and hard with progress of the disease. Hypersplenism invariably develops, the fall in thrombocytes being particularly dangerous.

Cirrhosis of the liver is associated with ascites, hypoalbuminaemia and disturbed liver function. The commonest symptom that brings the patient to the doctor is haemorrhage from the oesophageal varices. The patient either vomits the blood or passes a melaena stool. Pain over the spleen is sometimes a feature, due to infarcts. It should be remembered that after a haemorrhage the spleen may shrink temporarily. Ascites develops due to increasing pressure within the portal system and may lead to gross abdominal distension. *Veno-occlusive disease of the liver* is common in Jamaica where it is thought to be due to ingestion of Bush tea. It leads to widespread obstruction of the small and medium hepatic veins, with *early* development of gross ascites. Children under six years are commonly affected. A similar picture has been described in Southern Africa and India. The *Budd-Chiari syndrome* which involves the main hepatic vein is rare in children. However *portal vein thrombosis* is more common and is usually due to umbilical sepsis or repeated exchange transfusions via the umbilical vein.

Diagnosis
Barium swallow may reveal filling defects due to oesophageal varices. Oesophagoscopy may be a better method in skilled hands. Full blood count is required to determine the effects of repeated haemorrhage. Liver function tests are likely to be abnormal but the findings are not diagnostic as a rule. Splenic venoportogram delineates the portal system beautifully on X-ray but is a risky procedure. Liver biopsy usually establishes the diagnosis of the underlying liver disease.

Treatment
Blood transfusion may be required for a large acute haemorrhage or for anaemia due to chronic blood loss. Oesophageal bleeding may be controlled by intravenous vasopressin or by an intra-oesophageal balloon catheter. Eventually a by-pass operation will be required, in which the portal vein is joined to a systemic vein. The spleen is usually removed at the time of operation. Ascites are usually treated with diuretics such as frusemide and spironolactone. Careful control of fluid and electrolyte balance is essential to prevent hyponatraemia and hypokalaemic alkalosis. The prognosis in extrahepatic obstruction may be quite good, but if there is cirrhosis of the liver the prognosis is that of the liver disorder.

Tumours

Tumours of the liver are uncommon. Primary tumours include hepatoblastoma, hepatic carcinoma or sarcoma. These are malignant tumours which spread via local vessels to other parts of the liver, to the peritoneum, lymph nodes and lungs. Hepatomegaly and rapidly forming ascites are found. Haemangiomata of large size in the liver produce a bruit and may lead to heart failure due to the presence of an arteriovenous fistula. Hamartomas are benign malformations which contain both cellular and mesenchymal elements. Cysts both single or multilocular occur and may be associated with cysts in the kidneys, spleen and pancreas.

Metastatic tumours are relatively common, the extrahepatic source being a neuroblastoma, Wilm's tumour or lymphosarcoma.

Investigation
This requires intravenous pyelogram to exclude Wilm's tumour or displacement by an adrenal mass. A liver scan may help to localise the tumour. Splenoportography, coeliac axis angiography and cholangiography are useful additional investigations. In primary carcinoma of the liver and hepatoblastoma, alphafetoprotein appears in the serum and is diagnostic.

Therapy

Surgical excision is sometimes practicable after proper pre-operative preparation.

ABDOMINAL MASSES IN CHILDHOOD— A RADIOLOGICAL APPROACH

In any patient who presents with an abdominal mass and symptoms which cannot be diagnosed clinically, the following radiological investigations are suggested (in order):

1 Chest radiographs, frontal and lateral.
2 Erect and spine abdominal plates to confirm position of mass, gas distribution and free gas and fluid.
3 Ultrasound to differentiate solid from cystic masses. Either a grey-scale or real time study may be used to assess the relationship of the mass to the abdominal viscera. This is the safest of all investigations as it does not use ionising radiation and is non-invasive. However, the presence of gas may obstruct sound transmission.
4 Excretory urography and nephrotomography provides excellent anatomical delineation of the urinary system. Using the total body opacification technique it can differentiate vascular from avascular masses.
5 Nuclear Medicine Radioisotope Imaging is widely used in the investigation of liver, gall-bladder and splenic masses and to assess the vascularity of the mass.
6 Computed Axial Tomography is used to augment the previous three methods. It is often able to demonstrate very small masses but the paucity of perivascular and retroperitoneal fat limits its use in childhood. Where these methods are inadequate to make a conclusive diagnosis, then arteriography has a place.

Apart from ultrasound, all the above methods use ionising radiation and should be used with circumspection in children.

CHAPTER 16

THE GENITO-URINARY TRACT

THE KIDNEY

Even the smallest baby has approximately one million nephrons in each kidney. The newborn, and particularly the pre-term baby, may have problems with glomerular filtration and urinary concentration in the first few weeks of life but by 3–6 months most renal functions are comparable to adult levels when corrected for body surface area.

The specific gravity of the urine after birth is $\pm$ 1003. In the first week or two the premature may not be able to produce a more concentrated urine unless his solute load is increased. The full-term baby on water restriction can concentrate to 1010 (200 mOsmol/kg) or more. Full concentrating ability is achieved by three weeks, i.e. 1010–1020

The average daily urine excretion can be worked out roughly using the percentage method, the adult excretion being 600–2400 ml per 24 hours (average 1200 ml). Oliguria means that the child is passing less than 0.5 ml urine per kg of body weight hourly or less than 300 ml/m^2/day.

Examination of the renal tract

Too many adults suffer from chronic pyelonephritis for neglect of an examination of the urine in childhood. Too many recurrent fevers in childhood remain undiagnosed because the urine has not been cultured for bacteria. Failure to thrive, chronic ill-health and poor school performance may be due to underlying renal disease. Therefore *the examination of the urine of every patient should be routine, however trivial the complaint.*

History

The commonest complaints in childhood relate to bed-wetting, pain in the loin or over the bladder, burning on micturition, frequency and abnormalities of the urine. Parents are sometimes disturbed by the colour of the urine; in acute hepatitis it may become a dark yellow before the mother notices jaundice of the sclera; the darkening of urine on standing to a blackish colour may point to alkaptonuria; a red colour may be due to the presence of blood but could also be due to red pigments derived from beetroot or cheap sweets (eosin).

Recurrent fever, with or without rigors, should always suggest the possibility of a urinary infection. Recurrent abdominal pains, often vague but obviously related to the ureters or renal angle, may be a pointer. In males one should inquire about the stream of urine and, if possible, one should try to observe it. The nurse who collects the urine can often give valuable information.

The history may often be very misleading. Urinary infection may present with persistent jaundice in the neonate or as diarrhoea or vomiting in the older infant or child. Headache and visual disturbances may be the first lead to hypertension of renal origin.

Physical examination

In the newborn the cord should be examined carefully. Normally one vein and two arteries are present but if one artery is absent, congenital abnormality of the renal tract is more common.

Equally strange is the association of congenital renal anomalies with abnormalities of the ear. Normally the ear lines up with the nose whatever the position of the head. One should be suspicious of the low set ear, the abnormally shaped ear lobe, absent or extra lobes, or auricular sinuses. Other congenital anomalies of the eye, palate or heart may also be present. The face may look odd, as in Potter's facies in renal agenesis (p. 274).

The complexion may be sallow and signs suggestive of rickets (p. 74) may be present. Oedema of the face, limbs and sacrum should be noted and an increase in weight may indicate fluid retention. *The blood pressure should be examined even in the smallest infant.* See p. 124.

The sacral region is examined to exclude spina bifida which may or may not be associated with a neurogenic bladder. The sex organs should be very carefully examined for congenital anomalies.

In the male phimosis is often incorrectly diagnosed because of incorrect examination (Fig. 16.1). By pulling in the correct direction the true size of the opening can be assessed. The testicles and inguinal regions should be examined carefully and hernias should be excluded.

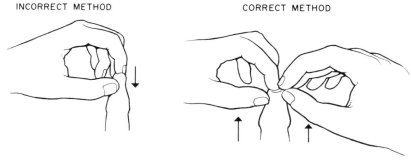

INCORRECT METHOD   CORRECT METHOD

If foreskin is pushed   If foreskin is grasped with both index fingers
downwards it makes   and thumbs and pulled upwards the true size
the opening look smaller   of the opening is apparent

Fig. 16.1 Examination of the foreskin for phimosis

In the female a good light is needed to examine the introitus, to ensure that the urethra is in the right place and to ascertain that no urine or other discharge is coming from the vagina.

Only now that the above examination has been completed, may the abdomen be examined! If the bladder is distended it can usually be felt, but distended ureters cannot usually be palpated. The kidney is very often palpable in the newborn and in conditions where the abdominal wall is very soft. With gentle but very firm pressure the lower poles of the kidneys may be palpable and, in some cases, the upper pole as well. The size, shape and consistency of renal masses should be noted, and whether or not they move on pressure from the renal angle or with respiration.

The collection of urine

Sterile urine in infants is obtainable by suprapubic puncture, provided that the bladder is palpable. It should be cultured immediately, and if there is to be any delay in sending the specimen to the laboratory, it should be kept on ice. Catheterisation should be avoided if possible, and only carried out under 'theatre' conditions. Often a 'midstream' or 'clean-catch specimen' will be found satisfactory. The 'midstream' urine can be passed directly onto a slide coated with bacterial culture medium. For ordinary examination plastic urine collecting bags which are pressed over the precleaned genitalia are very useful. The bag should be emptied and cultured as soon as possible because of the danger of contamination. Older children can usually supply a midstream specimen on request.

Tests of renal function

In children the most important tests of renal function, apart from a full blood count and radiological examination, are as follows:

Urinalysis
Normal urine should contain no reducing substances, acetone or bile pigments. After centrifuging there should be less than four white blood cells per high powered field, no red cells or casts. A urine pH of 5 would exclude a distal renal tubular acidosis. Less than 100 mg of protein should be excreted per 24 hours.

Glomerular function
The *plasma urea* rises when the glomerular filtration rate (GFR) falls, but the rise is not a sensitive measure of GFR and is affected by diet. The plasma creatinine is a better measure of GFR and is useful for long-term follow-up of patients in renal failure. In oedematous patients the *creatinine clearance* can be estimated on a 6–24 hour urine that has been

measured accurately, using the formula:

$$\text{Creatinine clearance} = \frac{\text{urine creatinine} \times \text{urine volume}}{\text{plasma creatinine} \times \text{hours of collection} \times 60}$$

This should be corrected for surface area:

$$\text{GFR} = \frac{\text{height of child (cm)}}{\text{plasma creatinine}} \times 0.45 \text{ ml*/min/1.73 m}^2$$

* If autoanalyser is used multiply by 0.55

Some centres measure GFR by estimating the rate of fall of ^{51}Cr EDTA after a measured intravenous injection. Each laboratory establishes its own method and normal values.

Tubular function
In some renal tubular disorders there may be glycosuria or amino-aciduria.

The ability of the kidneys to concentrate can be tested by measuring the specific gravity (SG) or osmolality of every urine specimen passed over a 24 hour period. The SG should vary from less than 1010 to more than 1020. A urinary osmolality greater than 760 mOsmol/kg indicates normal concentration. If impaired concentration is suspected 5–10 μg of intranasal desmopressin should cause the child to concentrate his urine normally within 9 hours.

Percutaneous renal biopsy
Needle biopsy is indicated for the diagnosis of active renal disease, especially if there is a fall-off in renal function or continued proteinuria, and as a guide to therapy and prognosis. The test should only be done after adequate training in a specialised renal unit. It is mandatory that immunofluorescent techniques and electron microscopy be available to examine biopsy specimens.

CONGENITAL ABNORMALITIES OF THE KIDNEY

Agenesis of both kidneys is obviously incompatible with life but sometimes only one kidney is affected. This and other congenital anomalies may be associated with a single umbilical artery. Potter's facies is seen in some cases and is characterised by low-set ears, prominent folds under the eyes and a small chin. Abdominal muscles may be absent (prune belly) and mega-ureters may be a feature. Agenesis may occur in a baby who appears in other respects to be entirely normal.

Hypoplasia of the kidneys may be unilateral or bilateral. It may or may not be associated with chronic infection. Bilateral cases lead to chronic renal failure, renal rickets and dwarfism. Unilateral cases may be compatible with a long life.

Horseshoe kidney

Horseshoe kidney occurs three times more often in boys than girls. The lower poles of the kidneys are joined by a bridge of renal tissue lying over the fourth lumbar vertebra. The ureters crossing the bridge may become obstructed and urinary stasis and infection occur. The bridge may be felt is some cases but pyelography is required to confirm the diagnosis (Fig. 16.2 H). Characteristically the calyces are directed *towards* the vertebral column. Surgical relief should be considered in symptomatic cases.

Polycystic disease of the kidneys

Two forms are described:

1 Infantile polycystic disease

This is inherited as an autosomal recessive disease. The kidneys are palpable and covered with tiny cysts radially arranged. Hepatic fibrosis and portal hypertension is a common association. Hypertension with secondary congestive heart failure may occur in the first few months of life. Urinary infection may occur and death result from uraemia, unless dialysis and transplantation are undertaken.

2 The adult form

This is inherited as an autosomal dominant disease. As there is far more functional renal tissue than in the infantile form, only 10 % of cases manifest themselves in childhood while 90 % present for the first time over the age of 40 years.

THE PELVIS AND URETER

Hydronephrosis

Hydronephrosis means dilation of the pelvis and calyces of one or both kidneys due to obstruction of urinary flow. It is unilateral when lesions lie proximal to the bladder, whereas it is bilateral in distal lesions (Fig. 16.2 E). The affected ureters and calyces become increasingly distended leading to progressive pressure atrophy of the kidney.

The obstruction may be associated with reduplicated pelvis or ureter (Figs. 16.2 B and C), kinking or stenosis of the ureter, neuromuscular dysfunction, or aberrant vessels crossing the ureter. Infections such as tuberculosis or bilharzia of the ureter must be considered. Rare but important causes of bilateral hydronephrosis in the male newborn are the presence of congenital urethral valve, hypertrophy of the verumontanum or a pin-hole meatus.

Symptoms are due to the obstruction to urinary flow. Abdominal

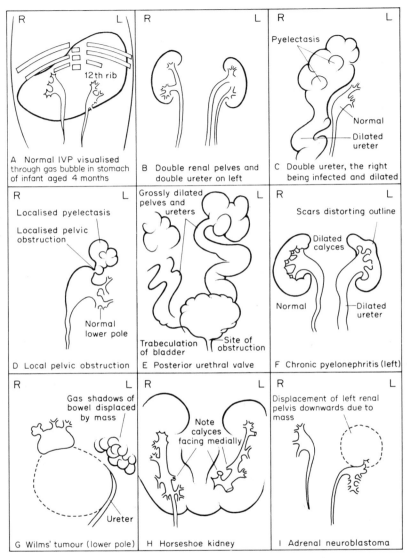

Fig. 16.2 Intravenous pyelograms in various renal diseases

pain or the presence of a palpable, cystic-like mass in the loin may be noted. The presence of dribbling or a poor stream may suggest bladder base obstruction or a posterior urethral valve. An easily palpable bladder after passing a goodly amount of urine would strongly support the latter.

Sometimes symptoms of infection predominate and the infant or child presents with a high fever, with or without urinary symptoms. Rigors and convulsions may occur. Failure to gain weight, sallowness and chronic ill-health may be a feature. The urine usually reveals proteinuria, pyuria and bacteriuria but these may be intermittent and will be discovered only by repeated examination of the urine. Occasionally haematuria may be the presenting feature.

Some cases may present for the first time with evidence of renal failure.

Diagnosis
Diagnosis of hydronephrosis depends on careful history and examination, careful observation of the child's urinary stream, *repeated* urinalysis, full blood count, blood urea, an intravenous pyelogram (Fig. 16.2) and renal echogram. A voiding cysto-urethrogram, isotope renogram and retrograde pyelogram may be helpful.

Treatment
Treatment depends on finding the cause and eradicating it. In difficult cases a urological consultation is advised.

Ureteric reflux

When the bladder contracts normally the lower ends of the ureters close so that all the urine in the bladder is directed via the urethra to the exterior. In some children, however, the urine refluxes back into the ureters, and is associated with recurrent urinary infection. Damage may occur in the presence of infection especially if it is associated with intrarenal reflux. This is a common cause of chronic pyelonephritis in young children and is now referred to as *reflux nephropathy*. The reflux can be demonstrated radiologically by means of a voiding cysto-urethrogram. Some cases are familial.

Treatment
Treatment is initially conservative. The patient should be treated with antibacterial agents until the reflux has ceased spontaneously. The voiding cysto-urethrogram may be repeated every 6–12 months and, if necessary, this treatment can be continued indefinitely. Surgery has little place in this disorder at present but may be necessary for young children with gross vesico-ureteric reflux and intrarenal reflux.

THE BLADDER

Congenital anomalies

Ectopia vesicae

This is the absence of the lower abdominal wall and the anterior wall of the bladder. The delicate, red mucous membrane of the posterior wall of the bladder may herniate through the opening. Nine out of ten cases occur in males and it may be associated with epispadias and inguinal herniae. In females the clitoris is cleft and the vagina exposed. Absence of pubic bones leads to a waddling gait.

Treatment consists of prophylactic chemotherapy and surgery. Plastic repair of the bladder may be attempted, or implantation of the ureters into an 'ileal conduit' may be necessary.

Patent urachus

This is a communication between the bladder and umbilicus. There may be discharge of urine from the umbilicus when the bladder is overfull but may remain asymptomatic throughout life. Treatment is rarely required. Partial obliteration of the urachus may be associated with a midline cyst, but this also rarely needs surgery.

Congenital posterior urethral valves

These lie near the verumontanum. They are valve-like flaps of mucosa in the prostatic urethra which open towards the bladder when a catheter is inserted, but shut when the patient tries to urinate. Complete obstruction leads to bilateral hydronephrosis and an early demise. Partial obstruction may occur and the course of the illness is greatly prolonged. It may present at any time with signs of urinary obstruction or infection. It should be suspected in any boy with a poor urinary stream, hesitancy or intermittency on voiding. A chronically distended bladder with residual urine on emptying may be found, though the residue may disappear because of ureteric reflux.

Diagnosis is confirmed by voiding cysto-urethrography in which the dilated prostatic urethra and the outline of the valves may be seen (Fig. 16.2 E).

Treatment is by prolonged suprapubic drainage, control of urinary infection and excision of the mucosal flaps.

Neurogenic bladder

This is characterised by urinary retention and hypertrophy of the bladder with periodic partial emptying or overflow. It differs from urinary retention due to obstruction by the ease with which manual pressure on the bladder causes emptying. Most cases in infancy are associated with meningomyeloceles but temporary neurogenic bladder occurs in meningitis, encephalitis, poliomyelitis and the Guillain-Barré syndrome. There is often an associated anal incontinence. Urinary infection and hydronephrosis are the rule in cases associated with meningomyelocele.

Treatment
Treatment consists of prophylactic antibacterial therapy. The mother

should be taught how to apply manual pressure to empty the bladder every 3–4 hours. Various surgical manoeuvres have been attempted, such as urinary diversion into an 'ileal conduit' or a bag. In girls intermittent urinary catheterisation, either by the mother or the child herself, is a useful alternative form of treatment.

Hypospadias

This is a condition in which the penile urethra opens on the under surface of the penis, scrotum or perineum. When the opening is proximal to the corona, the penis curves downwards due to the presence of a fibrous cord.

It is important to recognise the severer grades of hypospadias so that the patient may be directed to the urologist for plastic repair and not to the geneticist for chromosome studies. Severe cases may resemble hermaphrodites (p. 210) and require detailed investigation to determine their true sex.

Meatal ulcer

This is an ulcer at the junction of the urethra and skin of the glans and occurs usually within 18 months of circumcision. Friction and ammoniacal urine in contact with the unprotected corona may be factors in its production. Urination may be accompanied by screaming, and sometimes a few drops of blood may be passed. Neglect may lead to meatal stenosis.

Treatment
Treatment in the early stages is conservative. Nappies should be changed frequently and the skin of the glans protected by the application of a silicone barrier cream. The nappies must be washed, the soap removed by frequent rinsing and then given a final soak in an antiseptic such as benzalkonium (1 in 3000). Exposure of the affected penis to air and sunlight for half-hour periods two or three times during the day can only do good. If this is followed by neomycin cream for 2–3 days, healing is likely.

If cure does not take place within a week or ten days, meatotomy with repeated dilatation is advised. The wound is then treated as above.

Phimosis

Phimosis is a narrowness of the opening of the prepuce so that it cannot be drawn over the glans penis. In infants the prepuce is normally adherent to the glans but the secretion of a thick sebaceous material gradually loosens it. By five years of age the prepuce can be drawn over the glans without trouble or force. When, however, as a result of forceful manipulation, the prepuce gets stuck around the rim of the glans and cannot be pulled forward again, it is called *paraphimosis*. This usually occurs because mothers are taught by neighbours, welfare nurses and even doctors gradually to force the prepuce back. There are doctors who think it essential to dilate the 'narrow' foreskin, an error due to incorrect examination (see Fig. 16.1). It should be emphasised that if a child can urinate with a good stream, he does not have phimosis.

Labial adhesion

This is the female equivalent of phimosis except that it is much rarer. The lips of the labia minora are fused together and the only significance of the condition is that it may be confused with abnormal sex organs. In case of diagnostic doubt the lips are easily separated by blunt dissection with a probe. This leaves a raw area which should be dressed with tulles-gras until healed, otherwise fusion may again take place. If left alone, spontaneous separation will take place before puberty.

Hydrometrocolpos

This is the distension of the vagina and uterus with fluid other than blood or pus. It is due to an imperforate hymen and may be noted at birth as a bulging of the hymen. If the diagnosis is missed, it may be picked up at a later age as a mid-line abdominal mass. Incredibly some cases remain undiagnosed until after the menarche when the bulging hymen becomes blood-stained. Treatment is surgical—the sooner the better.

Hydrocele

Hydrocele of the tunica vaginalis is common at birth and disappears before two years of age. If it is associated with an inguinal hernia, surgery is indicated.

BED-WETTING (nocturnal enuresis)

A child who wets his bed beyond five years of age requires treatment. Statistics vary, but it seems that as many as 15 % of all children still wet their beds persistently at night at this age. At puberty figures as high as 3 % have been given and 0.6 % for young adults. There is often a strong family history of enuresis.

Two types are recognised though considerable overlap may occur between them.

1 Primary enuresis

The child with primary enuresis has never, or hardly ever, been dry. Most cases seem to be due to late maturation and they eventually become dry before puberty, though some persist into adolescence. A few have an underlying congenital anomaly or some other organic disease.

2 Secondary enuresis

This occurs in those children who have been dry for long periods, say a year or more, and then become wet again. There is often a history of a 'crisis' in the home such as the birth of a new baby, but sometimes it heralds the onset of some insidious disease in which polyuria occurs, such as chronic nephritis, diabetes insipidus or diabetes mellitus. In some cases it should be recognised that there is a heavy psychological overlay.

Management

A detailed history with emphasis on neurological and urological aspects and a full examination should always be undertaken. In particular sensation around the anus and perineum should be tested for. A rectal examination to test for anal tone and to exclude any masses near the base of the bladder should be performed. Every effort should be made to observe the child passing water lest his stream is poor, intermittent or dribbling. If the bladder was palpable before passing urine it should not be palpable afterwards.

The urine should be carefully examined to include specific gravity, chemical, microscopical and cultural examinations. If there is the slightest doubt about the possibility of organic disease, an intravenous pyelogram and voiding cysto-urethrogram should be done. A blood count, erythrocyte sedimentation and blood urea may be helpful. An EEG may be required to exclude nocturnal epilepsy.

Only when organic disease has been excluded can one talk of 'functional' disorder. Experienced practitioners usually do far fewer tests to reach this conclusion than their younger counterparts but may occasionally slip up as a result.

Treatment

Any organic disorder should first be eradicated if at all possible. Parents should be taught that urine control is a function that matures at different rates in different children. Early potting, disturbing the child from play to urinate, fatigue or excitement may aggravate the condition. The practitioner should try and sort out conflicts between parents and child and the anxiety and fear which the child has for himself.

Active encouragement with rewards such as a gold star for dry nights are helpful in some children. Punishment is likely to aggravate the disorder particularly when it becomes repetitive or meaningless.

Of drugs the best has proved to be the tricyclic antidepressant imipramine. The dose from five to ten years is 10–25 mg before retiring or at 6 pm. *Overdose may cause convulsions and dangerous heart irregularities*. Patients who respond will do so within one month and it is advised to continue therapy for at least six months.

When nocturnal epilepsy is suspected phenobarbitone 30–60 mg may be given in the evening.

The 'Enuresis Alarm Apparatus' consists of two aluminium sheets, one of which contains large holes. The two sheets are separated by a bed-sheet. The patient lies on top of this 'sandwich'. The aluminium sheets are connected to an electric bell. A few drops of urine on the sheets is sufficient to close the circuit and set off the alarm, which wakes the patient up and sends him staggering to the toilet. One should ensure that the mother knows how to use it properly. The method often works but not as often as enthusiasts claim!

GENITO-URINARY INFECTIONS

Infection of the urinary tract is common in childhood, particularly in girls. The infection may spread to the kidney via the blood, particularly in the neonate, or, more commonly, it may spread upwards through the bladder to the ureters and pelvis.

In practice the distinction between upper and lower urinary tract infection may be extremely difficult to make. The term 'cystopyeloneph-ritis' is a blanket word to denote infection of the whole urinary tract, though the term is commonly abbreviated to pyelitis or pyelonephritis.

Important factors in the development of urinary infection include congenital anomalies of the genito-urinary tract, urinary stasis, ureteric reflux and neurogenic bladder. The role of trauma, raised blood pressure, diseases such as diabetes mellitus, and immunological disturb-ances such as hypogammaglobulinaemia may be important in some cases.

Cystopyelonephritis (pyelitis or pyelonephritis)

1 Acute pyelitis

This is common throughout infancy and childhood. The commonest infecting organism is *E. coli*, which is usually the same serotype as that found in the patient's bowel. The enteropathogenic forms almost never attack the urinary tract.

Other organisms which may be isolated are haemolytic streptococci, *Streptococcus faecalis* and staphylococci. During the course of many illnesses such as typhoid, pathogenic organisms are excreted in the urine.

In recurrent and chronic cases, as a result of exposure to antibiotics and instrumentation, *Proteus, Pseudomonas* species, *Klebsiella aerogenes* and mixed organisms may be found.

Clinical features

The acute attack usually begins with high fever which may be associated with pain in the loin, frequency of micturition, rigors, delirium or convulsions. Non-specific symptoms may include anorexia, nausea and irritability. Meningism may be a misleading feature. A child previously dry at night may again wet his bed. Dehydration may result from diarrhoea, vomiting or excessive perspiration.

In infants there may be no localising features at all, or there may be fever, prolonged jaundice, irritability and convulsions.

It should be emphasised that urinary tract infection, like syphilis, is a great mimicker. It may masquerade as a fever of unknown origin, as meningitis, an acute abdomen, gastroenteritis or infective hepatitis.

On the other hand, diagnosis should never be made on the presence of loin pain, frequency or burning on micturition alone. Often such children have perfectly clear urines and other causes such as urethritis or threadworms should be sought for these symptoms.

Diagnosis

Careful examination of the urine, repeated several times if necessary, will usually establish the diagnosis. Proteinuria is usually slight, but the presence of pus cells and culture of the pathogenic organism spell a confident diagnosis. Often blood may be found during the first day or two of the infection but the absence of red cell casts usually excludes acute glomerulonephritis. The presence of white blood cell casts is proof of infection in the kidney itself.

It is worth staining a fresh drop of uncentrifuged urine with Gram's stain. If no bacteria are present the culture is likely to be negative. If organisms are seen there is probably infection, and treatment can begin immediately.

Bacterial count of a freshly voided mid-stream specimen, cultured within an hour, may be helpful. Counts of more than 100 000 bacteria per ml indicate infection, while counts under 10 000 do not. Between these two figures is a doubtful zone which demands a repetition of the test. In infants suprapubic aspiration of urine by needle puncture is justified.

Treatment

If the urine is acid, the infecting organism is probably *E. coli*. The urine may be alkalised by administration of sodium bicarbonate or potassium citrate, and a sulphonamide such as sulphamethizole administered for 14 days in full doses. This may be followed by one-third to one-half doses for 6 months or more, prophylactically. If there is no response by the time the results of urine culture are available (usually within 2–3 days), the antibacterial agent is altered according to the sensitivity tests. Useful drugs include trimethoprim-sulphamethoxazole (Septrin), nitrofurantoin (Furadantin), nalidixic acid (Negram) and various antibiotics.

It is advisable to check the urine weekly for pus cells and bacteria until the patient is cured; thereafter monthly for two years. If recurrence of the infection occurs, then further investigation including an intravenous pyelogram and voiding cysto-urethrogram are mandatory. In fact some authorities insist on these tests after the *first* attack.

Obstructive lesions, stones or ureteroceles should be referred for urgent surgical correction.

Patients with ureteric reflux are treated for prolonged periods with antibacterial drugs until annual repetition of the voiding cysto-urethrogram reveals resolution of the lesion. *Double micturition* is performed two or three times daily to ensure that the ureters and bladder are completely emptied. Urinary stasis invites infection.

2 Chronic pyelonephritis

This is a chronic or recurrent infection of the genito-urinary tract in which progressive coarse scarring of the kidney develops. There is usually a history of recurrent attacks of acute pyelitis as described above, but many cases are so insidious that they are detected for the first time on the autopsy table. The commonest cause is ureteric reflux with associated urinary tract infection. In young infants intrarenal reflux is particularly damaging (reflux nephropathy).

The same factors important in the acute case described above may be operative in chronic cases. The child may present with repeated acute attacks of urinary infection or his symptoms may be related to hypertension (headaches, visual disturbance, anorexia, cardiac enlargement) or renal failure (persistent proteinuria, polyuria, polydypsia and uraemia). Prolonged use of analgesics such as phenacetin can cause a similar picture (analgesic nephropathy). This picture, however, is distinguishable from renal biopsy specimens by some, but not all, pathologists. Intravenous pyelogram may reveal renal scars and dilated calyces (see Fig. 16.2 F).

Pyuria and bacilluria may be intermittent, necessitating repeated testing. With progress of the condition, inability to concentrate urine may become evident. Eventually the kidneys may be indistinguishable from those in chronic nephritis.

Treatment

Therapy is directed to slowing down the progress of the disease. Infection should be eradicated and repeated cultures done. Antibacterial agents are administered according to the results of sensitivity tests. They include sulphonamides, nalidixic acid, or one of the antibiotics ampicillin, cephalexin, carbenicillin, and gentamicin. Nitrofurantoin may sterilise the urine without eradicating the parenchymal infection. All these drugs may be used in greatly reduced dosage when renal failure sets in.

Surgical correction is required for obstructive lesions. Cases with ureteric reflux should be treated as above.

Serum electrolytes should be measured and any disturbances corrected. Acidosis is treated with a bicarbonate-citrate mixture.

The treatment of hypertension and uraemia is discussed on pp. 287 and 288.

Perinephric abscess

Perinephric abscess is usually due to a staphylococcal infection of the perirenal tissues. It may be due to trauma or extension from a renal abscess, or it may follow haematogenous spread.

The onset is with high fever, and rigors may occur. Pain in the renal angle radiates down the thigh, which is flexed due to psoas spasm. The urine is usually clear unless there is an associated pyelonephritis or renal abscess.

As the infection is usually aborted by antibiotics it is uncommon to see the full-blown picture. However, if an abscess forms it causes bulging in the loin and should be drained.

Tuberculosis of the kidney

The disease may be overshadowed by tuberculosis of other organs but it may dominate the picture. Renal pain, tenderness and enlargement may be present, with frequency and dysuria. Persistent pyuria with negative bacterial cultures should suggest tuberculosis. A positive tuberculin test in children under five years of age is highly suggestive, but is very rare.

Treatment
See page 325–326.

Bilharzia

See page 338–340.

THE NEPHRITIDES

Acute post-streptococcal glomerulonephritis [PSGN]

Acute glomerulonephritis is a non-suppurative disorder of the renal glomeruli characterised by the acute onset of haematuria, oedema of the face and body, oliguria, and variable hypertension. It is usually preceded 10–21 days earlier, by a group A type 12 beta-haemolytic streptococcal infection of the throat or type 49 in the skin. Infected scabies or impetigo may be a source of infection, or it may complicate scarlet fever. Soluble antigen-antibody complexes are formed which are trapped in the kidney, forming extracapillary 'humps'. The condition is known as acute post-streptococcal nephritis because the group A beta-haemolytic streptococcus is by far the commonest causative antigen. It is common in the tropics but unusual in the United Kingdom.

Clinical features
Classically the illness begins in a child between three and ten years of age, 10–21 days after a sore throat or other haemolytic streptococcal infection. Puffiness of the face may be the first complaint, or the mother may bring a bottle containing smoky, dirty brown urine for the physician's inspection. Sometimes the child is acutely ill with high fever, malaise, vomiting and headache. Oliguria with a small quantity of very

bloody, dirty brown urine may be present or, less commonly, total anuria. Two-thirds of patients develop some degree of hypertension. Occasionally increasing hypertension may lead to a crisis known as *hypertensive encephalopathy* in which severe headache, somnolence and vomiting is followed by epileptiform convulsions. Left-sided heart failure may be a feature.

On the other hand, some cases of acute nephritis are so mild that they are detected only after repeated urinary examination. It is likely that many cases are not detected at all.

Laboratory findings

The urine is diminished in quantity and contains variable quantities of protein and blood. Granular and red cell casts are invariably present. The casts may be missed if the urine is centrifuged too vigorously, as they are broken up by the spinning force.

The blood count may be normal though usually some degree of normochromic, normocytic anaemia is present. The sedimentation rate is usually raised but can be normal. The blood urea and serum potassium are usually at the upper level of normal, or slightly raised. The ASO (antistreptolysin O) titre is usually over 300 Todd units though it may be normal if the streptococcus is limited to the skin. Therefore to confirm the diagnosis it is best to send the AHT (antihyaluronidase titre) and anti-DNase B as well. Serum complement is low and returns to normal in six weeks. It is best to measure C3 which is very low and C4 which is moderately reduced, as they form the main alternative pathway and are easy to measure.

Throat swab may reveal type 12 beta-haemolytic streptococci in cases that have previously not been given antibiotics.

Renal biopsy is not usually necessary because the prognosis of post-streptococcal glomerulonephritis is usually good. It is done if a significant fall-off in renal function occurs or if proteinuria persists. In the acute phase there is diffuse swelling and proliferation involving the capillary endothelium, the mesangial cells of the capillary stalk, and the epithelial cells of Bowman's capsule. On recovery mesangial proliferation may be very prominent. Severe cases develop epithelial crescents which cause obliteration of the glomeruli and lead to progressive renal failure. The key words are proliferation, exudation and scarring. With immunofluorescent staining complement (C3), immunoglobulin G and other antigen-antibody complexes form a lumpy granular pattern on the basement membrane.

Differential diagnosis

The clinical picture of acute post-streptococcal glomerulonephritis is usually diagnostic. Recurrent attacks are unusual. The *haemolytic-uraemic syndrome* occurs before three years of age, and is associated with clear evidence of haemolysis. Thrombocytopenia usually develops in these cases. *Benign haematuria* is haematuria, in the absence of other symptoms of renal or haematologic disease (Focal nephritis, see below). *Acute pyelonephritis* may present with haematuria but the development of other features such as pyuria and positive bacterial culture soon settle the diagnosis.

Conditions such as sulphonamide crystalluria, bleeding disorders such as scurvy and thrombocytopenic purpura, renal calculi, renal vein thrombosis, tuberculosis, bilharzia and neoplasms can cause haematuria but are excluded by their associated features. A picture similar to acute glomerulonephritis occurs in *Henoch-Schönlein (anaphylactoid) purpura* (p. 104). The presence of a petechial rash concentrated mainly in the buttock area and the occurrence of joint pains may help to differentiate the two.

Prognosis
Over 95 % of patients recover without sequelae. Clinical improvement usually occurs in the first week with diuresis and disappearance of oedema. Microscopical haematuria may persist for several weeks. If the blood pressure is normal the child can usually get up from bed. Severe cases may take 6–12 weeks to settle down. A small percentage become chronic with persistent proteinuria, haematuria, hypertension and slowly progressive renal failure. Occasionally a patient may develop a picture resembling that of nephrosis (p. 288). There may be a long latent period between recovery from acute nephritis and the onset of the chronic phase. A persistent mild albuminuria may be the only warning.

Treatment
The child is initially put to bed and his urine, urine volume, temperature, pulse and blood pressure should be checked at each visit. Frequent blood urea and serum potassium measurements are required. The erythrocyte sedimentation rate (ESR) is *not* helpful in this disease.

As long as there is oliguria, the diet should consist mainly of starchy foods, salt-free butter, cream, honey and jam. Protein is limited to under 30 g per day for the first few days in order not to aggravate the tendency to uraemia. Fruits and fruit drinks are avoided initially because of their high potassium content (40 mmol/l) and no added salt should be given while there is oedema and hypertension. Initially fluids are restricted to 400 ml/m^2 per day, but water, fruit juices, weak tea and weak coffee may be given freely once diuresis occurs. The diet can be improved by the gradual addition of meat, fish, fruit, vegetables and dairy products.

Severe hypertension may be treated with frusemide 16 mg/m^2 by injection. Reserpine reduces the blood pressure in 1–2 hours and it may be repeated 12-hourly as required (*dose* 1.0–2.0 mg/m^2/dose i.m. or i.v. depending on the urgency of the situation). If necessary hydralazine hydrochloride (Apresoline) may be added in increasing doses (0.15 mg/kg/dose i.m. or i.v.). In an emergency sodium nitroprusside (i.v. infusion 0.5–2 μg/kg/min) or diazoxide (5 mg/kg/dose) may be used. Labetalol given intravenously is a good alternative. The blood pressure must be reduced in a controlled manner as blindness can result from a sudden fall from a very high pressure. When the blood pressure returns to normal, a combination of a beta blocker (e.g. propanolol) and a vasodilator (e.g. apresoline or prazosin hydrochloride) may be given orally for a few days. If convulsions occur, phenytoin or diazepam (Valium) may be given parenterally. Phenobarbitone is avoided because it is excreted almost entirely by the kidney, and therefore may accumulate to dangerous levels.

For left-sided heart failure, pulmonary congestion or anuria, frusemide is usually used but on rare occasions peritoneal dialysis may be considered. Frusemide also helps to reduce blood pressure and can help alleviate salt and water retention. Cation-exchange resins may be effective when given orally or as a retention enema in cases of hyperkalaemia.

To clear any residual streptococci from the throat, procaine benzyl-penicillin 600 000 units/m^2 intramuscularly, followed immediately by oral phenoxymethylpenicillin 140 mg/m^2 6-hourly, should be given for 5–7 days. As recurrences of acute glomerulonephritis are rare, prophylactic penicillin is not advised. Corticosteroids are not indicated in this disease, except in the very rare, rapidly progressive nephritis.

Any patient not following the typical course of acute glomerulonephritis should be referred for renal biopsy.

Acute nephritis is *not* an indication for tonsillectomy.

Focal nephritis

This is a form of non-purulent nephritis in which haematuria occurs at the height of an acute upper respiratory infection. There may be a single attack or the patient 'passes blood with every infection'. There is a rare form of focal nephritis which is familial and associated with deafness (Alport's syndrome).

The infection should be treated vigorously and recovery is prompt. However, microscopic haematuria or a slight proteinuria may persist and the development of chronic nephritis is a real danger.

The nephrotic syndrome

The nephrotic syndrome in children is characterised by generalised oedema, massive proteinuria and low serum albumin. The blood urea is normal but the serum cholesterol is raised. It is commoner in boys. Most patients are under five years of age at the onset of the illness.

In childhood the vast majority are of unknown aetiology. Kidney biopsy in 90 % of cases reveals 'minimal change lesions', which respond well to corticosteroids. In 9 % of children focal glomerulosclerosis is found. This group includes patients with a bad prognosis who usually do not respond to corticosteroids. Other proliferative forms of nephritis have been identified and include patients with a mixed picture of nephritis. These, too, do not usually respond to corticosteroids.

Other causes of the nephrotic syndrome include dissemminated lupus erythematosus, mercury poisoning, Tridione and penicillin hypersensitivity, but these are exquisitely rare in children. In parts of tropical Africa *Plasmodium malariae* infection is a common cause.

Clinical features

'Minimal change' type of nephrosis occurs commonly between the ages of two and four years. There is a gradual or abrupt onset of generalised oedema, associated with secondary hyperaldosteronism. Hydrothorax, ascites and hydrocele are common and may dominate the clinical picture. Symptoms may be limited to tiredness and lack of appetite.

Urine output is greatly diminished, the urine being loaded with protein. Hyaline, granular and cellular casts are found. There may be 6 g or more of protein in the urine daily. Blood is not usually found in the urine but sometimes transient microscopic haematuria may occur.

Plasma albumin often falls below 25 g/l. The blood urea remains normal. Plasma complement, which is low in acute glomerulonephritis, is normal in the nephrotic syndrome. The immunoglobulins are reduced, hence the liability of the patient to infection, notably pneumococcal peritonitis. Diarrhoea and vomiting are common.

The erythrocyte sedimentation rate is usually very high because of increased rouleaux formation and does not indicate the severity of the disease. Anaemia, if present, is usually mild.

Course

Minimal change nephrotic syndrome is a disorder characterised by remissions and recurrences. It is estimated that with modern therapy more than 90 % of children will recover completely, despite recurrences. The development of haematuria, hypertension or uraemia are bad prognostic signs which usually indicate one of the other causes of the nephrotic syndrome.

Treatment

Infection should be controlled by benzylpenicillin (300 000 units/m^2 i.m. twice daily) as the pneumococcus and streptococcus are normally sensitive. While oedema persists a low salt, adequate protein (40 g/m^2/day) diet is indicated. With diuresis the serum sodium and potassium levels fall and may require replacement.

Prednisolone is the favoured corticosteroid, the dose is 10 mg/m^2 6-hourly until there has been an adequate diuresis (usually about the tenth day), proteinuria disappears and the serum protein pattern returns to normal (about 3–4 weeks). Others give prednisolone as a single daily dose of 60 mg/m^2 or 2 mg/kg/day. Once the urine has been clear for three days to two weeks, the daily dose may be given as a single dose on alternate *mornings* (maximum 80 mg every 48 hours). This is then gradually tailed off over 6–8 weeks.

Should recurrence occur, the full therapeutic dose should again be given. If there is no response, renal biopsy should be done to determine whether further immunosuppressive therapy will be of value. Some corticosteroid-resistant cases have shown a good response to cyclophosphamide. Occasionally stopping all therapy has had a beneficial effect.

Diuretics such as frusemide and spironolactone may be helpful in the early stages of oedema when corticosteroids are introduced. The serum potassium levels should be watched carefully and supplements given when necessary.

ACUTE RENAL FAILURE IN CHILDREN

Acute renal failure means the rapid onset of severe oliguria or anuria, leading to uraemia, coma and death. It is usually classified into pre-renal, renal and post-renal causes, though considerable overlap may occur. The following are the commoner causes in children:

1 Pre-renal failure
(a) Hypovolaemic (blood, plasma or water loss, e.g. in motor accidents, burns or gastroenteritis).
(b) Hypotensive (shock due to septicaemia, poisoning, diabetic coma or congestive heart failure).

2 Renal failure
(a) Severe post-streptococcal glomerulonephritis.
(b) Severe Henoch-Schönlein disease.
(c) Gasser's haemolytic-uraemic syndrome.
(d) Fulminant ascending acute pyelonephritis.
(e) Acute tubular necrosis associated with persistent pre-renal failure, incompatible blood transfusion, crush injuries or carbon tetrachloride poisoning.

3 Post-renal failure
In this disorder, bilateral obstruction to the urinary tract is due to a lesion in the base of the bladder or urethra. It may present for the first time with uraemia. In infants a posterior urethral valve should be sought; in older children, especially in the tropics, bilharzia or tuberculosis should be suspected.

Treatment of acute renal failure
Pre-renal factors should be treated urgently with the appropriate intravenous fluids lest tubular necrosis supervenes. Central venous pressure should be monitored to avoid overhydration. In renal failure frusemide may be given both diagnostically or therapeutically in the presence of oliguria. An improvement in urinary flow is not necessarily a good sign as the quality of the urine may be poor. Obstruction to urinary flow should be relieved surgically.

Table 16.1 Approximate daily water, glucose, fat requirements in anuria for different weights

| Weight in kg | 6.5 | 10 | 23 | 40 | 70 |
Age in years	4 months	1	7	12	Adult
Water (ml)	80–120	100–150	200–300	300–450	400–600
Glucose (g)	40	50	100	150	200
Fat (g)	20	25	50	75	100
Protein (g)*	5	6.25	12.5	18.75	25
Approx. calories (kcal)	350	450	900	1350	1800
Approx. energy (kJ)	1400	1800	3600	5400	7200

Hycal is a flavoured liquid dextrose concentrate which provides 248 kcal/100 ml, for oral or intragastric administration. However it has a high water content which may lead to fluid overload. *Caloreen* is a synthetic glucose substitute and is less sweet than Hycal. Fluid overload is unlikely as it is in powder form.
* More protein may be offered if the patient is on dialysis
Adapted from: Catzel, P. *The Paediatric Prescriber* (5th Edition) Blackwell Scientific Publications (1981).

The aim of therapy in anuria is to prevent a rise in blood urea and serum potassium, and to maintain the blood volume and composition as near to normal as possible. The recommended intake is shown in Table 16.1.

Fats are no longer recommended in large doses, but *small* amounts of both fat and first-class protein may be given; (a medium egg contains 6 g protein and 100 ml milk contains 3.5 g; beef and chicken contain 22 g protein per 100 g portion).

The daily amount of urine is measured and this volume is given as additional water on the following day.

Hyperkalaemia is controlled by the oral or rectal administration of calcium resonium (*dose*: 8–15 g/m²). If the serum sodium is below 120 mmol/l then sodium resonium may be used in preference.

On this regime the urea level in the blood should not rise more than 3.4 mmol/l/day, but it may rise to 16 mmol/l/day in the presence of hypercatabolic states (trauma, burns and sepsis). *Peritoneal dialysis* should begin before the blood urea reaches 32 mmol/l, especially in small children. When the blood urea falls below 16 mmol/l a more adequate diet should be given.

Peritoneal dialysis should be continued intermittently if necessary for 4–6 weeks. If technical difficulties make this impossible the child should be referred for intermittent haemodialysis with a view to renal transplantation.

Chronic renal failure

Chronic renal failure is the end-stage of a number of diverse renal diseases such as pyelonephritis (reflux nephropathy), some cases of nephrotic syndrome, focal nephritis, Henloch-Schönlein disease, poly-cystic disease of the kidneys and many others. It is recognised by progressive inability to concentrate or dilute urine until eventually the specific gravity becomes fixed at 1010. It is accompanied by a slowly progressive uraemia.

The child may present with tiredness, lack of appetite, swelling, shortness of breath or headache. Thirst and polyuria may lead to bed-wetting. Electrolyte disturbances, dehydration and metabolic acidosis may be associated with hypertension, heart failure and uraemia. Pericarditis is a late sign and hiccoughs may be intractable. Some degree of anaemia is invariably present. Pruritus, purpura and pigmentation occur in advanced cases. Renal rickets and dwarfing may be present with or without renal glycosuria and amino-aciduria. The child is notoriously susceptible to infection.

Diagnosis
Diagnosis depends on a careful history and examination. The urine invariably shows some degree of proteinuria, and a few blood cells or large, broad casts may be present. Cultures should always be done to exclude secondary infection. The specific gravity may be fixed at 1010. Ability to concentrate and dilute urine is impaired, as is the creatinine clearance. The blood urea is raised to a variable degree.

An intravenous pyelogram should be done to exclude obstructive lesions which are surgically correctable. If the kidney is scarred and contracted, needle biopsy is contra-indicated in childhood.

Treatment
Treatment is directed at relief of the underlying lesion and conservation of the remaining renal function.

During the polyuric phase large volumes of fluids should be given to prevent dehydration. Initially the diet can be reasonably normal but as failure progresses restriction of fluid, salts and protein become necess-ary. The bulk of calories are obtained from Hycal and small amounts of fat if they can be tolerated. Protein should be reduced to about 10 g/day for children from 5–10 years of age. For metabolic acidosis 2–3 g sodium bicarbonate daily may be allowed.

Daily weighing may give one a good indication of sodium and water retention. Anaemia is common and it is doubtful if this should be treated unless the haemoglobin falls below 6 g/dl in children. Packed blood cells are used (10 ml/kg body-weight).

A diastolic blood pressure above 90 mmHg requires treatment. Vomiting and hiccoughs may respond to parenteral chlorpromazine, the adult dose being 25 mg intramuscularly.

Hyperkalaemia, often associated with hypocalcaemia and hyper-magnesaemia may damage the heart. A high serum potassium may be lowered with sodium or calcium resonium orally or rectally. Calcium gluconate may be given intravenously under ECG control.

Renal rickets may require very large doses of vitamin D (see p. 76). Restlessness should be controlled by *small* doses of short-acting barbiturates such as quinalbarbitone 15–30 mg/m² or chloral hydrate 150–300 mg/m².

Infections should be vigorously treated. Antibiotics such as penicillin and gentamicin are excreted entirely by the kidney and therefore should be given in greatly reduced dosage in the presence of oliguria.

Patients should be referred to specialised units for renal dialysis and renal transplantation. Continuous ambulatory peritoneal dialysis is proving a successful alternative to haemodialysis in some patients. The results of transplantation are better than in adults.

Renal tubular defects associated with rickets

Rickets due to renal tubular defects occurs in hypophosphataemic vitamin D resistant rickets and the De Toni-Fanconi syndrome. These disorders, together with rickets caused by chronic renal failure, are described on pp. 74–77.

Tubular disease associated with chronic renal disease

In chronic nephritis from any cause four defects of the tubule may present themselves:

1 Defect in concentration of water.
2 Electrolyte loss, e.g. sodium, potassium or calcium.
3 Acid-base disturbances.
4 Glycosuria and amino-aciduria.

These defects may dominate chronic renal disease and thus confuse the diagnosis, especially when evidence of glomerular disease is not clear-cut. Treatment is discussed under 'Chronic Renal Failure' (above).

Nephroblastoma (Wilms' tumour)

Two-thirds of cases of Wilms' tumour occur in the first three years of life. Commonly the mother notices an abdominal swelling, or fever and abdominal pain may be the leading features. Haematuria is surprisingly rare. Examination reveals a firm, non-tender mass attached to the kidney. Sometimes it may be remarkably large before it is detected.

Wilms' tumour is a developmental tumour (embryoma) of the kidney which contains both sarcomatous and tubular elements. It is the commonest malignancy of the genito-urinary tract in children.

X-rays may reveal a soft tissue opacity displacing the bowel in the renal area. This is confirmed by intravenous pyelography which shows distortion of the calyces by an intrarenal mass (Fig. 16.2 G, p. 276).

If Wilms' tumour is strongly suspected and the opposite kidney is normal, the patient is given a dose of actinomycin D pre-operatively and laparotomy done to confirm the diagnosis.

The tumour is usually encapsulated but may have invaded the renal pelvis, ureter, veins and neighbouring tissues. The larger the tumour, the more likely one is to find haemorrhage and necrosis. Frozen sections are examined by a pathologist and, if Wilms' tumour is confirmed, the tumour, or as much of it as possible, is removed. Before closing the abdomen, some units advise marking the limits of the tumour site with Cushing's silver clips as a guide to postoperative irradiation. If the tumour is well-encapsulated and completely removable irradiation is not necessary. This is especially true before the age of one year as the prognosis of these babies is very good.

The use of actinomycin D has improved the prognosis considerably and its use is advised even where liver and lung metastases are evident.

Differential diagnosis

Adrenal neuroblastoma may cause confusion with Wilms' tumour. However, constitutional symptoms are more marked in neuroblastoma, the mass pushes the kidney downwards, it tends to cross to the opposite side, and it tends to be harder and more fixed (Fig. 16.2 I). Secondary deposits to the liver or skull occur early, and VMA excretion in the urine is increased. *Congenital infantile cystic kidneys* form bilateral swellings and the X-ray picture is characteristic. *Retroperitoneal sarcoma* may cause diagnostic problems but is extremely rare.

Other tumours such as hamartomas, teratomas and haemangiomas are very rare. *Lindau-Hippel's disease* is characterised by cysts and adenomas of the kidney and pancreas associated with haemangiomas of the brain and retina. The condition is usually asymptomatic until adulthood.

CHAPTER 17

VIRAL INFECTIONS

The diagnosis of viral infection is based on the clinical picture and, when necessary, on laboratory tests. Attempts may be made to isolate the virus by culture of the appropriate secretion or excretion. In many cases the demonstration of an antibody response is appropriate, a rising antibody titre during the course of the disease being significant. Consultation with the local viral laboratory can be fruitful in unusual febrile illnesses.

The following viral infections can now be prevented by artificially induced immunity (active immunisation):

1 Poliomyelitis by oral vaccine.
2 Measles, mumps and rubella by injection.
3 Yellow fever by injection.

The following vaccines are used on special indication only:

1 Influenza by injection.
2 Rabies by injection.
3 Cytomegalovirus (under investigation)
4 Adenovirus by oral enteric-coated capsule.
5 Certain encephalitides.

THE EXANTHEMATA

The exanthemata are a group of viral infections which produce a characteristic rash at some stage during the illness.

Measles (rubeola)

Measles is an acute, highly communicable disease due to para-myxovirus, characterised by prodromal upper respiratory infection and a buccal enanthem (Koplik spots), which is followed by a dusky maculo-papular rash.

Clinical features
Ten days after contact with a case of measles the patient develops characteristic prodromal symptoms. There is a fever, conjunctivitis, running eyes and nose and a dry painful cough. The child feels and looks miserable. Two or three days later the pathognomonic Koplik's spots appear. These are usually seen on the buccal mucosa opposite the lower

molars, sometimes on the lower lip. They are tiny whitish spots surrounded by a red halo, and are best seen in bright daylight. The spots fade after about 12 hours but may last for 2–3 days.

Four days after the onset of these prodromal symptoms the temperature may rise to 40°C and a dusky macular rash appears behind the ears, on the cheeks and on the neck. It spreads downwards becoming increasingly maculopapular, reaching the lower chest in 24 hours and the tips of the fingers and toes by 48 hours. By this time the fever has broken, the child feels much better and can no longer be kept easily in bed. The rash starts fading on the face and disappears in the same order as it appeared. On disappearing a fine itchy desquamation of the skin may be noted.

In severe cases the rash becomes confluent and blotchy, and petechiae and ecchymoses may appear. Bleeding from the mouth and bowel may occur ('haemorrhagic' or 'black' measles).

In measles cervical lymph nodes are often palpable and the spleen may be tipped. Leucopenia is usual.

Diagnosis
Diagnosis may be confirmed by virus isolation, complement fixation or virus neutralisation tests, but this is rarely necessary as the clinical picture is so typical.

Differential diagnosis
In *roseola infantum* the fever disappears the same day as the rash appears. In *rubella* enlarged posterior occipital lymph nodes are usual and the rash less striking. In *rickettsial infection* the rash spares the face but excruciating headache is usually present. *Drug rashes* (phenytoin, phenobarbitone, sulphonamides, ampicillin) are not usually associated with fever, cough or conjunctivitis unless they were originally given for these symptoms. *Meningococcal septicaemia* is also not associated with cough and conjunctivitis. *Streptococcal rashes*, as in scarlet fever, are finer, feel like 'goose pimples' and are associated with strawberry tongue and circumoral pallor.

Complications
Pruritus is common. Otitis media and bronchopneumonia are probably due to secondary infections with streptococci, pneumococci and *Haemophilus influenzae*. Rarely giant cell pneumonia may occur. Tuberculin tests may become negative for six weeks or longer after an attack of measles due to depression of T-cell function.

Encephalitis is a rare complication (1 in 1000 reported cases), usually occurring 5–7 days after the measles rash appears. It may be associated with mild *or* severe measles. It is due to direct viral invasion of the nervous system which may cause demyelination. Occasionally encephalitis appears 5–7 years after measles (subacute sclerosing panencephalitis, see p. 179). This type has a grave prognosis.

Prevention and control

The patient should be isolated until his temperature has been normal for 48 hours. Contacts need not be isolated until days after being in contact with a known case, as they are not infectious during the incubation period of the disease, only during the prodromal period. Measles may be attenuated by giving a small dose (250 mg at one year, 500 mg at seven years) of Human Normal Immunoglobulin B.P. within 5 or 6 days of exposure. Double this dose is required for prevention.

Measles can also be prevented by active immunisation with a *live attenuated vaccine*. This is normally given at 15 months of age. In malnourished children measles is very severe and it is recommended that the vaccine be given as early as six months and repeated at 15 months of age. About one-third of patients have no reactions to the vaccine, one-third may have a slight fever and rash, and about one-third develop a mild attack of the disease. Most, however, do develop a solid immunity to measles for at least five years, perhaps life-long. It should be remembered that live attenuated measles vaccination is ineffective in the first 6–8 months of life as passively transferred antibodies from the mother are present. It is of interest that in Hindu cultures measles is attributed to a goddess and scientific treatment is not permitted.

Prognosis

In developed countries the prognosis is very good but in poorly developed countries an epidemic of measles may be disastrous.

Treatment

Nursing the patient in a partially darkened room is comforting when he has photophobia. An oral nasal decongestant such as Actifed helps reduce secretion. Fever is treated with antipyretics such as aspirin or paracetamol. Chloral syrup or elixir promethazine may be used as sedatives while Calamine lotion soothes the skin. Humidification of the atmosphere and mucolytics may soothe the dry hacking cough. Hypromellose eye-drops soothe the eye.

Antibiotics are ineffective in viral infection but should be used if secondary infection such as otitis media or pneumonia develop. They should not be given to *prevent* these complications because this invites the colonisation of antibiotic-resistant organisms.

German measles (rubella)

Rubella is a common, usually mild, infectious disease characterised by enlarged tender occipital, post-auricular and other lymphatic nodes and a rash. In older children joint swelling and purpura may occur. In early pregnancy it may be transmitted across the placenta and the infant may develop the *congenital rubella syndrome*. After birth viraemia is associated with the '*extended rubella syndrome*', and virus may be isolated from the baby's secretions for prolonged periods. It has been reported that rubella virus in Japan has an extremely low teratogenesis rate.

Rubella is caused by a togavirus which can be isolated from nasopharyngeal secretions, blood, urine and faeces during the acute phase of the illness. It has also been isolated from aborted fetuses.

Clinical features

14–21 days after contact, infected children develop mild prodromal symptoms. Characteristically, the occipital, postauricular and posterior cervical lymph nodes are enlarged and tender. Sometimes there is a generalised adenopathy and the spleen is often palpable. A fine pink enanthem may be seen on the palate, and the throat may be reddened. Twenty-four hours later a fine punctate or maculopapular rash appears on the face and spreads rapidly downwards. At the same time an erythematous flush may occur. The rash clears up on the third day. Fever, if present, begins at the height of the rash and rarely exceeds 38°C. A slight leucopenia may occur. Many cases are completely asymptomatic.

Rubella is an important disease because of its devastating effect on the fetus in early pregnancy. Up to 50% of infants of mothers infected early in pregnancy may develop the congenital rubella syndrome, the figure varying from epidemic to epidemic and from country to country. The common findings are congenital deafness, cataracts, congenital heart disease (especially patent ductus arteriosus), microcephaly, meningoencephalitis and mental retardation. Other skeletal, muscular and dental anomalies may occur. The virus is not strictly cytopathogenic, but retards the growth-rate of the affected cells.

In addition to these congenital anomalies, the baby may have a persistent viraemia due to a depression of immunoglobulin function and inability to inhibit viral growth ('extended rubella syndrome'). This results in fever, failure to gain weight, anaemia, thrombocytopenia, hepatosplenomegaly, jaundice, recurrent pneumonia, encephalitis and heart failure. The infant may shed virus from nasal and other secretions for 12 months or more after birth and should be regarded as highly infectious. He is the epidemiological carrier of the disease.

Mild cases of the congenital rubella syndrome may occur. The sole finding may be a unilateral cataract, a heart murmur or slight deafness which only becomes manifest when the child develops speech problems. Also the mother may have had a subclinical infection and the only evidence that she has had rubella is the demonstration of abnormal antibody titres.

Diagnosis

Diagnosis in pregnant women should be confirmed by serologic tests. Acute and convalescent sera should be tested for antibody response by haemagglutination inhibition or complement fixation. Rubella antibodies increase four-fold or more, two weeks after the onset of the illness. Rubella complement fixation antibodies are detectable three weeks after exposure. Rubella-specific IgM antibodies indicate recent infection. Virus can be cultured one week before the rash appears to five days after. However, it may take 3–4 weeks to culture the virus in the laboratory. In the newborn, virus may be isolated from nasopharynx, urine, faeces, tears and cerebrospinal fluid. Rubella-specific IgM in infant serum is diagnostic of *in utero* infection.

Differential diagnosis
In *scarlet fever*, although the rash may be similar to rubella, there is greater toxaemia and definite tonsillitis. Even mild cases of *measles* have Koplik spots, whereas the rubella enanthem is on the palate. *Roseola* is characterised by disappearance of fever on the day that the rash appears. *Drug rashes* are not associated with enlarged tender cervical lymph nodes. *Glandular fever* is associated with atypical lymphocytes in the blood and a positive Paul-Bunnell test.

Complications
Encephalitis, arthritis and peripheral neuritis may occur.

Prevention and control
Every girl between 11–14 years should be offered rubella vaccine. Pregnant females should avoid contact with the disease in the first 14 weeks of the pregnancy. The question of therapeutic abortion must be weighed according to the legal requirements of the country in which the physician practises. Definite proof of infection and the time at which it has occurred must be obtained by laboratory investigations.

Girls of childbearing age who receive rubella vaccine should avoid pregnancy for at least two months after the injection. No fertile female should receive vaccine without prior establishment of her immune status. The vaccine may not give permanent immunity.

Treatment
Treatment is symptomatic.

Roseola infantum (Exanthem subitum)

Roseola is an acute disease of infancy which is unique in that the temperature falls on the same day that the rash appears. It is thought to be due to a virus though no virus has been identified.

Clinical features
After an incubation period of 10 days (range 7–17 days) the infant suddenly develops a high fever. It may be ushered in by a convulsion. There are insufficient physical signs, no more perhaps than slight redness of the throat, to account for the fever. The white count may be high on the first day but there is a leucopenia on the second and subsequent days. On the fourth day, just when the parents are becoming panicky about the persistently high fever, it falls by crisis. A fine macular rash appears

and is best seen behind the ears and on the trunk. The rash disappears within 12–24 hours. In older infants puffiness of the eyes may occur. The disease occurs mainly between six months and two years of age, sometimes earlier, sometimes later. The diagnosis is clinical. The differential diagnosis is the same as for measles and rubella (p. 296). Recovery is usually uneventful though occasionally an encephalitic picture may develop.

Treatment
Fever should be reduced if over 38.5°C by means of aspirin or paracetamol and cool sponging. The latter is facilitated by giving chlorpromazine first to inhibit shivering.

Fifth disease (Erythema infectiosum)

Fifth disease is a mild disease occurring in circumscribed epidemics. It is probably due to a virus though none has so far been identified. It occurs in all ages.

After an incubation period of 6–14 days the patient may develop a rash on the cheeks which become unusually red ('slapped cheeks' rash). Macules which may become raised and resemble erysipelas appear, followed after a day or two by an erythematous maculopapular rash on the back of the hands and dorsum of both upper and lower limbs and buttocks. Subsequently it spreads to the flexor surfaces, but usually spares the trunk. After three or four days, and sometimes after several weeks, the rash fades in a very irregular 'lacey' manner. On exposure to a hot bath, cold or sunshine, the rash characteristically reappears. There are no characteristic laboratory findings and, more importantly, no known complications.

Differential diagnosis
The *butterfly shaped rash* on the face must be differentiated from *erysipelas, enterovirus infection, drug reaction* and *lupus erythematosus*, by the history and the mild but persistent course of the disease.

Treatment
Usually none is necessary. Calamine lotion can be used if the rash is itchy.

THE POXVIRUSES

Smallpox (Variola)

In 1979 the World Health Organisation declared that the disease smallpox had been eliminated from the earth. Travellers no longer require vaccination certificates against the disease and the practice of vaccinating babies is no longer necessary.

Chickenpox (Varicella)

Chickenpox is an acute, highly contagious viral disease, characterised by crops of macules, vesicles and papules with a centripetal distribution. It is caused by a herpes group virus called *Herpesvirus varicellae*. The same virus causes herpes zoster.

Clinical features
After an incubation period of 15 days (range 10–20 days) the child develops a low-grade fever, malaise and rash on the first day of the illness. The rash starts with a crop of macules which become papules and vesicles and begin crusting in rapid succession. The vesicles are thin-walled, superficial and surrounded by a red halo. While one crop dries up, successive other crops appear for four or five days The scabs dry up leaving a small pale depression. Scarring only occurs in lesions which have been secondarily infected as a result of scratching. The lesions predominate over the trunk, being fewer over the distal parts of the extremities (centripetal distribution). Lesions may appear on the mucous membranes of the mouth and may be found on the scalp. The height of the fever occurs when the rash is at its maximum.

Haemorrhagic varicella is a rare but severe form of the disease occurring in patients with poor immunological response, particularly children on corticosteroid therapy.

Diagnosis
The diagnosis is made on the typical clinical picture. Mild cases with only a few lesions may be missed, while very severe varicella may resemble smallpox. Complement-fixing antibody is present in the serum in the first week.

Differential diagnosis
This must include impetigo, papular urticaria (insect bites), scabies, rickettsial infection, eczema vaccinatum and herpes zoster.

Complications
Complications are rare and include encephalitis, hepatitis, secondary bacterial infection and pneumonia. Congenital varicella is due to intra-uterine infection. Fatal varicella may occur after corticosteroid administration.

Prognosis
Prognosis is excellent and an attack provides prolonged immunity.

Treatment
Treatment is symptomatic. The nails should be kept short to reduce the damage caused by itching. An antihistamine such as promethazine or trimeprazine orally may be helpful for itch. Calamine lotion may be used. For fever paracetamol or aspirin are effective. Antibiotics should only be used for secondary infection.

If a patient on corticosteroid or immunosuppressive therapy comes into contact with a case of varicella, he should be given a large dose of varicella-specific immunoglobulin in order to reduce the likelihood of infection.

Children with chickenpox should be kept out of school until the vesicles dry. The scabs are not infectious. Normally quarantine is not recommended as the illness is so mild, and it is safer to get the disease in childhood than in adulthood when it can be very unpleasant. High risk patients should receive varicella immunoglobulin and be isolated.

Molluscum contagiosum

Molluscum contagiosum consists of waxy, white or pale pink papules 2–10 mm in size, with central umbilication, due to a poxvirus. These lesions never occur on the palms or the soles. They are treated by shelling the molluscum body, which consists of white cheesy material. This is achieved by pricking the base with a scalpel and curetting, or squeezing between two fingernails.

Herpes zoster (shingles)

Herpes zoster is an acute infectious illness characterised by a vesicular rash confined to one or two dermatomes. It is unusual before the age of ten years. It occurs usually in patients who have previously had chickenpox, but occasionally occurs at the same time as chickenpox. Susceptible children who are inoculated with vesicle fluid from a patient with zoster may develop chickenpox.

Clinical features
After an incubation period of 7–12 days the patient feels pain and tenderness along the distribution of a peripheral nerve, usually on only one side of the body. Papules, which rapidly vesiculate, appear over the affected dermatome. Generalised malaise and fever may be present, while successive crops of vesicles may occur over a period of a week. In children the lesions usually dry and clear before the fourteenth day. The regional lymph nodes are invariably swollen.

Complications
Involvement of the supra-orbital branch of the trigeminus nerve may lead to corneal ulceration. Involvement of the seventh nerve may cause paralysis of the facial muscles on the affected side and vesicles in the ear canal (Ramsay Hunt syndrome).

Diagnosis
The pain which occurs before the rash appears may be confused with pleurisy, pericarditis or peritonitis. Migraine may be considered. Once the typical vesicular rash, which is limited in its distribution to a single nerve, appears the diagnosis becomes obvious. Herpes simplex may resemble zoster occasionally but pain is absent.

Prognosis
Prognosis is good. Post-herpetic pain has not been described in childhood.

Treatment
Treatment is symptomatic. The lesions may be dabbed with mercurochrome or an antiseptic powder. Secondary infection may require antibiotic therapy. Itch may be treated with a sedating antihistamine. Pain is rarely a problem in children. Topical idoxuridine has been used with success.

Herpes simplex

Primary herpes simplex occurs in patients who do not have circulating antibodies, while secondary herpes infection occurs in those that do and tends to be recurrent.

Primary infection in the newborn
This is a severe generalised disease, usually due to herpes simplex virus type 2, contracted from the mother who is non-immune. A week after birth symptoms resembling acute septicaemia may occur, i.e. vomiting, anorexia, high or low fever, jaundice, stomatitis or purpura. Sometimes a vesicular rash may be present anywhere on the mucous membrane or skin. Pneumonia or encephalitis may develop. Treatment is supportive. If pseudomonas infection supervenes gentamicin or carbenicillin may be given. Acyclovir or cytosine arabinoside may be considered in severe cases. The mortality may be high. Diagnosis is confirmed by isolation of the virus, by finding giant inclusion bodies on scraping of a vesicle and by the development of specific antibodies. Typical virus particles may be found on electron microscopy.

Primary herpes simplex infection in older infants and children
This is usually due to type 1 Herpes simplex virus and may cause herpetiform stomatitis, skin rashes above the waist, keratitis, rhinitis, dactylitis and encephalitis. It may complicate infantile eczema causing Kaposi's varicelliform eruption (p. 304). The type 2 strain is now regarded as the main cause of venereal infections after puberty, vulvovaginitis and rash below the waist, mainly on buttocks and thighs.

Herpetiform stomatitis
This is a very common form of the infection of young children. Although initially vesicles appear in the mouth, one usually sees the lesions *after* the vesicles have ruptured. This leaves a small ulcer 1–2 mm in diameter with a thin red halo around it. There may be only one or two lesions, or the whole mucous membrane of the mouth, tongue, gums and palate may be covered with them. The pharynx and fauces are usually spared, a feature distinguishing it from *herpangina*.

Severe infection including herpes hepatitis may occur in malnourished babies. Constitutional symptoms include high fever, inability to chew or swallow because of pain, dribbling of saliva and foul breath. The gums bleed easily. The condition tends to recur, because the virus almost always becomes latent. Subsequent lesions are always less severe because of immunity.

Treatment

The disease is self-limiting, the illness lasting a week. The mouth lesions may persist for 10–14 days. The mouth should be kept clean with pure glycerine or Oraldine after each meal. Analgesics are usually required for pain. In severe cases tube feeding may be needed to support nutrition.

Herpetiform lesions of the skin

1 *Herpes febrilis* or 'cold sores' ('fever blisters') are recurrent (secondary) lesions of the mucocutaneous junction of the mouth, nose or vulva which occur in association with other illnesses such as coryza, pneumococcal and meningococcal infection, sunburn, emotional stress and even menstruation. They always recur at the same site. Local treatment consists of dabbing the lesions with Friar's Balsam or mercurochrome.

2 *Herpetic whitlow* may occur in children with herpes stomatitis who transfer the infection by thumb-sucking. The lesions are very painful and may take 2–3 weeks to heal. They should never be incised.

3 *Eczema herpeticum* (Kaposi's varicelliform eruption) is due to infection of eczematised skin with herpes virus. The vesicles spread over the affected skin and several crops may recur over a period of a week. The patient may be extremely ill and death may occur from secondary infection or fluid and electrolyte disturbances. Treatment is supportive. Scratching must be prevented using physical restraints and sedation if necessary. Saline compresses or mercurochrome on the lesions may be helpful. Fluid and electrolyte balance and nutrition should be maintained.

Other herpetiform lesions

Herpes eye lesions

These include conjunctivitis and dendritic ulcers of the cornea. These may penetrate deeply and cause perforation, particularly if corticosteroids are administered. Although idoxuridine drops or trifluorouracil are effective in superficial ulcers they are not of much value for the deeper lesions. Some ophthalmologists advise scraping the ulcer and applying an antibiotic eye ointment to prevent secondary bacterial infection. Healing is determined with fluorescein eye drops.

Herpes encephalitis

This resembles other viral encephalitides (p. 177) but is more severe, the patient may present in deep coma and the condition is often fatal. It most commonly occurs in immunologically compromised patients.

RESPIRATORY VIRUSES

Most acute upper respiratory tract infections and many lower respiratory tract infections are caused by viruses and mycoplasma. These include the myxovirus, influenzae A, B and C, paramyxovirus, parainfluenza (1–4), respiratory syncytial virus (another paramyxovirus), adenoviruses (over 30 types) and the picornaviruses (coxsackie A: 24 types, coxsackie B: 6 types, and rhinoviruses: at least 100 types). Although there is much overlapping the following are associated most commonly with certain diseases.

1. *Respiratory syncytial virus* commonly causes acute bronchiolitis.
2 *Parainfluenza virus*, especially type 1, causes the majority of cases of croup. It may produce upper respiratory infections and bronchitis.
3 *Influenza A and B viruses* commonly cause upper respiratory infections during epidemics.
4 *Adenoviruses*, of which there are many types, tend to cause mild or symptomatic respiratory illnesses and conjunctivitis. Sometimes they may cause a fatal pneumonia. Type 12 may cause a very high lymphocytosis.
5 *Rhinoviruses* cause most coryzal infections.
6 *Coxsackie virus* infection is usually limited to the upper respiratory tract. Type A causes herpangina and tonsillopharyngitis. Both A and B types can rarely cause a non-specific undifferentiated illness. A21 ('Coe' virus) causes respiratory infection.

The clinical syndromes associated with these viruses will be found in Chapter 20. Apart from influenza A and B, no suitable vaccines are as yet available against respiratory viruses.

ENTEROVIRUSES

The enteroviruses are small particles with a single-stranded ribonucleic acid core. They may produce asymptomatic infection, non-specific febrile illnesses, or illness relating to the respiratory tract, gastrointestinal tract or central nervous system. Some enteroviruses may be associated with specific diseases, for example:

1 Paralytic poliomyelitis (p. 179) is due to one of the three polioviruses.
2 Herpangina and hand-foot-mouth disease is due to coxsackie A infection.
3 Bornholm disease, benign pericarditis and neonatal myocarditis is due to coxsackie B infection.

On the other hand, the same clinical picture may be produced by several viruses; for example, aseptic meningitis may be due to coxsackie group A or B virus or the numerous ECHO viruses. These three groups of viruses may also cause encephalitis, a febrile illness with rash, or acute respiratory illnesses. Specific strains may be isolated.

Viral hepatitis

See page 263.

Viral infections of the central nervous system

See pages 177–180.

MISCELLANEOUS

Mumps (epidemic parotitis)

Mumps is an acute contagious disease due to a paramyxovirus, characterised by painful enlargement of one or more salivary glands. It is spread by droplet or by contact with fomites contaminated by infected saliva. Epidemics occur at any time of year. Infants under six months are protected by maternal antibodies.

Clinical features
After an incubation period of 17 days (*range*: 14–24 days) children may have mild prodromal symptoms including fever, malaise, headache and neck pain. The parotid gland is the commonest salivary gland to be affected. Swelling starts at the angle of the jaw and spreads forward. It pushes the ear lobe forward and upward. Oedema over the affected part makes the swelling much easier to see than feel. The whole process settles in a week or less. The swelling of one gland is usually followed by swelling of the other within 24 hours, or both glands may swell simultaneously. The pain is aggravated by anything causing salivation, such as acid drops or lemon juice on the tongue. The opening of Stensen's duct, which lies on the buccal mucosa next to the second molar tooth, may pout and be inflamed. In one in ten patients the infection is limited to the submandibular glands. The opening of Wharton's duct in the floor of the mouth is red and swollen. Occasionally the sublingual glands are affected.

Complications
Meningoencephalitis is not uncommon and tends to be milder than that due to other common viral illnesses. Unlike other forms of encephalitis, the CSF glucose in mumps encephalitis may be lowered, causing confusion with bacterial meningitis. *Orchitis* is rare before puberty and occurs with or without concomitant salivary gland infection. The testis is

swollen and very tender. One-third of affected testes may atrophy. *Oophoritis* may cause pelvic pain and tenderness in females, but is rare. *Pancreatitis* may cause acute abdominal pain and vomiting and the serum amylase increases. It should be recalled that the pancreas is a 'salivary' gland and nearly always affected! *Diabetes mellitus*, which may be temporary or permanent, is an occasional complication in children.

Diagnosis
The swelling is usually typical but may on occasion be confused with enlarged lymph nodes. A *slight* rise in serum amylase is due to the parotitis, a *marked* increase to pancreatitis. There is usually a leucopenia unless complications ensue. This causes a polymorphonuclear leucocytosis. Virus can be isolated from the saliva, urine, CSF or blood early in the disease. A rising complement fixation antibody titre occurs.

Differential diagnosis
This includes *suppurative parotitis*, in which pus can be expressed from the duct. *Recurrent parotitis* is associated with sialectasis, in which the swollen ducts can be demonstrated by retrograde injection of lipiodol. *Salivary calculus* usually obstructs Wharton's duct and causes a painless, recurrent swelling of a submandicular gland. *Cervical adenopathy* may superficially resemble parotitis.

Treatment
An attenuated vaccine for the protection of mumps is available and may be given alone or combined with other viral vaccines, such as mumps, measles and rubella vaccine. It provides a solid immunity. Passive immunisation may be achieved with hyperimmune mumps human immunoglobulin.

For local pain and swelling analgesics should be given. Chewing should be kept to a minimum. Sour, acid or highly seasoned foods should be avoided. In severe pancreatitis the use of aprotinin (Trasylol) may be considered as it inhibits the proteolytic enzymes which escape into the blood stream. The dose is 30 000–60 000 units/m^2 by intravenous injection every hour for 8–12 hours, but its value has not been established beyond doubt.

Infectious mononucleosis (glandular fever)
Infectious mononucleosis is a mildly contagious disease caused by the Epstein-Barr virus, a latent herpesvirus of man, characterised by malaise, prolonged fever, sore throats, lymphadenopathy and splenomegaly. Hepatitis with or without jaundice may occur. Non-specific rashes occur in 20 % of patients on the 4th–10th day and may be morbilliform, scarlatiniform or petechial. If ampicillin is administered, which is often done erroneously, a maculopapular rash nearly always appears. Aseptic meningitis or encephalitis are rare manifestations.

Pericarditis should be watched for. About 90 % of young adults have antibodies to the disease. It seems likely, therefore, that asymptomatic infection is common in infancy and only becomes symptomatic in children from 2–10 years of age.

Diagnosis
Diagnosis is established by finding over 10 % 'atypical' lymphocytes in the peripheral blood and sometimes by a positive Paul-Bunnell (heterophil agglutination) test in the first week of the illness. Lymphocytosis appears from the fourth day onward. The use of rapid slide tests, such as the Hoff-Bauer test, may speed up the diagnosis. Rarely thrombocytopenia, anaemia or agranulocytosis may be found. Antibodies to E-B virus can be demonstrated by immunofluorescence or complement fixation tests. It is important to know that some tests for syphilis become falsely positive in the second week of infectious mononucleosis but become negative in about three weeks. Also false positive Paul-Bunnell tests may occur with other viral diseases and after the injection of animal serum (serum sickness).

Prognosis
The vast majority of patients recover completely. Rarely rupture of the spleen may occur. Occasionally hepatitis becomes chronic.

Therapy
Bed rest is suggested initially, the patient being allowed to rise continuously when he feels better. In very ill, toxic patients, especially with severe hepatitis or thrombocytopenia, prednisolone or ACTH may be given for a few days.

Cytomegalic inclusion disease

Cytomegalovirus is a herpesvirus. Cells infected by cytomegalovirus are epithelial or mesenchymal cells which enlarge and have both intranuclear and intracellular inclusions. Infection is acquired *in utero* or perinatally. The baby is usually light-for-date and at birth splenomegaly, hepatomegaly, jaundice, anaemia, thrombocytopenia and purpura may be present. On X-ray of the skull paraventricular calcification may be found, associated with microcephaly, hydrocephaly, mental retardation, optic atrophy and chorioretinitis. Diagnosis may be confirmed by virus culture and complement fixation tests and cytomegalovirus specific IgM.

Prognosis
Congenital cytomegalosis carries a high mortality rate and few neonates with obvious signs and symptoms recover completely. Permanent CNS damage is common. However, there is evidence that most babies have a subclinical infection and these cases have a good prognosis, probably because they possess maternal antibodies against the disease.

By the age of 60, 60–90% of adults have antibodies to the cytomegalovirus. Subsequent pregnancies are likely to be normal, but second babies can be infected due to reactivation of infection in the mother. Such infection is modified by the presence of maternal antibodies as these babies appear normal at birth. The long-term prognosis is not known.

Treatment

Treatment is symptomatic. The use of acyclovir for congenital cytomegalic inclusion disease is under trial.

Cat-scratch disease

The infective agent responsible for cat-scratch disease is unknown. Ten to thirty days after a scratch caused by a cat the child develops a low-grade fever and the lymph nodes draining the site of the scratch swell. A papule appears at the site of the original scratch. A purpuric rash or erythema multiforme develops in some cases. Rarely an encephalitis-like picture may occur.

Diagnosis may be confirmed by skin test using material prepared from an involved lymph node. The chlamydiae group antigen test may be positive.

Differential diagnosis

Cat-scratch disease must be distinguished from simple pyogenic adenitis, tuberculous adenitis, rat-bite fever, bubonic plague, lymphogranuloma venereum, Hodgkin's disease or lymphomas by the appropriate tests.

Treatment

The condition is self-limiting and almost always heals in 1–3 months. If the gland fluctuates it should be drained.

CHLAMYDIAE

The chlamydiae form a large group of Gram-negative obligate intracellular parasites with common group antigens.

Psittacosis

This disease is caused by *Chlamydia psittaci*. It is an ornithosis (bird disease) which is rarely seen in children under ten years. It should be suspected in any child with a 'flu-like illness or respiratory infection who sleeps in the same room as an ill bird. It responds to tetracyclines.

Trachoma and inclusion conjunctivitis

Both these conditions are caused by *Chlamydia trachomatis*. *Trachoma* occurs in tropical climates and is a chronic keratoconjunctivitis in which follicles and pannus formation are associated with scarring and blindness. *Inclusion conjunctivitis* usually presents ten days after birth as an acute purulent conjunctivitis which, if left untreated, can lead to scarring. The diagnosis can be made by examining a conjunctival swab for chlamydia. The inclusion bodies may also be demonstrated by immunofluorescent antibody stain in some centres.

Treatment

Tetracycline eye preparations may be combined with oral erythromycin or co-trimoxazole. In chronic cases of trachoma it clears the secondary infection but recurrences are common.

Chlamydiae may also cause urethritis, vaginitis, pruritis and pneumonia.

CHAPTER 18

RICKETTSIAL AND BACTERIAL DISEASES

RICKETTSIAL DISEASES

Rickettsiae are coccobacilli which cause febrile illnesses associated with rashes. They include typhus and South African tick-bite fever.

Typhus

Typhus may be *epidemic* (louse-borne) or *endemic* (murine). Epidemic louse-borne typhus is caused by *R. prowazekii* which is carried in the bowel of the louse. Children contract the infection through skin abrasions or inhalation of dried louse faeces. After an incubation period of about two weeks the child develops a high fever with rigors, frontal headache and general aches and pains. On the sixth day a fine rose-coloured rash appears on the chest. It then spreads to the rest of the body and limbs, including palms and soles, within eight hours, but avoids the face. Initially the rose-coloured spots disappear on pressure but soon they darken and no longer fade when pressed. In severe cases petechiae appear. Cardiac and renal damage may occur and the patient may die of uraemia.

The illness begins improving during the third week and recovery is usually complete. On the whole the illness is *less* severe than in adults. Recurrence can occur ten and more years after symptomatic infection (Brill-Zinsser disease).

Diagnosis
The severity of the illness and the occurrence of a non-fading rash may be confused with typhoid, meningococcal septicaemia, or measles. Diagnosis is confirmed by serological tests. The Weil-Felix test for OX 19 becomes strongly positive in the second week during the peak of the illness. The indirect fluorescent antibody test is very specific.

South African tick-bite fever

The South African variety of tick-bite fever is caused by *R. conori* var. *pijperi*, which is transmitted by Ixodid ticks. The incubation period is seven days from the time of the bite to the onset of symptoms.

The commonest site of the tick-bite is the scalp or exposed parts of the limbs, but infection can also be introduced through abraded skin or conjunctivae. There is often a primary sore with necrotic centre and tender swelling of the regional lymph nodes.

Seven days after being bitten the child complains of tiredness and increasingly severe headaches. Fever may be intermittent or remittent, photophobia is common and the patient may become delirious. A maculopapular rash develops in direct proportion to the severity of the illness and it may spread onto the palms and soles. The underlying skin may have a dusky cyanotic appearance. The rash may occur in daily crops for several days. Generalised lymphadenitis is usual but the tip of the spleen is felt in less than half the patients. Nevertheless, the left hypochondrium is tender. Myocarditis and arthralgia may occur.

The illness lasts 1–14 days but aesthenia and mental depression may persist for longer. Other complications are rare.

Diagnosis
The Weil-Felix tests are negative during the illness but become positive during convalescence. Either OX 2 or OX 19 or both are agglutinated. Skin biopsy of the papule may be helpful for identifying the Rickettsia.

Q fever

Q fever is often classified incorrectly as a rickettsial disease but is an infection caused by *Coxiella burnetii*. It is included here for convenience. The mode of spread is uncertain but may be by inhalation of the organism. Characteristically there is severe frontal headache, fever, chills and generalised weakness resembling influenza. Pneumonia and pleurisy may sometimes be a feature. Unlike rickettsial diseases described above, there is no rash. Consolidation and effusion may be found unexpectedly on X-ray of the chest. The illness may last 1–2 weeks and convalescence may be prolonged. Fortunately children rarely die of this disease. A complement fixation test is available for diagnosis.

Treatment of rickettsial diseases
The clothes and blankets used by patients during picnicking or camping should be ironed with a hot iron to destroy larval and adult ticks. Cattle dips to destroy ticks are used on farms. Infected animals should be protected with suitable insecticides.

The tetracyclines and chloramphenicol suppress but do not kill rickettsiae. It is suggested, therefore, that antibiotic treatment should not begin until after the fourth day of the illness so that the patient's own immune responses are stimulated. In patients with poor immune responses relapses are common. Treatment is continued until the temperature has been down for 48 hours, usually about five days, (*adult dose*: 1–2 g daily ÷ 4).

For the rest symptomatic therapy, maintenance of fluid and electrolyte balance, as well as of nutrition, are essential.

Prevention
Vaccines are available against most rickettsiae. In endemic areas boosters may be required every 6–12 months.

BACTERIAL INFECTIONS IN CHILDHOOD

Gram-positive infections of importance in childhood include streptococcal, staphylococcal and pneumococcal infections. Most of these are described under the names of the disease they cause, such as pneumonia.

Streptococcal infections

The most important streptococci in human infection include:

1 Group A beta-haemolytic streptococci (*S. pyogenes*) which is the commonest cause of acute bacterial pharyngitis. It is often cultured in skin infections, cellulitis, septicaemia, otitis media, pneumonia and meningitis. Non-purulent complications include acute rheumatic fever, Sydenham's chorea and acute glomerulonephritis.
2 Group B beta-haemolytic streptococci (*S. agalactia*) has come to the fore as an increasingly common cause of sepsis in the first three months of life. It may cause meningitis, otitis media, pneumonia and osteomyelitis in this age group.
3 Group D gamma-haemolytic (non-haemolytic) streptococci (*S. faecalis* or *enterococcus*) may cause endocarditis, urinary tract infection and peritonitis.
4 Non-typable alpha-haemolytic streptococci often referred to as *S. viridans*.

Streptococci release large numbers of antigens such as streptolysin O, streptokinase, hyaluronidase, deoxyribonuclease and Dick toxin. Antibodies to these substances form the basis of diagnostic tests. From a therapeutic point of view almost all beta-haemolytic streptococci remain very sensitive to benzylpenicillin G, especially *S. pyogenes*, *S. agalactia* and, to a lesser extent, *S. viridans*. *S. faecalis* is more likely to be sensitive to ampicillin, though widespread resistance to this and most other antibiotics may occur.

Scarlet fever (scarlatina)

Scarlet fever is an acute streptococcal infection of the throat in which a rash, due to an erythrogenic toxin, appears after about 24 hours.

The incubation period is less than one week, usually 2–3 days. There is a sudden rise in temperature with a very rapid pulse, nausea and vomiting, headache and prostration. The throat is red with petechiae on the soft palate. Follicular tonsillitis may be present with enlargement of lymph nodes. Within 24–48 hours a fine erythematous rash appears in the axilla and groins and spreads to the rest of the body below the chin-line. Circumoral pallor is present, contrasting with the flushed cheeks. *Pastia's sign* consists of hyperaemia of the transverse creases in the elbow which do not fade on pressure. Petechiae may be present. The rash fades in a week or less, leaving a branny desquamation. Two weeks later peeling of the palms and soles may be noted and this may be the only evidence of recent scarlet fever.

The tongue is at first coated with prominent papillae (white strawberry tongue). This desquamates leaving a red strawberry tongue.

Complications
Acute glomerulonephritis and *acute rheumatic fever* may occur in the second or third week, even with mild infections in about 1 % of patients.

Treatment
Benzylpenicillin G is the medicine of choice. Phenoxymethylpenicillin (*adult dose*: 250–500 mg 6-hourly) should be given for at least ten days to eliminate the haemolytic streptococcus. As the child usually feels better within 48 hours it is difficult to persuade mothers to finish the course. An alternative antibiotic is erythromycin which should be given for ten days.

Symptomatic therapy includes aspirin or paracetamol for pain, tepid sponging for high fever, and hot or cold compresses for swollen glands.

The urine should be checked daily for albumin in anticipation of glomerulonephritis. Functional heart murmurs may come and go, and should alert one to the possibility of rheumatic fever. Throat swabs should be taken from all close contacts and those that are positive should be treated with benzylpenicillin or erythromycin.

Streptococcal sore throat

The picture is identical to that of scarlet fever except that there is no erythrogenic toxin and hence no rash. Circumoral pallor, however, is often noted, contrasting with the reddened cheeks. Vomiting and fever may be the initial symptom in children and examination of the throat reveals a follicular tonsillitis or widespread tonsillopharyngitis.

The most dangerous complications are the development of quinsy, acute rheumatic fever or acute glomerulonephritis.

The treatment is as for scarlet fever.

Erysipelas

Also known as St Anthony's fire, erysipelas is a streptococcal febrile illness characterised by fever and a raised, hot, indurated lesion in the skin. The edge is serpiginous and recurrent attacks are liable to occur. Over the face it may have a butterfly shaped distribution. On fading it becomes branny and desquamates.

In the newborn the umbilicus is commonly attacked and the infant may be overwhelmed by the infection.

The swelling should be distinguished from cellulitis in which the border is not raised.

Treatment
Erysipelas is highly contagious therefore the patient should be isolated. It responds to penicillin and erythromycin.

Acute post-streptococcal nephritis

See page 285.

Acute rheumatic fever

Acute rheumatic fever is a complication of group A beta-haemolytic streptococcal infection. The illness is most common between 5 and 15 years, being rare before 4 years of age. It occurs in densely populated areas and in the underprivileged. It is rare in the United Kingdom.

Clinical features
Symptoms of acute rheumatic fever usually begin 10–21 days after a streptococcal infection, especially streptococcal sore throat, scarlet fever or infected scabies. The *major* manifestations of the disease are carditis, polyarthritis, chorea, erythema marginatum and subcutaneous nodules. The heart is usually affected in some degree (see p. 148). The most frequent signs of carditis are a sustained tachycardia and mitral and aortic valve murmurs which change during the course of the illness. Acute rheumatic carditis may lead on to chronic rheumatic valve disease and the risk of subacute bacterial endocarditis. The polyarthritis of rheumatic fever affects one or more of the large sized joints, commonly the elbow. Subsequently the pain leaves one joint to attack another ('flitting and fleeting'). Skin rashes are seen in 5 % of cases. Erythema marginatum consists of a map-like erythema with a thin red raised serpiginous margin and a pink central portion. The lesions vary in size and shape and the pattern changes continually. Rheumatic nodules may be felt in subcutaneous tissue overlying bony prominences such as the occiput and elbows.

The *minor* manifestations of acute rheumatic fever are a previous history of rheumatic fever, arthralgia, fever, a raised erythrocyte sedimentation rate and a polymorphonuclear leucocytosis. The C-reactive protein is strongly positive. Supporting evidence of group A beta-haemolytic streptococcal infection includes finding the organism on throat culture, a raised antistreptolysin O titre or antihyaluronidase titre. Recent scarlet fever, tonsillitis, erysipelas or infected scabies would be additional evidence of streptococcal infection.

Before accepting the diagnosis of rheumatic fever at least two major and one minor manifestation or two minor and one major manifestation should be present.

Treatment
Acute rheumatic fever is one of the few medical conditions in childhood for which enforced bed rest is advised. Penicillin or erythromycin may be

given in full doses every six hours for ten days to eliminate the haemolytic streptococcus. Thereafter smaller doses are given indefinitely to prevent recurrences. Salicylates should be given throughout the illness to reduce fever and the pain of the arthritis. The plasma salicylate level should be kept between 1.5–3.0 mmol/l (20–40 mg/100 ml). Congestive heart failure is treated in the usual way with sedatives, oxygen, digoxin and diuretics. Sometimes corticosteroids are given for heart failure in rheumatic fever. The activity of the disease should be judged clinically and by regular measurement of the sedimentation rate. The ECG and chest X-ray should be repeated as necessary. Acute rheumatic fever may last many months. Prophylactic penicillin should be given to all patients who have had acute rheumatic fever. Either intramuscular benzathine penicillin is given once monthly or oral phenoxymethylpenicillin 125–250 mg twice daily. This should be continued for at least five years, some authorities say for life.

NB Any patient with a history of rheumatic fever, or a family history of rheumatic fever, should be given penicillin prior to dental extraction, tonsillectomy, or other operation in order to prevent subacute bacterial endocarditis.

Sydenham's chorea (St Vitus dance)

Chorea is a *late* and unusual complication of rheumatic fever. By the time the patient gets chorea the acute manifestations of rheumatic fever have completely cleared. In half of the patients affected there is no antecedent history of rheumatic fever.

Clinical features
Chorea is commonest in girls of school age. The onset is insidious, the child becoming increasingly clumsy, often falls or drops objects and involuntary movements occur. The handwriting deteriorates and uncontrollable grimacing or smiling occurs. There may be involuntary clucking sounds, sighing or snorting noises. Choreiform movements are characteristically involuntary, jerky and unpredictable and may be more marked on one side. Occasionally there is marked hypotonia. The abnormal features disappear during sleep. Most patients recover completely in 3–6 weeks but recurrences are common.

Management
The patient is best treated in quiet surroundings as tension, anxiety or noise may aggravate the condition. Feeding difficulties may require the use of infant feeding cups or straws. The chorea in severely affected children may be controlled by haloperidol or tetrabenazine. The best medicine is probably an understanding mother or nurse. Penicillin is given as a rheumatic fever prophylactic.

STAPHYLOCOCCAL INFECTIONS

Staphylococci normally inhabit the skin. Pustules, furuncles and carbuncles may lead to staphylococcal septicaemia, abscesses in almost any organ, staphylococcal pneumonia and meningitis. The introduction of the isoxazolyl penicillins, *flucloxacillin, oxacillin, cloxacillin* and *dicloxacillin* have apparently brought this ubiquitous infection under control, though the victory may be a temporary one.

Clinical 'staph' syndromes

1 Skin infections including whitlows, folliculitis, furunculosis, carbuncles and impetigo.
2 Staphylococcal pneumonia which commonly causes pneumatoceles in the lung in babies (p. 362).
3 Staphylococcal septicaemia which leads to seeding of abscesses via the circulation.
4 Osteomyelitis due to infection of the metaphysis of bone (p. 382).
5 Staphylococcal enterocolitis due to overgrowth by resistant staphylococci in the bowel. This should be distinguished from 'food poisoning' due to a staphylococcal enterotoxin.
6 Staphylococcal sepsis.

Treatment

In all cases of staphylococcal infection the old surgical aphorism applies—'Where there is pus, let it out'. This will often cure the patient. In serious infections such as staphylococcal septicaemia, osteomyelitis, endocarditis or meningitis large doses of penicillin are required. It is safer to give an isoxazolyl penicillin until laboratory culture sensitivities are available. If the staphylococcus is *not* a betalactamase producer, then it is likely to be more sensitive to benzylpenicillin G.

Diphtheria

Diphtheria is due to *Corynebacterium diphtheriae* and is characterised by the formation of a membrane and the secretion of a powerful toxin. Infection is by contact with a patient or a carrier. The organism may be cultured from the affected part and is best grown on Loeffler's medium. Diphtheria is very rare in the United Kingdom; it usually affects children under the age of 14 years.

Clinical features

Faucial diphtheria: after an incubation period of 3 days (*range*: 1–7 days) the patient becomes ill with fever, headache and malaise. The throat is reddened and after 24 hours yellow spots, resembling acute follicular tonsillitis, appear on the tonsils. The spots rapidly coalesce to form a dirty-grey membrane which spreads beyond the tonsils onto the fauces, uvula and pharynx. The child becomes increasingly toxic, the pulse increases out of proportion to the temperature and the blood pressure may fall. Attempts to remove the membrane with a throat swab causes bleeding.

The membrane may spread up into the nose, or the nose may be the initial site of infection (*nasal diphtheria*). A serosanguinous or haemorrhagic discharge with a foul odour may be noted.

In many patients the membrane spreads down to the larynx causing obstruction (*laryngeal diphtheria*). In some cases the infection may be primary in the larynx and lead to laryngeal obstruction. Death from suffocation may occur unless a tracheostomy is done in time. There is often a brawny oedema of the neck which forms a 'collar' from ear to ear, presses on the jugular veins and causes facial congestion ('bull-neck diphtheria').

Complications
Peripheral circulatory failure due to shock may occur in the first 10 days. Myocarditis may also occur within 21 days of the onset. Paralysis of the palate, eye muscles, pharynx, larynx and respiratory muscles may occur between 2−8 weeks due to peripheral neuropathy.

Treatment
The patient should be isolated and, in anticipation of the complications, placed in an intensive care area where full supportive treatment, including tracheostomy and ventilation, can be given.

Specific treatment consists of diphtheria antitoxin in sufficient dose to neutralise the toxin. The patient should receive a test dose to test for sensitivity to antitoxin. In most patients 20 000−40 000 units should be enough but if there is no improvement in 24 hours, more should be given, half intramuscularly and half intravenously. Up to 120 000 units may be needed if there is severe disease which has lasted more than 48 hours. The diphtheria organism is very sensitive to penicillin and erythromycin and either one should be given to prevent further production of toxin.

Diphtheria is a dangerous and contagious infection. Cases should be notified to the Community Physician and expert epidemiological advice sought so that contacts can be traced and treated.

Prognosis
Even with the most sophisticated care the case fatality is about 10 %. The sooner antitoxin and penicillin is given, the better the chances of recovery.

Prevention
To prevent diphtheria, active immunisation of all infants is recommended. Diphtheria vaccine (Dip/Vac) is usually combined with tetanus and pertussis vaccine (DTP/Vac; Triple vaccine) and the first dose is given at 2−3 months of age, the second dose 1−2 months later and the third dose 2 months after that. For convenience a dose of

trivalent oral poliomyelitis vaccine may be given on each occasion.

Before entering school a booster injection of diphtheria-tetanus vaccine may be given.

Diphtheria has become so uncommon as a result of widespread immunisation, that many practitioners have never seen a case. It may reappear in the United Kingdom if higher rates of immunisation are not achieved.

Pertussis (whooping cough)

Pertussis is a highly contagious infection of childhood caused by a Gram-negative bacillus, *Bordetella pertussis*. It is characterised by a prolonged spasmodic cough terminating in a whoop and accompanied by vomiting. It is widely distributed and epidemics occur in densely populated areas every 2–4 years. The organism attaches itself to the ciliated cells of the respiratory tract leading to decreased ciliary activity with necrosis and sloughing of cells.

Clinical features
After an incubation period of 7–14 days the illness is ushered in by *catarrhal* symptoms. Anorexia, nasal discharge and sneezing are associated with a cough, which becomes increasingly severe over a period of ten days. This may merge with the second phase (the *paroxysmal* stage) in which the cough becomes paroxysmal. A staccato machine-gun-like cough is accompanied by congestion or cyanosis of the face and terminates with a sudden loud inspiratory crow (the whoop) and vomiting. The gastric contents contain thick tenacious sputum. The frenum of the tongue becomes ulcerated from rubbing against the lower teeth during spasms of cough. In infants the diagnosis may be missed because the characteristic cough is absent and the baby appears to have a series of cyanotic spells. Subconjunctival haemorrhages are common. Paroxysms of cough or cyanosis may be precipitated by excitement, eating, sudden changes in environmental temperature or inhalation of smoke. The cough is usually much worse at night.

After four weeks the *convalescent period* begins. The appetite improves, the paroxysms of coughing and vomiting get less. However, an intercurrent infection can cause a flare-up of the illness. Night cough may persist for many months or even years.

Diagnosis
The whoop, preceded by a paroxysmal cough, is diagnostic. In mild cases and in infants the whoop may be absent, making the diagnosis difficult. The lungs may be remarkably clear on auscultation unless bronchopneumonia supervenes.

Lymphocytosis occurs in the late catarrhal and early paroxysmal stage, the white count being in the region of 20 000–40 000 per mm^3 of blood or more. The blood sedimentation rate is low.

The organisms can be isolated from the nasopharynx using Bordet-Gengou medium during the catarrhal stage and in the first week of the paroxysmal stage. Fluorescent antibody staining of direct nasal swabs may be helpful.

Differential diagnosis

Epidemics of whooping-cough-like illness have been caused by *B. parapertussis* (which is distinguished from *B. pertussis* by culture) and by adenovirus (in which *B. pertussis* is absent). Atypical cases may be confused with tracheitis, bronchitis, bronchiolitis and interstitial pneumonia. Hilar glands pressing on a bronchus may cause a paroxysmal cough but no whoop. If the cough is of *sudden* onset, foreign body in the bronchus should be considered. If the cough is accompanied by steatorrhoea or excess sweating, cystic fibrosis of the pancreas should be excluded.

Complications

Otitis media, bronchopneumonia, atelactasis and emphysema may occur. Bronchiectasis is a serious complication. Excess vomiting may lead to emaciation and metabolic alkalosis with all its consequences. Cerebral haemorrhage during coughing spells may occur. Convulsions are common, especially in infants.

Prophylaxis

Infants carry over no immunity from the mother hence pertussis vaccine should be given from two months of age. It is usually given as the Triple vaccine (DTP/Vac).

During the 1970's several reports exaggerated the risks of encephalitis being caused by pertussis vaccine, resulting, in the United Kingdom, in a fall in the number of children being immunised. As a result the uptake for diphtheria, tetanus and polio immunisation also fell off and whooping cough became epidemic. Pertussis immunisation is contra-indicated if there is a history of previous severe reaction to immunisation.

Management

Infants should be protected from exposure to pertussis as far as possible. Antipertussis immunoglobulin injection may be given with an antibiotic such as ampicillin or erythromycin to eliminate the organism. These antibiotics are probably of little value in the paroxysmal stage.

Nutrition should be maintained with small frequent feeds. Vomiting may be reduced by small doses of cyclizine or phenobarbitone. If necessary parenteral fluids should be given to ensure that the viscid mucus remains reasonably soft. Sedation and oxygen are often required to reduce cerebral anoxia and convulsions. Cough medicines are of placebo value.

Prognosis
Usually good, except for small infants in whom complications may be severe and often fatal.

Tetanus (lockjaw)

Tetanus is an acute infection due to an anaerobic, spore-bearing organism, *Clostridium tetani*, in which the organism gains entrance via an open wound and secretes a neurotoxin (tetanospasmin). It is most likely to occur in areas contaminated by human and animal excreta.

Tetanus neonatorum is common in developing countries due to contamination of the umbilical stump.

Clinical features
The incubation period is usually 5–14 days but may last months or even years. The onset is insidious with increasing stiffness of the muscles of the face and neck. Trismus, difficulty in swallowing, increasing irritability and clonic convulsions occur. *Tetanic spasms* may occur early in the illness and are precipitated by the slightest stimulation. The head and spine are thrown into opisthotonos, the legs are extended, the arms often semi-flexed with hands tightly clenched. The spasm lasts 5–10 seconds and then the whole body relaxes. These become increasingly frequent, the body exhibiting board-like rigidity with decreasing periods of relaxation. Repeated facial spasm leads to a fixed grin (*risus sardonicus*). Asphyxia and cyanosis are due to spasm of the larynx and respiratory muscles. Excess sweating may lead to salt depletion.

Diagnosis
The history of sustaining a wound followed by the onset of trismus and tetanic spasms is usually diagnostic of *tetanus*. In *tetany* there is hypocalcaemia and neural irritability producing positive Chvostek and Trousseau's signs. *Rabies* is associated with the bite of a rabid animal, mental excitement, and hydrophobia due to pharyngeal spasm but without trismus. Strychnine poisoning should be excluded.

Prognosis and management
The shorter the incubation period and the deeper the wound, the worse the prognosis. The outlook for tetanus has vastly improved since the introduction of special intensive care units.

Therapy
Human tetanus immunoglobulin should be given intramuscularly at once as a single dose to neutralise any circulating tetanospasmin (if this is not available antitetanus serum, after a test dose, should be given). Wounds should be thoroughly cleaned and dead tissue excised. Penicillin is given in full doses. Tetracycline can be used in patients allergic to penicillin. Diazepam is given intravenously to reduce rigidity and spasm. Very high doses may be needed for patients with neonatal

tetanus. Tracheostomy should be performed early to permit bronchial toilet and by-pass the dangers of laryngeal spasm. Patients not responding to these methods should be paralysed and given intermittent positive pressure respiration. Water and electrolyte balance should be maintained intravenously and feeding may be given by nasal jejunal tube.

Prevention

Tetanus can be prevented by active immunisation. It is given in three doses in early infancy. It is usually combined with diphtheria and pertussis vaccines and given with the polio vaccine but it may be given separately. Neonatal tetanus can be prevented by immunising mothers during pregnancy. Children who have received an injury or a dog bite should be given penicillin and a tetanus vaccine booster, *provided that they have been fully immunised in infancy*. Booster doses should not be repeated more often than every 7–10 years. Patients with major wounds who have not received more than one previous immunisation should be given a full course of tetanus vaccination *and* human tetanus immunoglobulin.

Brucellosis

Brucellosis is also known as Malta fever, undulant fever and Bang's disease. It is an infectious disease of domestic animals, especially of cows (*Brucella abortus*) and goats (*B. melitensis*) which can be transmitted to man by drinking infected milk. It is mainly an intracellular organism and therefore difficult to eradicate. Children seem to be relatively immune to the disease. It usually presents as a 'pyrexia of unknown origin'. Prolonged observation reveals the undulant fever in which febrile periods lasting 1–2 weeks alternate with afebrile periods. Often the child feels well in the morning but comes home from school feeling ill. Abdominal or chest pain, sweating, cough, headache and constipation may be present. There may be lymphadenopathy and hepatosplenomegaly. Anaemia and leucopenia are often present and the ESR may be low despite fever. Diagnosis is usually confirmed by agglutination test, a rising titre during the illness being significant. The differential diagnosis is that of any PUO (pyrexia of unknown origin).

Treatment

Tetracycline may be given orally for 14–21 days. In severe cases it may be combined with streptomycin intramuscularly for 14 days. As relapses are common, the course of antibiotic may have to be repeated. Prevention depends on eradicating the disease in animals and in pasteurising cows' and goats' milk.

Gonorrhoea

Gonorrhoea is an acute purulent disease due to *Neisseria gonorrhoea*, a Gram-negative diplococcus. It may occur in the newborn as *ophthalmia neonatorum* which can cause blindness, while in older girls it presents as a purulent *vulvovaginitis*. It may occur in epidemics in institutions and may spread by sexual or non-sexual contact with contaminated articles, infected thermometers, toilet seats, towels or the insertion of foreign bodies into vagina or rectum.

Clinical features
After an incubation period of 1 week (*range*: 3–9 days) the patient, usually a pre-pubescent girl, complains of intense burning and itch, and the vulva is found to be swollen and red. There may be a yellow purulent discharge. The gonococcus can be found on Gram-stain or on culture, provided that the patient has not been given antibiotics prior to the test. The disease is very rare in boys and may present with a urethral discharge.

Differential diagnosis
Other organisms may cause a similar picture in young girls, but usually the infection is less intense. A foul-smelling discharge is often associated with a foreign body which young girls are liable to push into the vagina experimentally. Monilial vulvovaginitis may occur in diabetic children or as a complication of prolonged antibiotic therapy.

Therapy
Infections of this type are an ideal opportunity to investigate the patient's environment and to improve hygienic measures. Proper bathing and clean towels and underwear are advised. Penicillin usually cures 75 % of affected children if given in large doses (100 000 U/kg) intramuscularly together with probenecid (25 mg/kg) orally to maintain a high serum level. In resistant cases spectinomycin may be used. The local application of an oestrogen cream may be helpful by cornifying the columnar vaginal epithelium and thus increasing its resistance to infection.

The patient should be isolated until 24 hours after the discharge has disappeared. Contacts should be observed and if they develop infection it should be treated. When gonococcal infection is detected in children it is important to check for syphilis and illicit sexual contacts.

Syphilis

Syphilis is a systemic disease caused by *Treponema pallidum*, which may be congenitally acquired from an infected mother, or by venereal contact. There has been a marked increase in incidence of the disease over the last 20 years in adults, but in some Western countries it is still a rarity in childhood.

1 Syphilis in the pregnant mother

Syphilis is transmitted across the placenta to the fetus. All women should have serological tests for syphilis when they first attend for antenatal care or at the first available opportunity if they should conceal their pregnancy or not attend the antenatal clinic. Mothers with syphilis should receive a ten day course of penicillin which will also cure the infection in the fetus. Infants born to untreated or inadequately treated mothers should be treated for congenital syphilis and should also have a serological test for syphilis performed.

2 Congenital syphilis

General signs of congenital infection may be present at birth (see p. 42). Primary chancre does not occur. Signs of secondary syphilis appear on the skin and mucocutaneous junctions within the first few weeks of life. They include bullous lesions on the palms or soles, 'snuffles' which exoriate the skin of the upper lip and snail track ulcers in the mouth. Osteochondritis, nephrosis, pneumonia, hydrocephalus or acute meningovascular syphilis may occur also.

Late congenital syphilis may present several years after birth with *interstitial keratitis, condylomata, syphilides*, and *gumma formation*. Neurosyphilis also occurs but cardiovascular syphilis is rare.

3 Acquired syphilis

Syphilis may be acquired by kissing or sex play with an infected adult. Primary chancre is not common in children but the secondary and tertiary manifestations are similar to those found in adults.

Diagnosis

Infants born to syphilitic mothers should be tested for syphilis-specific IgM at birth. If this is present it indicates active infection. A positive test for syphilis in the first 3–4 months of life may be due to antibodies carried over from the mother via the placenta, in which case repeated testing will show a fall in titre. Screening tests used to detect antibodies to *Treponema pallidum* include the Venereal Disease Research Laboratory (VDRL) test and the Treponema Pallidum Haemagglutinating Antibody (TPHA) test. To confirm the diagnosis specific tests such as the Fluorescent Treponema Antibody-Absorbed (FTA-ABS) test or the Treponema Immobilisation (TPI) test may be used.

Treatment

The drug of choice is penicillin, whatever the stage of infection. For the neonate 50 000 U/kg of body weight (50 mg/kg) of procaine benzyl-penicillin G once daily for 10 days should be given. For the older patient the percentage method for estimating the dose may be used, based on the adult dose of 1 200 000 U (1.2 g) daily for 10 days. Benzathine penicillin may be given as a single intramuscular dose (*adult dose*: 1.8 g) to cure the disease. Serological tests should be repeated 3-monthly to establish cure.

The advice of the venereologist should be sought regarding management of the patient's mother and her contacts.

Tuberculosis

Tuberculosis is a chronic bacterial disease due to *Mycobacterium tuberculosis*, an acid-fast bacillus closely related to *M. bovis* of cattle and *M. avis* of birds. It is a very common disease whose incidence in highly developed countries has steadily decreased in the past half-century, but which has perhaps increased in many third-world countries. Public health measures and improved standard of living are probably of greater importance in the control of this disease than antimicrobial therapy.

Exposure to the tubercle bacillus does not necessarily cause the disease. Much depends on the *virulence of the organism*, the *resistance of the host* and the *age* of the patient. During adolescence girls are more severely affected than boys.

Intercurrent illnesses, such as measles, may cause a quiescent tuberculous lesion to flare up. The condition is common in patients with protein-calorie malnutrition.

Delayed hypersensitivity and immunity

Six to eight weeks after a primary infection with the tubercle bacillus the otherwise normal subject develops a delayed hypersensitivity (type IV) reaction to the micro-organism or its product, tuberculin. Modern tuberculin is a purified protein derivative (PPD) of the tubercle bacillus, and is used in diluted form for the intradermal Mantoux test or in concentrated form for the multiple puncture Heaf test. In individuals sensitised by *M. tuberculosis* a significant reaction (induration) to the Mantoux test occurs at the site of injection after 48–72 hours and in 4–7 days after a Heaf test. Lesser (insignificant) cross-reactions often occur in individuals sensitised by non-tuberculous ('atypical') myobacteria and BCG.

It is important to remember that other illnesses, particularly measles, steroids and *serious tuberculous disease*, may make an infected subject non-reactive to tuberculin, and a negative reaction does not exclude the diagnosis of tuberculous disease. The occurrence of hypersensitivity to tuberculin alters the patient's response to the infection leading to exudation and attempts to localise the infection. This immunity is not absolute and may not protect against re-exposure to a heavy infection with virulent organisms.

The role of age in tuberculosis

The newborn carries no protection against tuberculosis from his tuberculous mother, but should nevertheless be breast-fed if at all possible, particularly in developing countries. Isoniazid, 50 mg/day administered from the day of birth, will protect him against successful infection. The mother, of course, should receive the best drug regimen possible; rifampicin begins to affect tubercle bacilli one hour after administration.

Infection in children under five years *must* be treated because the very young have poor resistance of the disease.

Tuberculosis of the lung in infancy and early childhood tends to localise at the periphery of the lung, mainly in the lower zones (Ghon focus). The regional lymph glands become extensively involved and together with the primary lesions form the primary complex (Fig. 18.1). In older children the 'adult' type may occur, which localises at the apex or in the infraclavicular area. This does not cause tracheobronchial lymph gland enlargement but may cause extensive lung damage. Healing in children is mainly by calcification whereas in adults it is by fibrosis. Miliary tuberculosis is commonest in infancy.

Clinical features

Tuberculosis is a disease of extraordinary diversity which can attack almost any organ in the body. Like syphilis, it is a great imitator. *Tuberculous toxaemia* is characterised by fever, tachycardia, loss of appetite, night sweats and loss of weight. Many otherwise healthy infants may have no evidence of toxaemia and the illness may pass entirely unnoticed. Patients with severe malnutrition or impaired immune responses may show little toxic response to tuberculosis and may not react to tuberculin.

In *pulmonary tuberculosis* there is usually a history of contact with an infectious patient. There may be a cough, shortness of breath, consolidation, atelectasis and cavitation may develop. The presence of sputum and blood (haemoptysis) may be missed in children, as they swallow their sputum rather than cough it out. Pain in the chest may be evidence of pleurisy, especially if aggravated by a deep breath. In advanced disease the tubercle bacillus may attack the larynx causing hoarseness or stridor, or the pharynx causing dysphagia.

Tuberculosis of the gastro-intestinal tract may cause diarrhoea. Tuberculous peritonitis may be associated with abdominal pain, colic or ascites. There may be extensive peritonitis and intestinal obstruction may develop. Other organs involved may be the kidney and urinary tract, lymph nodes anywhere in the body (which may cause local pressure symptoms), bone and joint disease (with the formation of 'cold' abscesses). Invasion of the eye and skin by the tubercle bacillus lead to iridocyclitis, choroiditis and lupus vulgaris. Invasion of the pericardium may lead to pericardial effusion with subsequent constrictive pericarditis. Other manifestations of tuberculosis are *phlyctenular conjunctivitis* and *erythema nodosum*. These are probably allergic responses to the tubercle antigen.

Miliary tuberculosis is a generalised infection resulting from haematogenous tubercle dissemination. The onset may be sudden or insidious. Despite profound toxaemia there may be very few signs in the chest. The spleen may be enlarged 4–8 cm below the costal margin. Tubercles can often be seen in the retina a few millimetres away from the optic disc. They are usually about the same size as the disc.

Tuberculous meningitis is associated with miliary tuberculosis in about one-third of patients. During the first week of the illness the patient may become irritable, drowsy and anorexic. During the second week signs of meningism, papilloedema and cranial nerve palsies appear. In the third week the patient enters the final stage of the disease in which decerebrate rigidity, opisthotonos and Cheyne-Stokes respiration occur, terminating in death. Patients treated early in the course of the disease may make a complete recovery but morbidity and mortality become very high the longer treatment is delayed.

Diagnosis

Tuberculosis should be looked for in patients known to have been in contact with the disease. A delayed hypersensitivity reaction to *M. tuberculosis* may be found by skin testing with tuberculin. *Skin tests may be negative in the presence of active disease.* Acid-fast bacilli should be looked for in gastric washings when tuberculosis of the respiratory tract is suspected. It may be necessary to examine other specimens such as the urine, bone marrow or lymph glands. In addition to looking for tubercle bacilli, samples should be cultured and examined histologically. Chest X-ray may show a primary complex (Fig. 18.1), apical lesion or, in miliary tuberculosis, fine mottling throughout both lung fields. In tuberculous meningitis the CSF is under pressure and there may be an increase in cells, usually lymphocytes, with an increase in protein, and a fall in glucose. Tubercle bacilli may also be found in this form of the disease. There is usually radiological evidence of tuberculosis elsewhere.

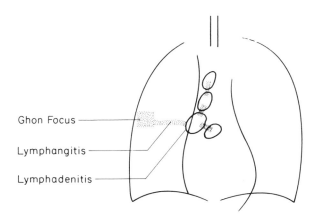

Ghon Focus

Lymphangitis

Lymphadenitis

Fig. 18.1 The primary complex

Treatment

All children with active tuberculosis and those who have been exposed and become tuberculin positive, as well as *all* children under the age of five years who are tuberculin positive, should receive antituberculous treatment. It is assumed that anyone under five years of age who has a positive tuberculin test has *active* tuberculosis even when there is no clinical or radiological sign of the disease. Child contacts of newly diagnosed infectious adults should immediately be treated with isoniazid and a tuberculin test delayed for three months when, depending on the result, the decision can be made to continue treatment for a further three months (if infected but not ill), or to stop treatment and give BCG. In every case an effort must be made to confirm the diagnosis.

Isoniazid should be combined with at least one other drug, or two in severe illness such as miliary tuberculosis, tuberculous meningitis, cavitating disease, or renal or osseous tuberculosis. This will generally overcome the problem of primary drug resistance (usually to isoniazid), which has fortunately not yet assumed serious proportions. Suitable companion drugs are rifampicin, ethambutol, ethionamide and pyrazinamide. Dosages are based on the mass of the patient and, whenever possible, all drugs are administered in a single dose once daily.

The length of treatment depends on the severity of the disease and the clinical response of the patient. Short-course therapy limited to six months is often sufficient when the combination of drugs includes rifampicin. In the case of tuberculous meningitis it is desirable to prolong the period of treatment and observation to 18 months or two years, although the administration of three drugs may usually be limited to the initial intensive phase of six months. Isoniazid alone, or in combination with ethambutol, may be administered thereafter. Serial changes in the CSF will influence the decision regarding the intensity and length of drug therapy.

In tuberculous meningitis it is no longer thought necessary to inject streptomycin intrathecally daily but the use of oral corticosteroids to reduce inflammatory exudate at the base of the brain is recommended. Corticosteroids are also sometimes recommended in highly toxic patients provided that they are fully covered by antituberculous drugs. They are said to speed up the absorption of tuberculous pleural and pericardial effusions and may be used in the form of eye-drops in phlyctenular conjunctivitis.

Mechanical disturbances, such as right middle lobe collapse due to erosion of enlarged lymph nodes into the bronchus, may require bronchoscopic suction of the granulation tissue to clear the airway.

Cold abscesses, such as psoas, retropharyngeal or supraclavicular, may require drainage. Whether tuberculous cervical lymph nodes should be excised or treated conservatively remains a controversial issue.

OPPORTUNISTIC INFECTIONS

Many bacteria, yeasts and fungi are non-pathogenic to the normal population. In the following conditions, however, the defences of the host may become compromised:

1 Inherited disorders—congenital asplenia, Bruton's disease or hereditary thymic dysplasia.
2 Acquired disorders.
   (a) Burns
   (b) Surgery, e.g. transplantation of organs, cardiac surgery, placement of catheters or shunts
   (c) Use of cytotoxic drugs
   (d) Prolonged use of corticosteroids
   (e) Chronic malnutrition.

The micro-organisms most commonly involved are *Pseudomonas aeruginosa*, *Staphylococcus epidermidis*, diphtheroids, *Bacteroides* species, *Serratia* species, *Mucor* species, *Candida*, *Cryptococcus neoformans* and many others. They can produce the most puzzling clinical pictures involving almost every organ of the body and, despite the most intensive investigations, the answers are not obtained until revealed by the scalpel of the pathologist or the culture plates of the microbiologist.

An 'Aide-Memoire'

Mnemonic	Disease	Day that rash appears after onset of symptoms
Really	Rubella	1
Very	Varicella	2
Sick	Scarlatina	3
Rogues	Roseola infantum	4
Must	Measles	5
Take	Typhus	6
Ease	Enteric fever	7

CHAPTER 19

PARASITIC DISEASES

PROTOZOAL INFECTIONS

Malaria

Malaria is a common tropical and subtropical disease characterised by paroxysmal fever, rigors and drenching sweats. It causes nearly a million deaths per year. It may be due to *Plasmodium vivax*, *P. falciparum*, *P. ovale* and *P. malariae*, all of which are carried by various species of anopheles mosquitoes. Some degree of immunity is conferred by sickle-cell anaemia, thalassaemia and G-6-PD deficiency. Some degree of immunity is transferred across the placenta to the fetus. *Congenital malaria* occurs in babies only if the mother is not immune. Occasionally a child may be infected by a blood transfusion donated by an infected but asymptomatic blood donor.

Clinical features
It should never be forgotten that malaria is often imported into non-tropical countries in travellers. The incubation period after being bitten by an infected mosquito is about two weeks for *vivax*, *falciparum* and *ovale* malaria, and about four weeks for *quartan* malaria (*P. malariae*). At first the fever may be continuous or intermittent, but within a week or two it settles down to the typical rhythmicity of the particular strain. Thus in the tertian fevers (*vivax*, *falciparum* and *ovale* malaria) fever, chills and rigors occur every 48 hours (i.e. on alternate days); in *quartan* malaria every 72 hours (i.e. every third day). These symptoms may be accompanied by headache, muscle aches, arthralgia, gastric distress and prostration. Each attack usually passes through four stages:

1 Rigors (shaking chills)
2 High fever
3 Drenching sweats
4 Apyrexial period.

The most dangerous form of malaria is that due to *P. falciparum* which is called *malignant malaria* because of its high mortality. It is particularly liable to attack the brain (cerebral malaria) causing meningismus, drowsiness, seizures, coma and death. It may present with an 'acute abdomen', with splenic pain or with acute hepatosplenomegaly and jaundice. Herpes lesions on the lips are common. Severe haemolytic anaemia, which may be fatal, occurs.

Other forms of malaria have few complications. Even without

treatment the paroxysms gradually diminish in intensity but may flare up each time the patient undergoes the stress of another illness such as bronchitis or pneumonia. *Chronic malaria* is often associated with debility and massive enlargement of the spleen, which may rupture as a result of relatively minor trauma. Hypersplenism may be a feature. Malaria due to *P. malariae* is sometimes complicated by a nephrotic syndrome.

Diagnosis
Malaria is confirmed by finding malaria parasites in the blood. Thick blood smears serve as a screening test and thin blood smears for detailed study (Fig. 19.1). Blood count usually reveals anaemia and leucopenia.

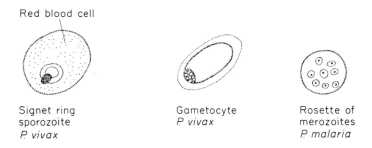

Red blood cell

Signet ring
sporozoite
P. vivax

Gametocyte
P. vivax

Rosette of
merozoites
P. malaria

Fig. 19.1 Malarial blood parasites

Treatment
Medicines which act on the erythrocyte cycle include chloroquine phosphate and amodiaquine which are given orally. In *cerebral malaria* chloroquine sulphate or quinine dihydrochloride should be given intravenously, together with appropriate therapy for shock when indicated. In *P. vivax*, *P. ovale* and *P. malariae* infection a course of chloroquine should be followed by a course of primaquine to eradicate exoerythrocytic forms. It should be remembered that methaemoglobinaemia and haemolytic anaemia may develop in Negroes with G-6-PD deficiency when exposed to primaquine, therefore this medicine should be given very cautiously in such patients initially. It should never be used together with quinacrine, quinine or sulphonamides.

Chloroquine-resistant strains of malaria usually respond to quinine or one of the newer antimalarial drugs.

Chemoprophylaxis
For the *prevention* of malaria the medicines of choice are chloroquine and amodiaquine. A useful slow-acting preparation is pyrimethamine (Daraprim), which is give once weekly.

It should be remembered that after leaving an area where tertian malaria can be contracted this dose should continue for ten weeks. In areas where *P. vivax* is endemic, a course of primaquine should be given to prevent relapses.

Malaria control

Control of the mosquito by means of insecticides is the main method for controlling the disease. Breeding grounds should be drained and larvicides used as required. Active treatment of infected patients should be carried out. Control of malaria is complicated by insecticide-resistant strains of mosquito and of plasmodia that have become resistant to antimalarial medicines.

Toxoplasmosis

Toxoplasmosis is a parasitic infection of man and animals due to an intracellular protozoon *T. gondii* (Fig. 19.2). It is spread by undercooked meat and by cats. Two forms are recognised, congenital and acquired. *Congenital toxoplasmosis* can be transmitted across the placenta only in women who acquire the infection for the first time during pregnancy. Perhaps one third of fetuses acquire the infection and only a small proportion of these are severely infected. Some abort and some are born prematurely or at term. Symptoms usually begin shortly after birth and include feeding difficulties, fever, maculopapular rash, hepatospleno-megaly and convulsions. Microcephaly, microphthalmia and hydro-cephaly may be present. Almost all cases shows some degree of chorioretinitis and skull X-ray reveals calcification in two-thirds of affected patients. Those that survive may be mentally retarded, partially blind and spastic. The mother can be reassured that subsequent pregnancies will be safe as far as toxoplasmosis is concerned.

Acquired toxoplasmosis is usually asymptomatic, but severe forms with fever, malaise and generalised lymphadenopathy may occur. The spleen may be enlarged and there may be a persistent maculopapular rash. Rarely meningo-encephalitis, hepatitis, myocarditis, myositis or pneumonia may occur, especially in patients on immunosuppressive therapy. Chronic toxoplasmosis may be asymptomatic and may be

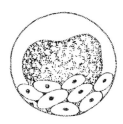

Fig. 19.2 *Toxoplasma gondii* in a mononuclear cell

detected by the unexpected finding of choroidoretinitis on ophthalmo-scopy. Lymphocytosis is usual in these patients. In fact lymphoid proliferation may be so marked as to resemble lymphosarcoma.

Diagnosis
X-ray of the skull may reveal the characteristic calcification around the ventricles. Two antibodies may be found in the serum:

1 A persistent antibody which remains positive for decades and is detected by the Sabin-Feldman dye test or by an indirect fluorescent antibody test, in both mother and baby.
2 A short-lived antibody which is detected by a complement-fixation test, gelatine diffusion test or fluorescent test for specific toxoplasma IgM. A positive test indicates recent infection and remains positive for a year or two only.

Treatment
The decision whether to treat or not may be difficult as many patients already have irreparable brain damage at birth. For acquired infection spontaneous cure is common therefore treatment should be considered only for severe cases, toxoplasmal meningitis or for *active* choroidoretin-itis. The drug treatment of choice at present is pyrimethamine 15 mg/m^2/day for 3–4 weeks. At the same time sulphadiazine in standard doses is given, also for 3–4 weeks. Folic acid 5 mg or Leucovorin 1 mg daily should be given to prevent anaemia during therapy. Twice weekly blood counts should be done. The role of clindamycin has yet to be evaluated.

Giardiasis

Giardiasis is an infestation due to a flagellated protozoon, *Giardia lamblia*. The vegetative form is passed in diarrhoeal stools whereas the cystic form is found in formed stools (Fig. 19.3).

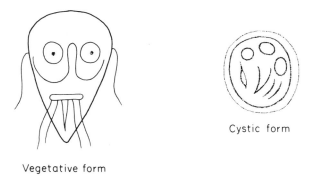

Cystic form

Vegetative form

Fig. 19.3 *Giardia lamblia*

The condition may be asymptomatic but with heavy infestation the patient has bouts of diarrhoea or even steatorrhoea. Sometimes blood and mucus may be present, producing a dysentery-like picture. The appetite is often voracious.

Treatment
Metronidazole is the drug of choice, the adult dose being 200 mg orally, three times daily for 7 days. Cure should be confirmed by microscopic examination of the stools 1–2 weeks after therapy.

Amoebiasis

See page 254.

Pneumocystic carinii pneumonia

See page 365.

ROUNDWORM (NEMATODE) INFECTIONS

Ascariasis

Ascaris lumbricoides, the great roundworm, is probably the commonest worm infestation in the world. It is also the largest, being 20–40 cm long (Fig. 19.4).

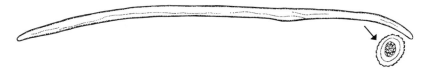

Fig. 19.4 *Ascaris lumbricoides*

The eggs may be ingested at any age and the larvae hatch in the small intestine and penetrate the mesenteric veins and lymphatics. They pass through the portal circulation to enter the pulmonary artery and pulmonary vascular bed. From here they penetrate the alveolar epithelium, moult within the alveoli, and after about ten days emigrate up the bronchial tree to the pharynx where the majority are swallowed and settle in the jejunum, where they copulate and lay eggs. These are passed with the faeces.

Clinical features
Ascariasis may be entirely asymptomatic, the eggs being found on routine examination of the stools. Moderate infestation may cause recurrent abdominal pains or vague abdominal discomfort. Nausea and

vomiting may occur. The worm may be passed through the mouth or by rectum, much to the horror of the young patient.

Complications
Allergic reactions in the lung during their migration is a common cause of Löffler's syndrome (p. 365). Ascariasis may rarely cause serious lesions in the eye, brain and other organs. Heavy infestation may cause intestinal obstruction. The parasite may enter the pancreatic or biliary ducts causing acute pancreatitis or jaundice. Obstruction of the appendix with signs of acute appendicitis may occur.

Diagnosis
The eggs can usually be identified in the faeces; in Löffler's syndrome in the blood-stained sputum. Sometimes worms are seen during a barium meal, outlined by the contrast medium.

Treatment
Piperazine citrate (*adult dose*: 4 g) as a single dose in the morning is usually curative. If the patient tends to be constipated a dose of bisacodyl may be given at the same time to ensure the expulsion of the worm. Overdose of piperazine in children causes ataxia, also known as 'worm wobble'. As the larvae are not affected by medicines, it may be necessary to repeat the dose a few weeks later when the larvae have grown to adult size.

Intestinal obstruction usually requires surgical intervention to remove the obstructing bolus of worms.

Prevention
Children should be taught not to defaecate indiscriminately. Proper sewerage disposal is important. Food grown in night soil should be properly cooked.

Threadworms

Threadworms or pinworms (*Enterobius vermicularis*) are tiny worms, the female being about 10 mm long and the male 5 mm or less. They should not be confused with *Strongyloides stercoralis* which is also referred to as a 'threadworm'. The female carries more than 10 000 eggs in her uterus. She migrates to the anus at night where she lays many eggs. This causes local itching with resultant finger-mouth contamination. Alternatively the eggs hatch around the anus and the larvae migrate back into the colon. They mature in the caecum.

Symptoms
The infestation may be asymptomatic. Pruritus ani and reinfection is common. Restless sleep may be due to the itch. 'The night cries of little girls' due to the migration of the worm across the hymen have been described. Vaginitis and masturbation due to local irritation may occur.

Diagnosis
Diagnosis is confirmed by finding the threadworms around the anus. They are best seen at night by torchlight. Eggs around the anus may be taken up onto transparent adhesive tape and identified under the microscope.

Treatment
Pyrvinium pamoate, a red dye, 150 mg/m^2 should be given orally as a single dose in the morning. It may cause nausea and vomiting. Alternatively piperazine citrate 600 mg/m^2 twice daily may be given for a week, repeated again two weeks later. Pyrantel pamoate and mebendazole are equally effective single dose treatments. Hygienic measures include the wearing of tight underpants to prevent scratching of the anus. The nails should be kept short and scrubbed with a nail brush after each bowel action. It is recommended that the whole family should be treated simultaneously. However re-infection may occur from air-borne eggs. 'Night cries' may be cured by gently lifting the worm off the hymen with a pair of forceps.

Visceral larva migrans

Children with pica may sometimes become infected by the roundworms *Toxocara canis* and *T. catis*, harboured by pet dogs and cats. After the eggs have been ingested the larvae hatch in the duodenum and jejunum, then penetrate the mesenteric vessels to enter the liver and sometimes the lungs. Rarely the brain, eyes, kidneys and heart are invaded. The larvae are unable to complete the cycle in humans and thus cause intense reactions to the internal organs of the host.

Symptoms
The condition may be asymptomatic but abdominal distension, anorexia, fever, cough and wheezing may occur. Occasionally neurological signs, convulsions and blindness may be found. A granulomatous lesion in the eye may be mistaken for a retinoblastoma.

Diagnosis
Marked eosinophilia up to 90% is present, and there is hypergammaglobulinaemia. The diagnosis is best made on liver biopsy. X-ray may reveal pulmonary infiltrations.

Treatment
Diethylcarbamazine (Hetrazan) 60–120 mg/m^2 three times daily for two weeks. Pica often accompanies iron deficiency which should be treated. Antihistamines and corticosteroids may be required for eye lesions and heavy pulmonary infestation. Dogs should be dewormed at frequent intervals.

CESTODES

Tapeworms

1 Taenia solium (pork tapeworm)

This widely distributed segmented flatworm attaches to the mucous membrane of the small bowel by hooklets around the head. The infection is acquired by eating infected pork. The ova may hatch out in the child's intestine and enter the circulation causing cysticercosis (Fig. 19.5).

Clinical features
Abdominal pain, recurrent diarrhoea and voracious appetite may be associated with failure to gain weight. Segments of the worm 1–2 cm long may be passed in the stools or crawl out of the rectum. Cysticerci may lodge in the brain causing convulsions, hydrocephalus or signs of meningitis. They may lodge in the eye. Nodules, which eventually calcify, may be felt in the muscles.

Diagnosis
Diagnosis is confirmed by finding flat segments or eggs in the stool. Eosinophilia is not a feature.

Treatment
Niclosamide, (*adult dose*: 2 g) is given as a single dose in the morning to replace breakfast. Two hours later a saline purge should be given to prevent cysticercosis. If the purgative is not given the gravid segments are digested releasing large quantities of eggs into the intestine. Cysticerci which cause symptoms, for example in the brain or eye, should be excised surgically.

2 Taenia saginata (beef tapeworm)

Taenia saginata resembles *T. solium* but is much longer (Fig. 19.5). It is more likely to cause intestinal obstruction. Occasionally paraesthesia and squint occur due to absorption of neurotoxin. Cysticercosis is rare and treatment is with niclosamide.

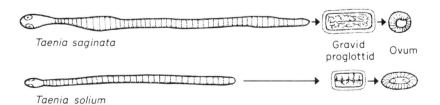

Taenia saginata

Gravid proglottid   Ovum

Taenia solium

Fig. 19.5 Tapeworms

3 Hydatid disease (Echinococcosis)

Echinococcosis is a worldwide disease caused by the tapeworm *Echinococcus granulosa* which infests dogs, cats and other carnivores, and uses man as an intermediate host. After a child ingests the eggs they hatch out in the small bowel, penetrate the intestinal wall and enter the circulation. Surviving cysts usually settle in the liver or lung where they develop into slowly expanding cysts. Scolices may bud off from the inner layer of the cysts.

Clinical features
Hydatid cysts may either cause pressure symptoms or allergic responses to the contained fluid. In the liver, hepatomegaly occurs and the cyst may often be palpable. The cyst may press on the bile ducts and cause jaundice, or it may press on the diaphragm. Urticaria and marked eosinophilia may be associated with the leak of hydatid fluid into the tissues or rupture into the bronchus. Coughing or asthma may occur and the sputum may contain daughter cysts and pieces of the cyst. In the brain convulsions and focal neurological signs may occur. Renal involvement causes haematuria. A cyst in the bone is very painful.

Diagnosis
The finding of daughter cysts in the sputum, ascitic fluid, urine or CSF is diagnostic. Eosinophilia may be marked or absent. The Casoni skin test is positive in over 80 % of patients but false positives and false negatives occur. The most reliable and sensitive serological test is the indirect haemagglutination test. An ultrasound scan may demonstrate cysts in the liver. Large cysts may be seen in the lung on chest X-ray. The cysts can calcify.

Treatment
Cysts which cause symptoms should be removed intact. Hydrogen peroxide should first be injected to sterilise the cyst, lest the cyst rupture and seed daughter cysts. Allergic reactions should be treated with adrenaline injection, corticosteroids and antihistamines.

TREMATODES (flukes)

Schistosomiasis

Schistosomiasis or bilharzia is a blood fluke infestation of world-wide distribution. Its intermediate host is the river snail; its definitive host is man. The disease is commonly acquired by children swimming in polluted waters.

Clinical features
An itchy rash, consisting of red papules which mark the site of cercarial

invasion, appears within a few hours of swimming and subsides in 2–3 days (*Kabure itch*). *Bilharzial fever*, also known as *Katayama disease*, appears 4–10 weeks after exposure to infected water. The fever is irregular, associated with a normal pulse, and may last several weeks. General lassitude, weight loss and anorexia are common. Allergic symptoms including urticaria, angioneurotic oedema, arthralgia and polyarthritis occur. During its cycle through the lung the fluke may cause an irritating cough and produce a patchy bronchopneumonia. Mild to moderate hepatosplenomegaly, with or without lymphadenopathy, may be encountered.

At this stage an intense eosinophilia (up to 65 %) may be found, and a diligent search may reveal parasites in the urine and stool.

Months or even years later the patient may present with urinary symptoms, notably *dysuria with terminal haematuria*. Ova of *S. haematobium* may be found amongst the blood cells in the urine. Infection with *S. mansoni* and *S. japonicum* produce predominantly a chronic diarrhoea, the stools containing blood and mucus (Fig. 19.6).

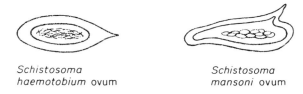

Schistosoma
haemotobium ovum

Schistosoma
mansoni ovum

Fig. 19.6 Schistosomiasis ova

Complications
Fibrosis of the terminal ureters and bladder leading to hydronephrosis, bacterial infection and renal failure may occur. Hypertension is uncommon. Cirrhosis of the liver, portal hypertension and ascites have been attributed to *S. mansoni* infestation. Cor pulmonale due to pulmonary fibrosis may occur leading to right heart failure. Malignancy of the bladder is a late complication.

Diagnosis
The finding of ova in the urine or stool is diagnostic. A positive complement fixation test is suggestive but not diagnostic. The finding of calcification in the lower ureter or bladder on X-ray is highly suggestive. The best test is rectal biopsy which may reveal both *S. mansoni* and *S. haematobium* ova. Occasionally a liver biopsy may be justified.

Prevention
By eradication of infected snails or discouraging children from swim-

ming in rivers known to be contaminated. Public health measures and sanitary disposal of excreta is essential.

Prognosis
Early treatment can achieve cure. Once dense fibrosis has set in treatment is complicated and may require prolonged therapy, such as dilatation of ureters, or transplantation of ureters. In advanced disease drug treatment, by causing the death of a large number of worms, may aggravate cirrhosis of the liver and ascites.

Therapy
Treatment for schistosomiasis includes metrifonate for *S. haematobium* and oxamniquine for *S. mansoni*. A new drug is praziquantel for both types. Patients with fibrotic lesions of the ureters are likely to require dilatation or other appropriate urological procedures. In portal cirrhosis with portal hypertension, palliative surgery should be considered.

CHAPTER 20

THE RESPIRATORY TRACT INCLUDING EAR, NOSE AND THROAT

The respiratory tract in children should always be regarded as a single unit. Obstruction to the larynx will cause marked retraction of the lower chest wall, while a severe lung disease such as bronchiectasis is often associated with chronic sinusitis. Any separation of the upper respiratory and lower respiratory tract must be regarded purely as a matter of convenience.

UPPER RESPIRATORY TRACT INFECTIONS

The upper respiratory tract includes all structures above the larynx, i.e. the air passages of the nose, the sinuses, the posterior nasal space and pharynx. The vast majority of infections of these structures are due to viruses with the notable exception of *C. diphtheriae* and group A beta-haemolytic streptococci. Of the viruses, influenza virus A and B, parainfluenza, respiratory syncytial virus, adenovirus, rhinovirus and coxsackie A and B viruses can cause upper respiratory infections. All except the coxsackie viruses can also attack the lower respiratory tract and cause croup, tracheobronchitis, bronchiolitis and bronchopneumonia in children.

The common cold (coryza)

In children the common cold (acute nasopharyngitis) is a more serious illness than in adults because secondary infection by group A streptococci, staphylococci, pneumococci or *H. influenzae* lead to complications such as otitis media, mastoiditis or sinusitis. Colds are commonly caused by adenoviruses, which are spread by droplet infection. A child may often suffer three or more attacks per year.

Clinical features
In infants there is usually a low grade fever with nasal obstruction, thin nasal discharge, restlessness and feeding difficulty. Nasal obstruction is sufficient to cause respiratory distress, and rib retraction may be noted. Sometimes the cervical lymph nodes enlarge. The ear drums are congested and otitis media may develop. Parenteral diarrhoea or vomiting may occur. The illness should not last more than three days unless complicated by secondary infection.

Older children complain of nasal and pharyngeal irritation. Sneezing is common. A thin nasal discharge appears which rapidly becomes purulent. Tears may pour from the eyes, which often become swollen. Loss of appetite is common but not invariable. Mouth breathing aggravates the dryness and soreness of the throat. Fever is slight after infancy. Symptoms usually clear in 3–4 days.

Diagnosis
Coryza is a clinical diagnosis and it is not necessary to isolate the virus. However, it must be realised that the same symptoms precede a number of acute illnesses in childhood, especially measles, whooping cough and mumps. A child who is said to have a 'continuous cold' or 'is never free from colds' probably has an allergic rhinitis and eosinophils are found in the nasal discharge. Nasal discharges are common in infants and should not be referred to as *snuffles* unless excoriation of the upper lip occurs and spirochaetes can be detected in the discharge by dark field microscopy. The term *snuffles* implies congenital syphilis. A bloody nasal discharge suggests diphtheria or an impacted foreign body in the nostril.

Complications include otitis media, mastoiditis, sinusitis, cervical adenopathy, laryngitis and/or croup, and spread to the lower respiratory tract (bronchitis, bronchiolitis or bronchopneumonia).

Treatment
The first aim should be to relieve nasal congestion. In babies nasal suction should be carried out with a rubber bulb to which a soft rubber or plastic catheter is attached. This should be done *before* feeds and at night, in order to reduce restlessness due to the blocked nose. If this is not entirely successful 0.25 % ephedrine nose drops for infants or 0.5 % for older children is suggested. Some practitioners like oral nasal decongestants such as pseudoephedrine hydrochloride 30 mg per 5 ml. Dose at one year in 2.5 ml and at seven years 5 ml three or four times daily. There are dozens of 'cold' preparations on the market, often containing several ingredients such as analgesics, antipyretics, antihistamines, cough suppressants and even cough stimulants. Such polypharmacy is to be deplored in modern medicine.

Babies with colds are best nursed prone so that the nasal secretions can more easily drain onto the bed rather than into the throat. A humidified environment prevents the mucus from drying out and is particularly useful if the infant has a dry cough. Cough suppressants and expectorants are not recommended as they are likely to do more harm than good. The same applies to antibiotics as these have no action on viruses. They should be used however if purulent complications develop.

Acute pharyngitis

This term refers to acute inflammation of the pharynx when this dominates the illness. However, acute pharyngitis may also be part of any upper respiratory tract infection, measles, rubella or other infections. It is a matter of definition whether acute tonsillitis should be regarded as an entity separate from acute pharyngitis or whether one should perhaps use the term *acute tonsillopharyngitis.*

Viral pharyngitis

Fever, malaise, headache and nausea are associated with a sore throat of moderate intensity. There may be hoarseness, cough and rhinitis. Follicular tonsillitis resembling that due to streptococcal infection may be present. The illness may last a day or two or may persist for a week.

Streptococcal pharyngitis

The illness tends to be more acute with high fever, headache, abdominal pain and vomiting. Within a few hours the throat becomes painful, the tonsils frequently become red and swollen and in the older child covered with exudate. The latter tends to be creamy and when rubbed with a throat swab does not bleed, a feature which usually distinguishes it from diphtheria. In children under three years exudate is less common but the tonsils, pharynx and soft palate are inflamed and petechiae may be noted on the uvula. Cervical lymph nodes often swell and are tender. Circumoral pallor is common. Unlike viral pharyngitis, one does not get rhinitis, hoarseness or cough in streptococcal infection. However, scarlet fever, acute glomerulonephritis and acute rheumatic fever (p. 315) may complicate the illness, as may otitis media, sinusitis, quinsy and retropharyngeal abscess.

Diagnosis
Throat swab may reveal a group A beta-haemolytic streptococcus and the antistreptolysin O titre in the serum rises in the untreated patient. Early treatment with antibiotics may inhibit this reaction. If complications such as rheumatic fever or acute nephritis occur, it tends to remain high for several weeks, otherwise it returns to normal in about ten days.

Viral cultures are not usually done. The white blood count is not helpful in distinguishing viral and streptococcal infection as, in the early stages there may be a polymorphonuclear leucocytosis in both.

Differential diagnosis
Diphtheria, infectious mononucleosis and *agranulocytosis* all cause sore throats with membrane formation. They are distinguished by throat culture, blood count and Paul-Bunnell tests. *Herpangina* is more likely to cause herpetiform lesions on the pharynx and faucial pillars. *Streptococcal infection* often causes acute abdominal pain and vomiting, but other causes for an 'acute abdomen' such as acute appendicitis should always be kept in mind.

Treatment

Penicillin G is the antibiotic of choice in streptococcal infections, and a response may be expected in 24–36 hours. A throat swab should be taken prior to therapy in all cases and if a haemolytic streptococcus is isolated it is recommended that the penicillin be continued for at least 10–14 days, in order to eradicate the organism and thus reduce the incidence of rheumatic fever. Sometimes *Staphylococcus aureus*, which produces penicillinase, may be cultured in addition to the streptococcus and it inhibits the action of the penicillin on the haemolytic streptococcus. In such cases cloxacillin should be given in addition to phenoxymethylpenicillin in order to eliminate both organisms. Warm saline gargles are comforting for older children. Paracetamol or aspirin may be given for pain but adequate fluid intake should be given to prevent aspirin toxicity. Swallowing is painful therefore soft foods, clear soup, ice-cream and jellies are usually preferred.

Retropharyngeal abscess

Retropharyngeal abscess lies between the posterior pharyngeal wall and the prevertebral fascia. It is usually secondary to follicular tonsillitis but may occur after an injury to the throat, for example by a sharp object.

There is high fever, difficulty in swallowing, excess salivation and gurgling respiration. The head is held in extension but despite this breathing becomes laboured.

On examination a bulge of the posterior pharyngeal wall is noted. It should be palpated with the patient in the Trendelenburg position and with a suction apparatus handy in case it bursts. If it is fluctuant it should be incised under general anaesthesia in a properly equipped theatre. Delay may be dangerous as the abscess may spread and cause *oedema glottidis*. Occasionally it burrows into the oesophagus, the mediastinum or the neck. Rarely subluxation of the upper cervical vertebrae may occur. In all cases penicillin G should be given as streptococci are the chief causative organisms. Subluxation of the neck should be treated by extension and immobilisation.

Quinsy

Quinsy is a peritonsillar abscess rarely seen nowadays. It is preceded by an attack of tonsillitis. The pain in the throat gets worse, there is trismus due to pterygoid spasm, and dysphagia. Neck stiffness is often present. The affected tonsil is swollen and inflamed and the uvula is displaced on one side.

Treatment

Penicillin may abort the infection but usually the abscess must be incised as soon as it fluctuates. It is usual practice to remove the tonsils 4–6 weeks after the inflammation has subsided.

Sinusitis

The frontal sinuses do not pneumatise until 2–4 years of age, but the maxillary antra and the posterior ethmoid cells are present at birth, though small. The sphenoidal sinus varies in size at birth and rarely becomes infected before five years of age.

Infection of the sinus commonly occurs in coryza and other acute viral upper respiratory infections. It may be asymptomatic or there may be a feeling of stuffiness ('head cold') and headache. Sphenoidal sinusitis may cause suboccipital headache, anterior ethmoidal infection may cause pain over the eyes or temple, while posterior ethmoiditis may cause pain over the distribution of the trigeminal nerve and mastoid area. The pain is intensified if the ostia are obstructed. Pus may be seen in the superior or middle meatus, depending on which sinus is affected. Peri-orbital cellulitis usually accompanies ethmoidal infection. Complications include otitis media, cavernous sinus thrombosis, meningitis and abscess formation. Diagnosis can usually be confirmed by X-rays of the sinuses.

Treatment

Penicillin or other appropriate antibiotic should be given in full dosage. Ephedrine nose-drops may be used to shrink the nasal mucous membranes. Oral nasal decongestants are often successful. If this does not ensure drainage then surgical drainage may be necessary.

Chronic sinusitis

Persistent sinusitis may be due to an underlying anatomical defect such as deviation of the nasal septum, hypertrophied adenoids, focal infection, allergy or underlying immunological deficiency.

It may manifest itself by a persistent or intermittent postnasal drip, mouth breathing, throat clearing or cough. Headaches and tenderness over the affected sinus may be detected. Sneezing and thin nasal discharge is usually due to an underlying allergy. There is often an associated 'bronchitis' (sinobronchitis). X-ray may reveal thickened mucous membranes or total opacity of one or more of the nasal sinuses. The lung plates may show bronchitic changes.

Treatment

The chronic use of nose drops and oral nasal decongestants probably contributes to the chronicity of sinusitis, by damaging the ciliary blanket. If simple treatment is not successful within a few days, the patient should be referred for ENT consultation. Two popular methods of treatment include the Parkinson 'head-down' position with instillation of nasal solution, and the Proetz displacement method. Surgery may be considered in selected cases.

The chronic tonsils and adenoids problem

Waldeyer's ring consists of the lingual tonsil, two faucial tonsils, the adenoids and lymph tissue on the pharyngeal wall. They form a defence against infection, but repeated infection may lead to hypertrophy, abscess formation and/or fibrosis. Hypertrophied tonsils may appear enormous, often touching in the mid-line, yet they may cause the minimum of trouble. Hypertrophied adenoids, often associated with swelling of the nasopharyngeal mucosa, invariably cause nasal obstruction and mouth breathing. This leads to a vicious circle of infection, swelling, re-infection and more swelling of the adenoids. The obstruction may extend to the Eustachian tubes causing recurrent pain in the ears and otitis media. The so-called *adenoid facies* may be due to any disorder causing nasal obstruction. The nose is pinched, the eyes dull and the mouth open. The affected child often looks stupid and retarded, an appearance aggravated by his constant mouth breathing and drooling. Orthodontic problems are common. The child has difficulty in swallowing saliva and when he chews meat he is liable to spit it out because of difficulty in swallowing. Speech is somewhat muffled. Many of the symptoms attributed to 'chronic T's and A's', however, may well be due to an underlying allergy.

Laboratory findings
Throat swabs should be cultured for both group A beta-haemolytic streptococci and for staphylococci, as the latter may be producing penicillinase and negating treatment with penicillin G. Cloxacillin should be used together with penicillin G in such patients. Positive cultures are found in perhaps one-quarter of patients. In babies *E. coli* is sometimes found.

Nasal swabs should be examined for eosinophilia and, if the history and examination warrants it, full skin testing for allergy to inhalants should be done. Lateral X-ray of the nasopharynx may reveal a soft tissue mass at the site of the adenoids.

The tonsillo-adenoid-cardiac hypertrophy syndrome
In some cases of nasopharyngeal obstruction due to enlarged tonsils and adenoids right-sided cardiac hypertrophy may occur. It is probably due to anoxia and acidosis causing pulmonary vasoconstriction, pulmonary hypertension and pulmonary oedema. Suspicious symptoms include stridor on lying down, attacks of sleep apnoea and somnolence by day. In these patients removal of the tonsils and adenoids may be curative.

Indications for tonsillectomy
1 Recurrent tonsillitis more than four times annually in any child over four years of age, who has had adequate penicillin therapy on each occasion.
2 Persistent sore throat despite treatment, especially if the jugulodigastric gland at the angle of the jaw is enlarged and tender.

3 After an attack of quinsy.
4 Massively enlarged tonsils, *provided that they cause symptoms*, such as in the tonsillo-adenoid-cardiac hypertrophy syndrome.
5 Rarely for diphtheria carriers in whom antibiotics are unsuccessful in eliminating the infection.

Contra-indications for tonsillectomy
1 Underlying allergy. Tonsillectomy may aggravate allergies in some patients.
2 Recurrent colds and chronic health problems are rarely due to 'tonsils'.
3 Patient under three or four years of age.
4 Large tonsils without symptoms. It should be remembered that tonsils tend to increase in size to about 10–12 years of age, and then steadily involute.
5 Tuberculous cervical adenitis is no longer regarded as an indication. One does not excise a Ghon focus in the lung—why excise a tuberculous focus in the tonsils?
6 Rheumatic fever and nephritis are not indications unless intensive antibiotic therapy fails to eliminate the haemolytic streptococcus. Even so, one should look for other carriers of the haemolytic streptococcus in the family who may be infecting the child repeatedly. The carrier should be treated.
7 Parental insistence on tonsillectomy is not an indication!

Indications for adenoidectomy
1 Adenoid facies due to enlarged adenoids and *not* due to nasal allergy or non-adenoid nasal obstruction.
2 Recurrent otitis media due to Eustachian tube obstruction.
3 Deafness due to enlarged adenoids.
4 Some cases of chronic sinusitis.
5 The tonsillo-adenoid-cardiac hypertrophy syndrome (see above).

It is customary to remove both tonsils and adenoids at the same operation (T's and A's) though a few lone voices insist that each should be assessed separately on their merits. If there is not adequate improvement after adenoidectomy, a lateral X-ray of the skull should be done to determine whether all adenoid tissue has been removed.

A word to the wise—never judge a tonsil by its appearance or size. Never decide on tonsillectomy during an acute infection—the tonsils may be normal in 2–3 weeks time.

Complications
Incomplete removal of tonsils leads to hypertrophy of the remaining tissue, hence the layman's view that the tonsils have grown again. A *membrane* always forms in the tonsillar bed after tonsillectomy and should not be confused with diphtheria. *Post-tonsillectomy haemorrhage* may occur shortly after operation due to an arterial tie coming loose, or

it may occur several days later due to erosion of a vessel by infection. Rarely dislocation of the atlanto-axial joint occurs due to softening of the ligaments. The patient may present with *torticollis* ('wry-neck'). Before the days of widespread poliomyelitis immunisation *bulbar palsy* was a real threat. With modern anaesthesia pneumonia and lung abscess should not occur.

Stridor

Stridor is a harsh crowing noise occurring on inspiration in infants, due to obstruction anywhere from the epiglottis to the bifurcation of the trachea. It is associated with retraction of the supraclavicular, intercostal and subcostal spaces. In mild cases stridor may be limited to noisy breathing and hoarseness whereas in severe cases there is a loud crowing noise and marked sternal retraction. In older children hoarseness and aphonia is usually present. The term croup should be limited to the loud 'brassy' or barking cough due to tracheitis. It may or may not be accompanied by stridor. Stridor and croup should be distinguished from the whoop of pertussis in which a single inspiratory noise (the whoop) follows the typical spasmodic cough. In asthma there is a wheezing sound which is predominantly expiratory, not inspiratory.

Causes of stridor
Stridor is produced by any disorder which causes narrowing of the laryngeal inlet and trachea:

1 Infections, notably viral (parainfluenza 2, adenovirus, measles and respiratory syncytial virus) and bacterial (*H. influenzae* and *C. diphtheriae*).
2 Spasmodic croup.
3 Foreign body.
4 Congenital anomalies of the larynx such as laryngeal web, laryngomalacia or tracheomalacia. In the latter condition the laryngeal or tracheal cartilage is soft and collapses on inspiration.
5 Pressure on the trachea by an anomalous aortic arch, aortic vascular ring, by enlarged upper mediastinal glands, retropharyngeal abscess or goitre.
6 Laryngospasm due to hypocalcaemia.
7 Papilloma or other tumours of the vocal cords.

Clinical features
The clinical picture will depend on the underlying cause, but inspiratory stridor and some degree of rib retraction is common to all types. In *laryngeal diphtheria* (p. 317) the patient is extremely toxic and progressive laryngeal obstruction and cyanosis may develop early in the disease. A fatal outcome is common.

Haemophilus influenzae produces an extremely severe form of *acute epiglottitis* with high fever, toxicity and prostration. Progressive dysphagia, dyspnoea and stridor develop with alarming speed. The pharynx should *not* be inspected as it may precipitate *total* obstruction. *The patient should not be forced to lie down for the same reason.* Lateral X-ray of the neck will reveal the diagnostic swelling of epiglottis. Facilities for emergency intubation should be available at all times. The white blood count is markedly raised.

Viral croup varies in intensity and is often quite mild. Slight redness of the throat and variable fever may be present. Hoarseness is marked. The white blood count is usually normal. Often the infection spreads down the trachea and bronchi (*acute laryngotracheobronchitis*) and the patient becomes progressively ill, dyspnoeic and restless. It is, however, far less explosive than bacterial croup.

Spasmodic croup (laryngitis stridulosa) usually occurs in highly strung children of 1–3 years of age. It wakes them in the early hours of the morning. It may be preceded by an upper respiratory infection but often the child goes to bed apparently normal. He wakes with a barking cough, his respiration is noisy and he is very alarmed by the illness. There is little or no fever and the throat is clear. The next day he is usually well enough to go to school.

Congenital web, laryngomalacia and other anatomical deformities of the larynx usually cause noisy breathing which is aggravated by the slightest infection, including the common cold. Laryngomalacia (floppy larynx) may persist for 18 months or more, and is usually more distressing to the parents than to the patient. It tends to disappear with the growth of the larynx. In some cases, however, respiratory obstruction or serious chest deformity can result and therefore the illness should never be treated lightly. The diagnosis is made by direct inspection of the larynx. *Aortic rings* or other vascular anomalies are suspected when the usual causes for stridor are not apparent. X-ray of the chest or a barium swallow may be diagnostic but sometimes a left heart catheterisation may be required to establish the diagnosis.

Laryngospasm due to hypocalcaemia is usually associated with signs of rickets and the serum calcium is usually below 2 mmol/l of blood. Attacks are brief but may occur many times during the day.

Treatment

Treatment depends on the underlying cause. Often some improvement is obtained by extending the head and positioning the infant on his side. Humidification with a continuous warm air humidifier and oxygen are required in most patients.

In *diphtheria* (p. 317) and *acute laryngotracheobronchitis* laryngeal intubation may be life-saving and should be done too soon rather than too late. Penicillin and antitoxin should be given as indicated. *Spasmodic croup* usually responds dramatically to an intravenous injection of hydrocortisone.

Acute epiglottitis due to *H. influenzae* is treated urgently, with large doses of ampicillin, 5 g/m^2/24 hours (or chloramphenicol 1–2 g/m^2/day) and an endotracheal tube or tracheostomy tube should be inserted if necessary. In *viral infections* an endotracheal tube or tracheostomy may also be required. For *hypocalcaemia* intravenous calcium may be given. *Foreign bodies* should of course be removed.

Indications for intubation
1 Cyanosis, progressive dyspnoea and reduced air entry on auscultation.
2 Marked increase in heart rate with pulsus paradoxus above 20 mmHg (2.7 kPa).
3 Increasing restlessness despite oxygen administration.
4 Dilatation of the pupils—a late sign!

Warning: prolonged intubation may cause laryngeal stenosis.

THE EAR

The ear may be very small (*microtia*), very large ('bat ears', *macrotia*) or absent (*anotia*). Low set, malformed ears are often associated with congenital malformations of the renal tract or face (see p. 272). *Accessory auricles* are usually very small. Atresia of the external auditory canal requires investigation to assess whether the internal ear is normal.

Trauma to the external ear causes haematomas which, if not evacuated, may organise and cause a 'cauliflower ear', so common in boxers and wrestlers.

Pain in the ear

Babies often rub their ears, which the layman attributes to 'teething', but this is unlikely at two or three months of age. The ear is supplied by branches of the fifth, ninth and tenth cranial nerves, as well as the second and third cervical nerves. Pain may be referred to the ear from the teeth (but only the third molars!), the temporomandibular joint, the sinuses, the pharynx and the upper cervical spine. Herpes zoster of the fifth cranial nerve causes pain in the ear in its pre-eruptive phase. Pain may precede Bell's palsy by 8–24 hours. Impacted wax on the ear drum, which receives fibres from the vagus nerve, may cause a reflex cough which disappears when the wax is syringed out. Sudden changes in barometric pressure causes sharp pain which can be relieved by yawning or swallowing, as this equalises the pressure on both sides of the tympanic membrane. In babies crying has the same effect in relieving ear pain on take-off or landing.

Wax in the ear

At birth the ear drum is obscured by vernix caseosa which disappears by the end of the week when the ear drum can more easily be viewed (Fig. 20.1). Cotton-buds tend to push wax towards the tympanic membrane and should not be recommended. Most ears tend to be self-cleaning but some children seem to produce excessive amounts of wax. It is hard to explain why sometimes one ear may be perfectly clean and the other totally blocked by a plug of dark wax. In most cases wax is easily syringed out but the following points of technique are important:

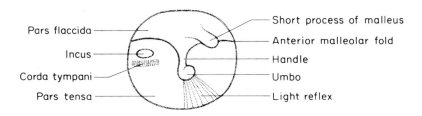

Pars flaccida

Incus

Corda tympani

Pars tensa

Short process of malleus

Anterior malleolar fold

Handle

Umbo

Light reflex

Fig. 20.1 The normal anatomy of the ear drum

1 In small children the ear lobe should be pulled backwards to straighten the auditory canal, while in older children it should be pulled upwards.
2 The nozzle of the syringe should be smaller than the canal so that the fluid can run out easily. Warm tap water or 1 % sodium bicarbonate is suitable.
3 The nozzle of the syringe, and hence the stream of fluid should be directed against the posterior wall of the canal, *never* straight at the wax.
4 If the wax is stubborn, a few drops of 'Cerumol' should be inserted into the canal and the opening closed for 10–15 minutes with cottonwool soaked in petroleum jelly. This prevents the Cerumol from running out. Thereafter the syringing should be repeated. Many practitioners are adept at removing wax with a Jobson-Horne probe.

Foreign bodies
Insects sometimes fly or crawl into children's ears and can be floated out with a few drops of warm olive oil. Most foreign bodies can be lifted out gently by means of forceps. Occasionally a general anaesthetic may be required if the child is uncooperative or the foreign body too large.

Infections
Furuncles in the ear canal are extremely painful especially if the ear lobe is moved. Fever and enlargement of the pre- and postauricular lymph

nodes often occurs. The furuncle should be incised if it is ripe, otherwise cloxacillin or benzylpenicillin should be given with a view to aborting the infection.

Chronic infections tend to smoulder. They are commonly due to pseudomonas, proteus, klebsiella, candida or aspergillus infection. They are often very itchy. Debris should be syringed gently and a wick soaked in a suitable antimicrobial such as gentamicin. For dry and itchy lesions drops containing an antimicrobial and corticosteroid such as clioquinol may be used. Ototoxic drops should be given for short periods only and are contra-indicated if there is a perforated ear drum.

'Swimmer's Ear' is due to loss of protective waxes in the ear. There may be maceration of the canal wall with secondary infection by pseudomonas or *Aspergillus niger*. The ear should be dried thoroughly after swimming and propylalcohol drops inserted. Thereafter lanolin may be inserted as a protective coat inside the canal.

Otitis media

Babies are especially liable to middle ear infection because the Eustachian tubes tend to be horizontal, the baby lies supine and drainage is hindered. Obstruction by lymphoid tissue during upper respiratory infection or allergy aggravates the infection. *Acute otitis media* may complicate systemic infections such as measles, rubella, coryza and influenza. The commonest organisms cultured are *Diplococcus pneumonia, Haemophilus influenzae* and beta-haemolytic streptococci. There is high fever, pain and restlessness. The ear drum is red initially, but later pus accumulates, the drum bulges and the landmarks are lost. Parenteral diarrhoea or vomiting is common, and there may be meningismus or convulsions.

Treatment
Fever and pain should be reduced by tepid sponging and paracetamol elixir. Ampicillin or benzylpenicillin are usually effective. Diluted nose-drops or oral nasal decongestants may help drainage from the Eustachian tube. A bulging drum should be incised under anaesthetic but many practitioners prefer conservative therapy for 48 hours before considering surgery. Sometimes the patient is seen for the first time after the drum has burst. In that case an ear swab should be sent for culture and sensitivity, and penicillin therapy begun. The ear canal should be swabbed clean repeatedly otherwise the pus will macerate the skin.

Complications
1 *Recurrent attacks* of otitis are common. The drum becomes thickened and dull, the landmarks often being obscured. Retraction of the drum may occur. Careful examination for underlying causes, especially enlarged adenoids and allergy, should be made and treated when found.

2 *Secretory (serous) otitis media* is a sterile exudate in the middle ear due to obstruction of the Eustachian tube. It may occur during the course of a 'head cold' or following acute otitis media. It may be due to a large adenoidal pad blocking the entrance to the Eustachian tube. The exudate may become tenacious and is referred to as *glue ear*. The mobility of the ear drum is reduced. *Treatment* consists of inserting a grommet, which is a flanged teflon tube via an anterior radial myringotomy in order to ventilate the middle ear (Fig. 20.2). There is an immediate improvement in hearing and the grommet extrudes spontaneously in 4–12 months.

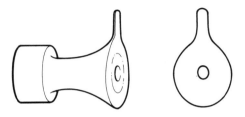

Fig. 20.2 A teflon grommet

3 *Acute mastoiditis* (rare). Despite active antibiotic therapy, infection may spread to the mastoid air cells, or it may infect the bone causing osteomyelitis. There is a recurrence of fever with swelling, redness and tenderness over the mastoid process. Infection may spread to the dura causing meningitis and even brain abscess. The treatment of acute mastoiditis consists of intense antibiotic therapy. If there is no improvement in 48 hours there is likely to be osteitis of the bone. Mastoidectomy is indicated under continued antibiotic cover.

4 *Chronic otitis media* is often associated with chronic mastoiditis. There is a chronic painless discharge through a permanent defect in the ear drum. A *cholesteatoma* is a mass of debris containing cholesterol crystals which develops in the middle ear and destroys the ossicles. Bone deafness is present. These children should be treated by the otolaryngologist with a view to tympanoplasty and reconstruction of the ossicles.

Myringitis is an inflammation of the ear drum which accompanies many viral infections such as roseola infantum, rubella and measles. There may be an associated otitis media or otitis externa. As one is not sure in many cases whether the infection is bacterial or viral in origin, penicillin is usually given. One form, however, which is almost certainly viral is *bullous myringitis*. One or more vesicles or bullae appear on the drum and it is extremely painful until the blob bursts. Auralgicin ear-drops provide some comfort.

Deafness

Neonatal deafness can be detected by special instruments; which are used as screening tests in many neonatal units. Complete hearing loss is rare and a great deal can be done to utilise the residual hearing which is available to the infant. Any hearing loss of over 15 decibels in the normal speech range is likely to lead to retarded speech development (deaf-mutism). This should not be confused with speech retardation due to mental deficiency, brain injury or infantile autism. An audiologist should be consulted in cases of doubt.

Hearing loss should be suspected in small babies who do not respond to loud noises or do not quieten when spoken to. Older infants who do not turn their head when called from behind may be deaf. Failure to say a few words by 18 months of age may be due to deafness. Faulty speech development ('jargon speech') or retarded speech development may be due to partial deafness, but could also be due to cerebral palsy or mental retardation. A normal child can put three words together in meaningful sentences by two years of age, a deaf child cannot.

Treatment

Rubella in pregnancy can be prevented by immunising all girls by 13 years of age. Aminoglycosides, like gentamicin, should only be given for short courses and the plasma levels should be monitored. Bacterial upper respiratory tract infections, notably acute otitis media, should be adequately treated. The deaf child should be referred for ENT opinion for proper assessment and referral to the appropriate authority. Hearing aids, lip-reading and special education may be required.

Hearing loss—a check list

1 *Nerve deafness* (Eighth cranial nerve and its connections to the organ of Corti and the brain):
   (a) Hereditary, usually X-linked disorders.
   (b) Infections: congenital rubella syndrome, measles, mumps or meningitis.
   (c) Neonatal hyperbilirubinaemia.
   (d) Trauma to petrosal bone.
   (e) Tumour, e.g. acoustic neuroma.
   (f) Toxins causing reversible deafness such as quinine or aspirin or irreversible damage, e.g. streptomycin and other amino-glycosides.
2 *Conduction deafness*:
   (a) Wax or foreign bodies blocking ear.
   (b) Perforation of tympanum due to trauma or infection.
   (c) Acute otitis media and serous otitis media.
   (d) Chronic otitis media and cholesteatoma.
   (e) Congenital atresia or stenosis of the canal.

THE NOSE

Nose-bleeds

Epistaxis is commonly due to trauma (including nose-picking) in children and involves the venous plexus in the anterior nares. It can usually be stopped with a plug of cotton-wool in the nose. If infection is present an antibiotic cream such as Naseptin may be applied two or three times daily.

Bleeding in the posterior nasal cavity is often due to more serious causes such as disorders of the clotting mechanism, or leukaemia. Packing of the affected side with long 6 mm strips of gauze soaked in 1:1000 adrenaline solution may be required while the underlying disorder is treated. The gauze strips should be replaced daily. A sedative should be given if the child (or his parents) is frightened.

Nasal allergy

Hay fever (p. 113) and perennial rhinitis are usually associated with excess sneezing, tear formation and swelling of the eyes and nasal mucosa, when the patient comes in contact with allergens especially inhalants such as pollens. The mucosa is usually swollen and pale and may obstruct the nose sufficiently to cause mouth-breathing. The swelling may be so marked as to produce polyps. The diagnosis is confirmed by finding eosinophilia in a nasal smear and in the blood.

Treatment
Desensitisation to the offending antigen by intradermal injection is successful in many patients. Oral antihistamines provide symptomatic relief. They may be combined with oral nasal decongestants such as pseudo-ephedrine. Nasal polyps should be removed surgically (see Chapter 8).

THE LOWER RESPIRATORY TRACT

Foreign bodies

Foreign bodies may lodge in the larynx, trachea or bronchus. A sharp object like a broken piece of a toy may lacerate the mucosa and cause local infection. Peanuts and other vegetable matter are notorious for lodging in the right middle lobe bronchus and causing a widespread inflammatory reaction.

Foreign bodies which completely obstruct a bronchus will cause resorption atelectasis of the parts distal to it. Sometimes a 'ball valve' obstruction occurs so that air enters the alveoli but cannot get out again. This results in obstructive emphysema. The affected lobe is over-aerated and during expiration the mediastinum shifts to the unaffected side.

Clinical features

When the foreign body is inhaled, choking, gagging and breath-holding may be observed. Stridor, hoarseness, cyanosis or wheezing may occur, depending on the site of lodgement. Signs of atelectasis or obstructive emphysema may be found over the affected lung. Delay in seeking medical help may lead to infection, pneumonic consolidation and abscess formation in the affected lobe. The physical signs are those of the underlying lesion.

Screening of the chest (Fig. 20.3) will reveal radio-opaque foreign bodies. Non-opaque foreign bodies are inferred by the finding of atelectasis of the affected lobe if the obstruction is complete, or obstructive emphysema, shifting of the mediastinum to the opposite side with expiration and flattening of one of the diaphragms if there is a ball-valve obstruction. It is often possible to take films in expiration and inspiration for comparison. Do not confuse the sail shadow of the thymus (Fig. 20.4) with those of atelectasis on p. 368 (Fig. 20.6).

Treatment

One should not attempt to make the patient cough lest the foreign body impacts in the larynx from below. Arrangements should be made for removal of the foreign body under anaesthesia as soon as possible.

Prevention

Cheap plastic toys which often contain loose beads or sharp parts should be banned by law. Children should be warned not to run and eat, especially peanuts, at the same time. Back-slapping should be discouraged.

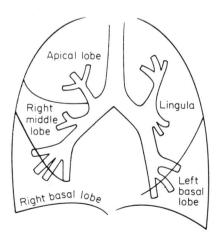

Fig. 20.3 Chest X-ray showing the main lobes and fissures (full inspiration)

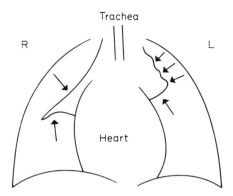

Trachea

R

L

Heart

Fig. 20.4 Chest X-ray showing the 'sail shadow' of the thymus. Note the indentation of the ribs on the left border of the thymus gland.

Congenital malformations

Tracheo-oesophageal fistula is suspected in a newborn baby who salivates excessively and chokes on his first feed (see p. 238). Tracheal stenosis and atresia are rare anomalies. Tracheomalacia is a form of stridor due to collapse of an abnormally soft trachea during inspiration. The azygos lobe is an anomaly due to failure of the azygos vein to migrate medially so that it 'cuts' a vertical fissure in the right upper lobe. Accessory lobes, hypoplastic and absent lobes may occur but are uncommon. Anomalous drainage of the pulmonary veins into the vena cava or right atrium has been described. Congenital cysts may cause problems in diagnosis.

Acute bronchitis and tracheitis

Acute bronchitis is an acute infection of the large tubes of the lung (i.e. the trachea and bronchi) due to either a viral or a bacterial infection. It may start with an upper respiratory infection 'which goes to the chest' or it may form part of another illness such as measles. It may start in the trachea and spread down the bronchial tree (acute tracheobronchitis) or may be limited to the trachea or the bronchi. In babies and infants the larynx is often involved (acute laryngotracheobronchitis).

Clinical features
The illness is ushered in with cough and fever which becomes progressively worse. The cough is dry and unproductive and may have a brassy or barking quality when the trachea is predominantly involved (tracheitis). There is marked substernal discomfort. After 48 hours the cough becomes productive and the sputum purulent. Children swallow sputum and are liable to vomit as a result. Gradually the illness subsides

but it takes 7–10 days or more before the child is well enough to return to school.

Physical findings initially are those of 'just being ill'. The breath sounds become coarser and bilateral rhonchi are usually heard. These may be sonorous or low-pitched due to plugs of mucus and inflammatory debris in the large bronchi, or they may be high-pitched and wheezy due to bronchospasm. Children with recurrent wheezy attacks usually turn out to have asthma.

Treatment

During the 'dry' phase of the illness, humidification of the atmosphere by suitable nebulisers is comforting. Mucolytics, if given at the onset of the illness, may ensure a fluid sputum. Antibiotics have little place in the acute illness but should be given for complications such as otitis media or bronchopneumonia.

Children with repeated attacks of bronchitis should have an X-ray of the chest to exclude foreign body or other underlying pathology such as tuberculosis or bronchiectasis. The sinuses also should be X-rayed. A nasal swab should be examined for eosinophils to exclude allergy. The blood proteins, especially the immunoglobulins, should be estimated to exclude agammaglobulinaemia, while a sweat test should be done for suspected cystic fibrosis. The sputum, obtained by gastric aspiration in infants and by coughing in older children, should be cultured for *Mycobacterium tuberculosis*. A blood count may reveal a neutropenia in 'viral bronchitis' and a neutrophil leucocytosis in 'bacterial infection'. This is, however, not a very reliable distinction.

Acute bronchiolitis

Acute bronchiolitis is a disease of infancy occurring in winter epidemics. The commonest cause is the respiratory syncytial virus but parainfluenza virus, adenovirus and *Mycoplasma pneumoniae* have been implicated in some epidemics. The most dangerous age is from 1–6 months.

Clinical features

The infant is acutely ill with fever, dyspnoea and rapid shallow respiration. There may be surprisingly little cough. Air entry to both lungs is decreased and fine crackling crepitations may be heard. Marked inspiratory rib retraction is usually present but cyanosis is variable. Sometimes an expiratory wheeze may be present. Generalised emphysema is present due to air trapping so that the diaphragm and liver may be depressed. X-ray of the chest reveals over-inflated lungs with patches of atelectasis, increased bronchovascular markings and flattened diaphragms.

Diagnosis

In some cases the virus responsible for the infection can be rapidly identified using immunofluorescent antibody tests on pharyngeal aspirate.

Treatment
A humidified oxygen tent should be used. Dehydration and electrolyte disturbances are common and should be corrected, as should acidosis when present. Antibiotics should be given if the patient is ill and it is not possible to make an aetiological diagnosis. Erythromycin is perhaps the antibiotic of choice as it covers *H. influenzae, M. pneumoniae* and the pneumococcus. A tranquilliser such as diazepam may be helpful. Severe cases may require intratracheal intubation and continuous positive airway pressure (CPAP).

The pneumonias

Pneumonia may be classified according to anatomical distribution or according to cause.

Anatomical diagnosis (where is the lesion?)
1 Lobar pneumonia.
2 Lobular pneumonia.
3 Bronchopneumonia.
4 Interstitial pneumonia.
5 Bronchiolitis.

Aetiological diagnosis
1 Bacterial infection (pneumococcus, streptococcus, staphylococcus, *Haemophilus influenzae, Klebsiella pneumoniae, Legionella pneumophila* and tubercle bacillus.
2 Viral infection and *Mycoplasma pneumoniae.*
3 Chlamydia (p. 309).
4 Rickettsiae (p. 311).
5 Fungi (candidiasis, histoplasmosis and coccidioidomycosis) (p. 364).
6 Protozoa (*Pneumocystis carinii*) (p. 365).
7 Metazoa (ascaris as a cause of Löffler's syndrome).
8 Aspiration (paraffin, oily nose drops, zinc stearate).

Clinical features
In infants pneumonia from any cause varies in severity. It may develop insidiously with an upper respiratory infection 'which goes to the chest'. It may begin acutely with high fever, dyspnoea, cough, and if there is pleuritic pain, a grunting respiration. Diarrhoea and vomiting may be misleading features. It may present as an 'acute abdomen' due to referral from the pleuritis along T6–12. Meningismus may be due to apical pneumonia. Convulsions may occur, but lumbar puncture usually reveals a clear fluid.

On physical examination there may be a few signs though usually the occurrence of dyspnoea, grunting, flaring of the ala nasae and rib retraction is strong evidence of underlying pulmonary disease. In bronchiolitis or bronchopneumonia, widespread crepitations may be heard while in lobar pneumonia the classical signs of consolidation are sometimes but not always present. In children and infants, it is always necessary to confirm the diagnosis by means of an X-ray of the chest (Fig. 20.5).

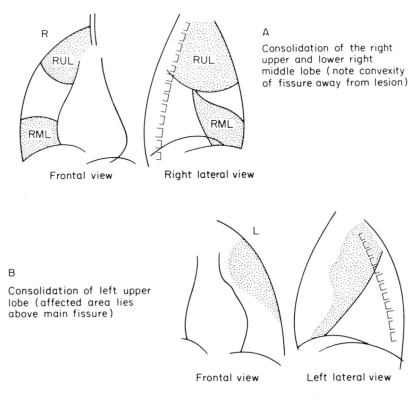

A

Consolidation of the right upper and lower right middle lobe (note convexity of fissure away from lesion)

Frontal view   Right lateral view

B

Consolidation of left upper lobe (affected area lies above main fissure)

Frontal view   Left lateral view

Fig. 20.5 Chest X-rays showing consolidation of the lungs

Pneumococcal pneumonia

Pneumococcal pneumonia is due to *Streptococcus pneumoniae* infection and is probably the commonest form of pneumonia in children, types 1, 6, 14 and 19 being the usual culprits. It is commonest in late winter and early spring. In infants it is usually bronchopneumonic in type, while in older children it tends to involve a single lobe. A frequent dry barking cough, fever, cyanosis and rigors may occur at the onset of the illness or there may be a prodromal illness resembling a 'cold' lasting 24–48 hours. Dyspnoea, flaring of the ala nasae, rib retraction and respiratory distress are usually noted. In infants the clinical signs may be minimal. If dullness to percussion is present it usually means fluid, whereas in older children dullness on percussion is due to consolidation of the underlying lung. Fluid in older children produces *stony* dullness. Auscultation may reveal fine crepitations and reduced breath sounds over the affected side. Expiratory sound may be prolonged and tubular breathing may be heard. The classical signs of consolidation may be present. When the patient begins to recover the signs change and coarse crepitations are heard while the cough becomes productive. The picture in older children is similar to that in adults.

Laboratory findings

The white blood count is markedly increased and polymorphonuclear leucocytes predominate. A low white count either indicates that the diagnosis is wrong or that the illness is a particularly grave one. The pneumococcus may be isolated from the blood in one-third of patients, as well as from the pharynx or from pleural fluid.

X-ray of the lungs in infants usually reveals a patchy infiltrate over both lung fields, whereas in older children consolidation of one or two lobes may be found. A small pleural effusion is common. X-ray signs of consolidation are often present before the physical signs appear and may persist for weeks after apparent recovery.

Complications

Empyema is a purulent exudate into the pleural cavity. It may lead to the formation of a thick fibrinous exudate on the pleural surfaces. Occasionally other infections such as pericarditis by direct extension may occur. Rarely peritonitis and osteomyelitis complicate the illness.

Treatment

Streptococcus pneumoniae is very sensitive to benzylpenicillin G, 125 000 U/m²/day four times daily i.m. being more than adequate. Improvement occurs in 24 hours though treatment should continue for several days. In recent years a number of penicillin-resistant strains of the organism have been cultured and some show multiple antibiotic resistance.

Adequate fluid and nutrient should be given. High fever can usually be controlled by tepid sponging. Analgesics such as paracetamol (140–280 mg/m² orally) should be given for pain. Initially pethidine may be required if the pain is severe. Empyemata should be drained surgically.

Streptococcal pneumonia

The clinical picture of streptococcal pneumonia may resemble that of pneumococcal pneumonia. Sometimes the infection is mainly interstitial and therefore there may be few signs to percussion or auscultation. In addition to a polymorphonuclear leucocytosis, the antistreptolysin O titre may be raised. X-ray may reveal lobar, bronchial or interstitial infection.

Treatment
Treatment is the same as for pneumococcal pneumonia.

Staphylococcal pneumonia

Two-thirds of patients with staphylococcal pneumonia are less than a year old. Epidemics may occur in nurseries, pathogenic organisms usually being coagulase positive staphylococci. Skin infections in the patient or in adult contacts are common. The characteristic features are the rapid progress of the illness, its toxicity and the tendency to produce pneumatoceles, pneumothorax and empyema. The pneumatoceles may become so large that they fill one hemithorax and cause a mediastinal shift to the opposite side. Marked respiratory distress and a shock-like state may accompany the illness.

X-ray reveals bronchopneumonia of varying extent and density. Pneumatoceles of varying size are usual and may occur on one or both sides. Rupture of a pneumatocele causes a pneumothorax or a pyopneumothorax. A bronchopleural fistula is a dangerous complication.

Therapy
The course of the illness is a stormy one. Oxygen is usually required and nutrition should be given parenterally for the first few days. The antibiotic of choice is one of the isoxazolyl penicillins such as oxacillin or cloxacillin which may have to be continued in large doses for several weeks. Empyemata should be drained surgically. Rupture of a pneumatocele should be anticipated as it may cause sudden collapse due to the formation of tension pneumothorax. A needle attached to an underwater tube should be inserted to reduce the tension. This may be followed by closed surgical drainage.

H. influenzae pneumonia

H. influenzae pneumonia is usually lobar in distribution. It tends to be more insidious in onset and more prolonged than pneumococcal pneumonia. Diagnosis is confirmed by finding *H. influenzae* type b in the nasopharynx or in the blood. The X-ray findings are those of lobar consolidation. Complications are common including pericarditis, empyema, septic arthritis and meningitis.

Treatment
The antibiotic of choice is ampicillin $4\,g/m^2/day$ or more by injection. Multiple antibiotic resistance is becoming common.

Klebsiella pneumonia

Klebsiella pneumoniae, previously known as Friedlander's bacillus, is now classified as a coliform bacterium. Although uncommon as a cause of pneumonia it causes a very serious infection. It produces a lobar pneumonia which rapidly breaks down to form multiple irregular cavities. Empyema is a common complication. X-ray shows consolidation with bulging of the fissure due to swelling of the lobe. Multiple abscesses may be noted within 48 hours. Diagnosis is confirmed by culture of the purulent secretion, the blood or pleural fluid.

Treatment
Gentamicin or amikacin are often recommended but the cephalosporin cefuroxine may also be used as it is also effective against staphylococcal pneumonia with which this disease may be confused. Treatment should be prolonged but despite this cavities may persist and resection may ultimately be required.

Warning: Any infant who has recurrent attacks of pneumonia should be investigated for gastro-oesophageal reflux, cystic fibrosis or immunological defects.

Legionnaire's disease

Legionnaire's disease, first discovered at the 58th Annual Convention of the American Legion in July 1976, is a respiratory infection due to an aerobic Gram-negative bacillus *Legionella pneumophila*. It is not uncommon in children, affecting males more than females (3:1).

Clinical features
Fever, malaise, muscle-pain, headache, abdominal pain, vomiting, rigors, chest pain and mental confusion may occur. Examination reveals an acutely ill patient with relative bradycardia, fever and crepitations. There is a neutrophilia, proteinuria, haematuria, and hyponatraemia of less than 130 mmol/l. X-ray shows patchy bronchopneumonia and there may be a pleural effusion.
   Diagnosis may be confirmed by an indirect fluorescent antibody test and by pleural fluid culture.

Treatment
Erythromycin (*adult dose*: 2–4 g daily) for 4–8 weeks as resolution may be slow.

Tuberculous pneumonia

See pages 325–328.

Mycoplasma pneumonia

Primary atypical pneumonia is an acute, self-limiting respiratory disorder characterised by malaise, fever, cough and pulmonary infiltrates. The cause is *Mycoplasma pneumoniae* (Eaton agent).

Clinical features

About 90 % of patients with *M. pneumoniae* infection are asymptomatic. The rest develop an upper or a lower respiratory infection. The incubation period is about two weeks, the onset is insidious with headache, chills and fever. Sore throat and a dry cough are common. Later the cough becomes productive with variable amounts of blood-streaked sputum. The remarkable feature of the illness is the paucity of clinical signs despite clear-cut radiological signs of pulmonary infiltration. It is most dense at the hilus, becoming less dense towards the periphery. Sometimes one lobe clears up while another lobe becomes affected. Recovery usually occurs in ten days.

Diagnosis

Diagnosis may be confirmed by culturing the *M. pneumoniae* in pharyngeal swabs and sputum and by serology (complement-fixation tests, haemagglutination inhibition tests and immunofluorescent techniques). Peak cold haemagglutinin titres occur in the third week, but are not specific in children. There may be a lymphocytosis.

Treatment

Treatment is symptomatic. Erythromycin destroys the mycoplasma but does not seem to alter the course of the illness. It does however prevent spread of the infection. Complications are unusual.

Fungal infections

Fungal infections tend to produce chronic lung lesions. *Actinomycosis* produces lung abscesses and chronic draining sinuses which contain typical 'sulphur granules'. Usually both lower lobes are involved. Treatment requires the use of massive doses of benzylpenicillin G, 5–10 mega units/m² daily for 6–8 weeks.

Other fungal infections are extremely rare except in patients with depressed immune responses due to extensive radiotherapy, corticosteroid or chemotherapy. *North American blastomycosis* may mimic viral infection, miliary tuberculosis or staphylococcal pneumonia. Treatment is with parenteral amphotericin B. *Histoplasmosis, coccidioidomycosis, nocardiosis* and *sporotrichosis* may also involve the lung during the course of their infection. Larger works should be consulted by the interested reader.

Interstitial plasma cell pneumonia

Pneumocystis carinii is a protozoon which can cause pneumonia in small newborn infants and children with altered host resistance following immunosuppressive therapy or as the result of a genetic defect. The source of the infection may be a contaminated incubator or atmospheric contamination.

Clinical features
The onset is usually insidious with cough which leads to respiratory distress over a period of 2–3 weeks. Cyanosis, tachypnoea and a bluish-white facial colour is noted. Fever is usually absent and there are few or no abnormal signs on percussion or auscultation. X-ray usually reveals hyperexpanded lung fields with a granular pattern. Hilar infiltration is present. Diagnosis is best confirmed by tracheal aspiration or by biopsy of the lung.

Treatment
Human immunoglobulin and pentamidine injection have been successful. Recently co-trimoxazole has been recommended.

Löffler's syndrome

Löffler's syndrome is an unusual allergic response to a variety of antigens, such as *Toxocara canis*, *T. cati* and *Ascaris lumbricoide*, which pass through the lungs during their life cycle and cause eosinophilic infiltration, with or without bronchospasm. There may be fever, cough and dyspnoea with paucity of lung signs. X-ray, however, reveals localised or generalised infiltrations or lobar consolidation. Blood count invariably shows an intense eosinophilia, often over 60 %. Hyperglobulinaemia and a positive heterophil agglutination test may be found.

Treatment
The allergic response may be controlled by antihistamines or, in severe cases, by corticosteroids. The underlying nematode infestation should be treated.

Aspiration pneumonia

In the newborn aspiration of amniotic debris, meconium or infected material may occur and require urgent bronchial toilet and antibiotic therapy.

Inhalation of milk may occur in tracheo-oesophageal fistula (p. 238) and in weak, debilitated infants. Patients with bulbar palsy are in great danger of aspiration. Inhalation of zinc stearate dusting powder causes an intense pulmonary reaction with bronchospasm.

Ingestion of paraffin (Kerosene) is almost invariably associated with aspiration (often aggravated by gastric lavage). There is fever, cough and drowsiness. Signs of consolidation develop early, usually within 24 hours. Treatment consists of magnesium sulphate to speed up expulsion of the paraffin, and benzylpenicillin G for the pneumonia. Oxygen and humidification are often helpful. In severely ill patients corticosteroids have been recommended to reduce the inflammatory response. Gastric wash-outs are contra-indicated in paraffin poisoning.

Lipoid pneumonia may be due to the use of oily nose-drops in babies or the inhalation of fish liver oil by a struggling infant. The latter is especially irritating to the lung and may cause a diffuse fibrosis. Cough and dyspnoea are usually present. Signs of bronchopneumonia may be present. X-ray reveals perihilar infiltration spreading towards the periphery of the lungs.

Treatment is symptomatic. Frequent change of position is recommended.

Prevention

Oily nose-drops should be avoided. Medicines should never be forced down the throat of a struggling child. Vitamin A and D should be given in water-miscible form. Castor oil and mineral oil should be banned. Infants who regurgitate easily should be nursed prone.

Atelectasis

Primary atelectasis means failure of the alveoli to expand. It is seen only in the newborn, especially babies of low birth-weight.

Secondary atelectasis or re-absorption collapse is usually due to obstruction of the affected bronchi. The obstruction is most commonly due to inhalation during an anaesthetic, but there may be many causes:

1 Obstruction of a bronchus by foreign body, mucus, aspirated material, or tuberculotic granulomatous tissue.
2 Lesions in the wall of the bronchus such as tuberculotic or fibrotic lesions.
3 Pressure on the lungs or bronchi from outside:
   (a) Impaired respiratory excursion such as occurs in bulbar poliomyelitis, cerebral palsy, Guillain-Barré syndrome, spinal muscular atrophy and other neurological diseases.
   (b) Chest deformity due to severe rickets or kyphoscoliosis such as in Morquio-Brailsford syndrome.
   (c) Diaphragmatic paralysis.
   (d) Pleural effusion, pneumothorax or diaphragmatic hernia preventing expansion of the lung.
   (e) Compression on a bronchus by enlarged lymph nodes, tumours or cardiac enlargement.

Clinical features

Symptoms depend on the size of the collapsed lung. Small areas are asymptomatic. Large areas cause dyspnoea, rapid respiration, flaring of the nostrils and cyanosis. Collapse of the apex causes the trachea to be displaced towards the same side. Collapse of a basal lobe causes mediastinal shift or elevation of the ipsilateral diaphragm. There is diminished air entry over the affected lobe with decrease in vocal fremitus. The percussion note may be dull or it may be unchanged because the remaining lobe undergoes compensatory emphysema.

Diagnosis
Diagnosis is confirmed by radiology (Fig. 20.6). Small areas of collapse associated with small areas of emphysema is characteristic of cystic fibrosis. A lobar collapse may resemble consolidation though usually concavity of the affected fissure is noted in collapse and the lobe is reduced in size.

Displacement of the trachea or mediastinum to the affected side may be noted, unless compensatory emphysema of the unaffected lobe occurs.

Therapy
Prevention may be achieved by proper breathing exercises before and after anaesthesia, and proper ventilation during the anaesthetic. Postural drainage and percussion of the chest helps to shift mucous plugs. Coughing should be encouraged and not suppressed. Antibiotics are usually required for secondary infection. The underlying causes should be treated when possible.

Pleurisy

Pleurisy is an inflammation of the pleural sac. It may be a primary disease but is more commonly secondary to pulmonary disease, such as lobar or bronchopneumonia, or tuberculosis. It may be dry or wet. Dry pleurisy is characterised by severe pain which may be localised over the chest or may be referred to shoulder or abdomen. It is aggravated by movement of the chest or diaphragm and causes the child to grunt with each respiration. A short, sharp, painful cough is usually present. On examination the affected side of the chest shows diminished movement. In diaphragmatic pleurisy pain may be referred to the shoulder and the abdominal wall may be rigid. There may be decreased air entering the lungs as a result of the diminished movement on the affected side, and a *pleural friction rub* may be heard. This is usually a harsh sound synchronised with respiration. It usually disappears in 24–48 hours and this is attributed to fluid separating the inflamed surfaces. The condition may resolve completely; it may form a dense fibrotic layer which literally splints the lung; or it may progress to form a pleural effusion.

X-ray of the chest may reveal a clear-cut shadow at the site of the inflammation or there may be a diffuse irregularly shaped shadow. There may of course be evidence of underlying lung pathology such as lobar pneumonia or tuberculosis.

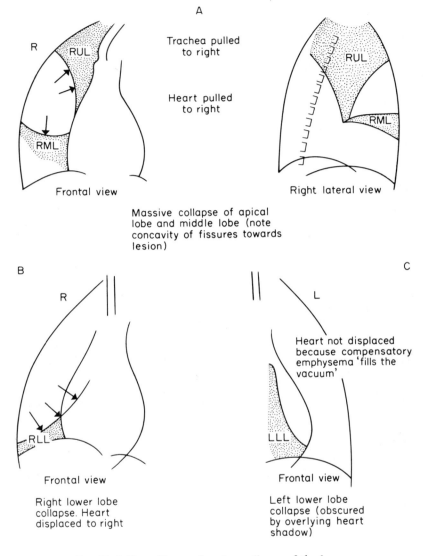

A

Trachea pulled
to right

Heart pulled
to right

Frontal view

Right lateral view

Massive collapse of apical
lobe and middle lobe (note
concavity of fissures towards
lesion)

B

Frontal view

Right lower lobe
collapse. Heart
displaced to right

C

Heart not displaced
because compensatory
emphysema 'fills the
vacuum'

Frontal view

Left lower lobe
collapse (obscured
by overlying heart
shadow)

Fig. 20.6 Chest X-rays showing collapse of the lungs

Treatment
Pain may be relieved by salicylates and by strapping the chest to reduce
movement. Antibiotics should be given for underlying bacterial
infection.

Empyema

Empyema is a collection of pus in the pleural cavity, which is especially likely to complicate pneumococcal, staphylococcal or *H. influenzae* pneumonia. It should be suspected when a child with pneumonia responds poorly to therapy or there is a recurrence of fever and dyspnoea. The signs which develop may be similar to those of pleural effusion (see below). There may be marked pleural thickening with loculation of the pus. The pus may collect between the fissures.

Blood count usually reveals a marked increase in polymorph leucocytes.

Treatment

Initially antibiotics are given once a specimen of the empyema fluid has been sent for culture and sensitivity. Local instillation of antibiotic may speed up the sterilisation of the fluid and encourage reabsorption. Large collections of pus should be drained. If the exudate is fibrinous, streptokinase may be instilled to dissolve these deposits before they cause thickening of the pleura. Sometimes surgical drainage is required but usually repeated needle aspirations are adequate in children.

Pleural effusion

Wet pleurisy or pleural effusion may consist of exudate, transudate, blood or chyle in the pleural cavity.

Exudates are inflammatory in origin and may represent an early empyema (see above) or it may be sterile as in polyserositis, partially treated pneumonia, neuroblastoma and tuberculosis.

A *transudate* is a clear, sterile, yellow fluid with a low specific gravity (hydrothorax). It may be found in congestive heart failure, acute nephritis, nephrosis or malnutrition.

Blood in the pleural sac (haemothorax) is usually due to trauma, diseases of the blood clotting mechanism or neuroblastoma. *Chyle* is usually due to obstruction to the thoracic duct. It is the commonest cause for a fluid collection in the chest of neonates, and is due to rupture of the thoracic duct.

Clinical features

Absent or diminished movement on the affected side with stony dullness over the effusion is found. Above the effusion an area of tubular or amphoric breathing may be heard, whereas over the effusion itself the breath sounds are reduced or absent. The degree of dyspnoea and cyanosis depends on the size of the effusion.

X-ray confirms the presence of a collection of fluid in the chest.

Treatment

The underlying disease should be treated. The chest should be tapped for diagnostic purposes and to relieve the pressure from a large effusion. In tuberculosis the use of corticosteroids for a few days may speed up the resorption of the fluid, provided that the drug is covered by anti-tuberculosis therapy.

Pleurodynia

Also known as Bornholm disease and epidemic myalgia, pleurodynia is characterised by the sudden onset of the acute, severe pain in the lower chest or abdomen. There may be fever, dyspnoea and headache. The pain may strike with great suddenness and children have been known to double up in the middle of a class during an attack. It may simulate pleurisy or an 'acute abdomen'. It is caused by a coxsackie B virus.

Treatment
Treatment consists of bed rest and analgesics. Strapping of the chest may be helpful.

Bronchiectasis

Bronchiectasis is a chronic disease characterised by localised or generalised dilatation of the bronchi, with progressive fibrosis and destruction of the affected lung.

In cystic fibrosis the bronchiectasis is generalised, tubular and associated with widespread areas of emphysema and atelectasis.

Bronchiectasis of the saccular type may be a complication of foreign body in the lung, acute viral or bacterial infection or chronic lesions such as tuberculosis.

In a small percentage of cases bronchiectasis is associated with sinusitis and dextrocardia (Kartagener's syndrome) and is due to abnormal ciliary action.

Clinical features
A chronic loose cough, which is aggravated by change of posture (lying down or getting up) or by exercise is usually present and becomes progressively worse. Dyspnoea, anorexia and loss of weight develop at some stage of the disease. Halitosis due to the presence of copious foul-smelling pus and debris in the dilated bronchi is often a feature unless the patient learns to cough up the material completely. Haemoptysis is less common than in adults.

Clubbing of the fingers and cyanosis may develop early and becomes progressively worse. The chest signs vary from time to time but coarse rales, which do not disappear on coughing, can usually be heard. A low-grade fever is present.

Laboratory findings
Various Gram-positive and Gram-negative organisms are cultured depending on what antibiotics the patient has been treated with. Resistant organisms often become a problem. There is usually a chronic

anaemia. On X-ray of the chest heavy basal markings are commonly found. In some areas cyst-like spaces may be found. The sinuses are often affected. Bronchography with the insertion of contrast medium into the affected lobes may be used to define the exact areas that are affected, prior to surgery.

Treatment
Antibiotics should be given according to sensitivity tests on sputum cultures. They may be given orally and by aerosol. Postural drainage should be carried out two or three times daily to prevent stasis. This is perhaps the most important part of the treatment.

Attention should be paid to infected sinuses, tonsils and adenoids. Surgery should be considered for lesions localised to one or two segments or to one or two lobes, which do not respond to conservative treatment. It should never be used in cystic fibrosis because the lesions are too extensive.

Lung abscess

Lung abscesses may be single or multiple. They are commonly due to bronchial obstruction, the distal portion of the lobe or segment becoming atelectatic and infected. An abscess forms when the infected tissue becomes necrotic. Sometimes it opens into a bronchus, the pus is coughed up and it heals by fibrosis. Sometimes the abscess becomes encapsulated by a thick wall. The organisms most commonly cultured are staphylococci and *Klebsiella* organisms which cause single or multiple abscesses. Anaerobic or mixed flora are often found. Tuberculosis and certain fungi produce chronic, multiple lesions. Host resistance plays an important role in the formation of abscesses. A common cause for lung abscess is aspiration of foreign bodies like peanuts, or aspiration of infected material during anaesthetic.

Clinical features
The history of inhalation of foreign body, or of a recent anaesthetic, may precede the onset of fever, which is usually intermittent or hectic in type. Cough is often present but may be unproductive. If the abscess is near the surface of the lung pleuritic pain may be present. It may rupture into a bronchus producing spontaneous cure. Haemoptysis may occur. Clubbing can develop very rapidly in some patients. X-ray may reveal circular lesions with or without fluid levels.

Treatment
Vigorous antibiotic therapy may sometimes abort an abscess. Underlying causes such as foreign body or agammaglobulinaemia should be treated when present. Sometimes the abscess points into a bronchus and can be opened under direct vision and aspirated. Postural drainage should be carried out 4-hourly to encourage emptying and

closure of the cavity. Surgery to remove an infected lobe is rarely indicated.

Pulmonary function tests

Pulmonary function tests in young children can be done in specially equipped respiratory units. They help to distinguish *obstructive* diseases such as bronchial asthma from *restrictive* lung diseases such as that resulting from kyphoscoliosis.

The forced vital capacity (FVC) is the maximum volume of air that can be forced out of the lungs after maximum inspiration. The forced expiratory volume in one second (FEV_1) is the volume of air expired in the first second while performing the FVC.

In *obstructive* disease the FVC is normal or reduced and the arterial P_{CO_2} increased or normal. The FEV_1 is always decreased. The P_{O_2} may be normal or decreased. In *restrictive* lung disease the FVC and P_{O_2} are decreased while the P_{CO_2} is increased. Although the FEV_1 is reduced the FEV_1/FVC is within normal limits. In most patients a satisfactory diagnosis can be made on the FVC and the FEV_1. See the Spirogram in lung disorders (Fig. 20.7).

The P_{O_2} and P_{CO_2} may be measured from blood sampled from the radial artery using a 25-gauge needle. For repeated sampling a percutaneous arterial line should be placed. In newborns the radial or umbilical artery may be used.

Oxygen therapy

Arterial oxygen tension should be kept between 8 and 10 kPa (60 and 90 mmHg). Nasal catheters or nasal prongs maintain the concentration of oxygen entering the respiratory tract at 40 % with a flow of 2 l/min. Oxygen tents, unless well-sealed, maintain a concentration of less than 30 %. In premature babies oxygen therapy can damage the lungs and eyes (retrolental fibroplasia). Arterial oxygen tension therefore should be maintained between 8–12 kPa (60–90 mmHg) to avoid hyper-oxaemia. In carbon monoxide poisoning hyperbaric oxygen at 1–2 atmospheres (100–200 kPa) is highly effective, the patient recovering in half-an-hour.

Humidification

In asthma and other conditions where there is a tendency for mucus to dry out, humidification of the air is recommended in order to prevent dehydration of the air passages. For large airways, for example after tracheostomy, humidification with particles of $10 \, \mu$m diameter is suggested. For small airway problems ultrasonic nebulisers should be considered as very fine particles are possible. It is thought that mouth-breathing is superior to nose-breathing for inspiring these fine particles into the bronchioles.

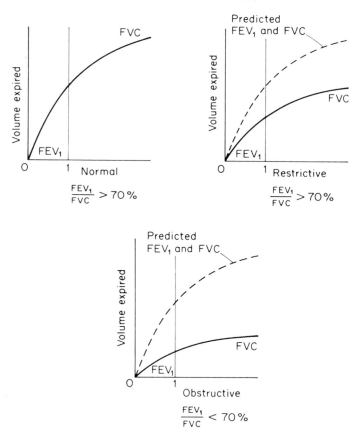

Fig. 20.7 Spirogram of lung disorders

RESPIRATORY FAILURE

Respiratory failure may be defined as any condition which causes a persistent increase in arterial P_{CO_2} of 7.5 kPa or more associated with hypoxaemia (P_{ao_2} less than 8.0 kPa). It may be caused by:

1 Lung diseases such as severe bronchial asthma, severe laryngeal stridor, cystic fibrosis, respiratory distress syndrome, pneumonia, pulmonary oedema or cor pulmonale.
2 Foreign body in the lung.
3 Cyanotic heart disease.
4 Disorders of the central nervous system such as head injury, bulbar poliomyelitis, Guillain-Barré syndrome, myasthenia gravis, amyotonia congenita.

Treatment

The underlying disorder should be corrected when possible, so that the oxygen and carbon dioxide tension can be restored to normal. Ventilation may be of two types:

1 Assisted ventilation, in which the slightest effort by the patient triggers the machine to complete the respiratory cycle.
2 Controlled ventilation in which the machine breathes for the patient. It controls the rate and depth of respiration. Usually the patient is given morphia or neuromuscular blocking agents to prevent him from taking over respiration on his own.

Ventilators are of two types:

1 Volume cycled ventilators such as the Angström which delivers preset volumes of gas to the lung and are useful in asthma and pulmonary oedema.
2 Pressure cycled ventilators, such as the Bird, in which gas flow ceases as soon as the preset pressure is reached.

Artificial respiration in children

The airway should be cleared, the head extended with forward traction on the mandible and mouth-to-mouth respiration commenced immediately. In babies it may be sufficient in using mouth-to-mouth respiration for the operator to fill his cheeks with air (or even lead an oxygen tube into his mouth) and to blow gently into the baby's lungs. For older children, however, the operator should take a deeper breath and blow somewhat harder. It is convenient to practise these manoeuvres on appropriately sized models which are available. Some of the models such as 'Resusci-Anne' are highly sophisticated and some are available with electronic gadgetry which register correct and incorrect actions by the operator.

Mouth-to-mouth respiration should be continued indefinitely unless unequivocal signs of death such as *rigor mortis* sets in. A fixed dilated pupil is a sign of death provided that the patient is not suffering from belladonna, atropine or imipramine poisoning. Prolonged unresponsive hypothermia is significant. As long as the heart beats the operator should persist with his efforts until help arrives or the patient can be placed on a ventilating machine.

Drowning

Drowning means death of the patient after submersion in water. The term *near drowning* is used to denote survival after submersion in water. The most serious consequence of near drowning is hypoxaemia which may occur as a result of acute laryngospasm or may follow aspiration.

The initial procedures are the same whether the patient drowns in fresh or salt water:

1 Initiate mouth-to-mouth breath *immediately*. If there is no effective circulation a second assistant should intiate closed cardiac massage.
2 As soon as suction apparatus is available the throat should be suctioned and a stomach tube passed to empty the stomach while artificial respiration is continued.
3 Oxygen should be administered, under pressure if necessary, to overcome low lung compliance.
4 Fluid and electrolyte disturbances should be assessed and treated. Metabolic or respiratory acidosis, haemoglobinuria and ventricular fibrillation require vigorous treatment.
5 In sea-water aspiration, large volumes of protein-containing fluid may be lost from the lungs (secondary drowning) and should be replaced by plasma.
6 Sedatives should be given if the patient is conscious and agitated. The role of corticosteroids is not settled. Prophylactic antibiotics are advisable especially if the water is known to be contaminated.
7 Pulmonary oedema may require intermittent positive pressure respiration.
8 Hypothermia should be treated.

Accidental hypothermia

When rescuing victims of immersion or exposure to cold, priority should be given to thin children and those that seem the quietest. The body should be immersed in a hot bath at 41–45°C with the limbs and head held out of the water. In all cases heat loss should be prevented by removing wet clothes, drying the skin and covering the patient in dry blankets.

In the case of suspected cardiopulmonary arrest mouth-to-mouth respiration and closed chest cardiac massage should be carried out at half the normal rate.

If the core temperature is less than 30°C, colonic lavage and intravenous infusions at 40°C may be given. Peritoneal dialysis with warm fluids may also be tried. It is said that atrial fibrillation may be ignored but ventricular fibrillation requires urgent cardioversion.

The onset of shivering is said to be a good prognostic sign.

CHAPTER 21

SKELETAL AND ORTHOPAEDIC DISORDERS

CONGENITAL ANOMALIES

Complete absence of all four extremities is called *amelia*, while the absence of one extremity is *ectromelia*. Absence of the proximal parts of the extremities so that the hands and feet arise direct from the trunk is called *phocomelia* or *seal limbs*. Thousands of such patients were born with these abnormalities due to the use of thalidomide during pregnancy and many are with us still, but chorionic bands may be a factor in some cases.

Intra-uterine amputations, partial or complete, may occur. Sometimes deep circular grooves may be seen encircling a limb or one or more digits. The cause is not understood.

Absence or deformity of individual bones such as the radius or fibula may occur, with or without other congenital anomalies, for example the *Holt-Oram syndrome*, which consists of hypoplastic thumbs, skeletal anomalies of the limbs and an atrial septal defect. Skeletal deformities are also found in Fanconi's Apert's and Marfan's syndromes (pp. 97, 155 and 124). Increase in the number of digits, *polydactyly*, is common. The extra digit may be a pedunculated tag of tissue on the ulnar border of the hand. Fusion of the digits (*syndactyly*) occurs or there may be a complete absence of one or two digits and their metacarpal bones, especially the third and fourth, such as occurs in *lobster claw hand*. This may be symmetrical and involve both hands and feet. *Congenital trigger thumb* or *fingers* may be found. *Gigantism* or *dwarfism* of individual digits or limbs may occur. Sometimes *hemi-hypertrophy* or *hemi-atrophy* of the whole of one side of the body may occur; or a limb may hypertrophy due to the presence of a large cavernous haemangioma or lymphangiectasia.

Bow legs (genu varum) and knock knees (genu valgum)

Bow legs and knock knees are common causes for parental concern. Bow legs are almost universal in babies, the appearance being exaggerated by the distribution of fat on the lateral side of the calves. It tends to disappear with growth and the legs may go through a phase in which knock knee is present. This rarely lasts beyond $2\frac{1}{2}$–3 years. When knock knee is associated with over-weight there is sometimes laxity of both knee and ankle ligaments present. The patient should be encouraged to lose weight otherwise pain in the limbs may become a distressing problem later. Knock knees tends to persist beyond puberty in fat patients. In all children with such problems torsion of the tibia or femur should be excluded by comparing the plane of the ankles and knees.

Club feet (talipes equino-varus)

One should carefully distinguish true club foot in which deformity of the tarsal bones is present, and deformities due to an abnormal fetal position of the foot. The latter is easily corrected by manipulation and disappears within a week or so. Severe club foot is a more difficult problem. If conservative measures fail then aggressive surgery may be required as early as 6–12 weeks of life to obtain the best results.

Congenital dislocation of the hip

This can often be diagnosed at or soon after birth and, with proper treatment, can be cured in a few weeks or months. If diagnosis is delayed until the toddler begins walking then treatment is prolonged, unpleasant, and the results are not always satisfactory. It should be routine to examine the hips of every newborn baby at birth. Full abduction and external rotation is usually possible. If this is limited the disorder should be suspected. *Ortolani's sign* is a clicking sound heard from the hip at the end of passive abduction. It is due to the subluxated head of the femur slipping back into the acetabulum. On adduction it slips out again with a click. The creases of the thighs may be asymmetrical. The diagnosis should be confirmed by X-ray of the hips.

Dislocation of the hip should also be looked for in older children with cerebral palsy and spastic paraplegia in which severe adductor spasm causes the dislocation. Bilateral dislocation may occur in hypothyroidism causing a waddling gait and lordosis.

Flat foot (pes valgus)

Flat foot is almost universal before three years of age and requires no therapy. In the infant it is due to 'filling-in' of the arch of the foot with plantar fat. If there are no symptoms no treatment is required. When flat foot is secondary to spasticity or hypotonia surgical intervention may be indicated.

Cleidocranial dysostosis

Cleidocranial dysostosis is a rare, dominantly inherited disorder in which membrane bone fails to develop. The clavicles are absent permitting the anterior shoulders to meet in the mid-line. The skull is poorly ossified and there is delay in teething and development of ossification centres.

Craniofacial dysostosis (Crouzon's disease)

See page 155.

Sprengel's deformity

Sprengel's deformity is a rare disorder in which one scapula is small, elevated and fixed. There is limitation of movement at the affected shoulder girdle. Treatment is orthopaedic. An abnormal scapula may be associated with the *Klippel-Feil syndrome* in which the neck is very short due to absence or fusion of several cervical vertebrae, and there is a web which runs from the ear to the shoulder. It should be distinguished from *platybasia* in which there is flattening of the base of the skull. This results in kinking of the medulla oblongata over the odontoid process (C2).

Arthrogryposis multiplex congenita

This is a disorder in which fibrous ankylosis of some or all of the joints of the limbs occurs. As a result fixed contractures in flexion or extension occur. The limbs are small contrasting with the large fusiform or cylindrical joints. The muscles are atrophic. Treatment is orthopaedic.

Osteogenesis imperfecta congenita

This is a rare, dominantly inherited disorder, in which multiple fractures occur *in utero*. The mother often hears the bones snap. The baby is born with severe deformity due to multiple fractures in varying stages of healing. In addition deep blue sclera and lax ligaments are noted. The teeth are poorly formed and deafness occurs due to 'otosclerosis'. Excess sweating and constipation occur.

Less severe forms, *osteogenesis imperfecta tarda*, may occur. Fractures first appear *after* birth due to the thinness of the bone cortex.

Treatment
There is no specific treatment. Parents need guidance about the risks of recurrence and advice on how to protect their children from *unnecessary* trauma. Fractures are treated with the minimum immobilisation. As in so many disorders with variable expression, the severity of the disease tends to be similar to that already found in the family.

Achondroplasia

Achondroplasia is a form of dwarfism which may be inherited as a dominant autosomal character or may be the result of a mutation. The condition is recognisable at birth as the infant has short limbs but a normal sized trunk. The head by contrast is large. Milestones and intelligence are usually normal. The gait is waddling, laxity of the ligaments is present though the elbow and knee joints may show limitation of extension. The fingers are short and arranged in pairs of equal length ('trident hand'). X-ray reveals that the tubular bones are short and thick, the epiphyseal plates are irregular, and the ends of the long bones very broad.

Treatment
There is no treatment. Achondroplastic females can only deliver by Caesarian section. Many of the children have become famous as clowns in circuses. Their ability to jump from the sitting to standing position is quite startling.

POSTNATAL ORTHOPAEDIC DISORDERS

Non-accidental injury
See Child Abuse, page 388.

Caffey's disease (infantile cortical hyperostosis)

Caffey's disease is a curious disorder occurring *in utero* and in the first few months of life. It is characterised by laminated cortical thickening of the jaw, facial bones, clavicle, scapula, ribs and long bones. They are tender to the touch and the overlying tissues are thickened. The skin is freely mobile. Fever and a raised blood sedimentation rate is commonly present. The patient may be acutely ill. The local glands never swell. Recovery is the rule but may take several weeks or even months. The diagnosis is confirmed by X-ray of the face, jaw, scapula and extremities. The condition must be distinguished from bone malignancies, hypervitaminosis A (which does not affect the jaw), non-accidental injury and osteomyelitis.

Treatment
The disease is self-limiting. Severe cases benefit by corticosteroids which are given until the fever has settled for 48 hours. Recurrence is common. Antibiotics are not indicated.

Juvenile rheumatoid arthritis (Still's disease)

Juvenile rheumatoid arthritis embraces a number of clinical syndromes involving chronic inflammatory joint disease and is mentioned in this chapter for convenience. It is uncommon and the cause is unknown.

Clinital features
The disease may present at any time after early infancy, sometimes as a 'pyrexia of unknown origin'. The temperature can be as high as 40°C and is often associated with a pale pink maculopapular rash which comes and goes. The child appears toxic and may have enlargement of the lymph nodes, liver and spleen. Subcutaneous nodules may sometimes be felt over bony prominences. The nature of the illness declares

itself when the patient develops arthralgia or polyarthritis. Joints usually affected include the knees, ankles, wrists and interphalangeal joints, but other joints such as the cervical spine may be involved.

Juvenile rheumatoid arthritis can also present with arthritis of one or two joints only. In these children there may be little in the way of systemic illness and the disease runs a chronic course. *Iridocyclitis* may occur and should be looked for by slit lamp examination.

Girls are particularly susceptible to a form of the disease where several joints are severely affected leading to joint deformity and loss of function.

Diagnosis

There is no specific test for juvenile rheumatoid arthritis and a definitive diagnosis may be impossible in the early stages of the disease. The blood shows a neutrophil leucocytosis and a high ESR. Immunoglobulin M rheumatoid factor is absent except in older children with 'adult disease'. Antinuclear antibody may be present particularly in patients with iridocyclitis. Synovial biopsy may be required to make the diagnosis if only one joint is affected. Radiological changes may be absent in the early stages of the disease; soft tissue swelling and periarticular osteoporosis may be seen, but by the time other X-ray changes are found the diagnosis is obvious.

Differential diagnosis

Septic arthritis and osteomyelitis should be excluded by blood culture, aspiration and, if necessary, tuberculin skin testing. Arthritis due to viral infections such as rubella, adenovirus and infectious hepatitis should be excluded by serological tests. In anaphylactic purpura arthritis may preceed the abdominal pain and skin rash. In rheumatic fever there is evidence of a preceeding streptococcal infection. Arthritis may be the first manifestation of ulcerative colitis or Crohn's disease. Other collagen disorders such as systemic lupus erythematosis and neoplastic diseases such as leukaemia and neuroblastoma may also cause confusion.

Treatment

Soluble aspirin is the drug of choice. If a high dose is required blood salicylate levels should be measured to prevent overdosage. Gastro-intestinal discomfort can be minimised by using enteric coated aspirin (Nu-Seals aspirin). Ibuprofen and naproxen may also be used. If the child is severely affected long-term treatment with penicillamine or gold should be considered. Patients with persistent systemic symptoms may require corticosteroid therapy.

Regular physiotherapy is essential to alleviate pain and prevent loss of function and deformity. Occasionally orthopaedic advice is necessary. The paediatrician should supervise the affected patient closely and attend to his emotional and physical needs at home and at school.

Prognosis
The long-term outlook is generally much better than in adults. In most cases the disease 'burns' itself out after a number of years. About one-third of patients will be left with a chronic handicap.

Juvenile osteochondroses

A number of degenerative diseases of the epiphyses occur. They probably all have the same underlying pathology. In *Perthes' disease* avascular necrosis of the femoral head occurs between four and eight years of age. It is four times commoner in boys than in girls. It is occasionally bilateral. Initially there is an intermittent limp which becomes constant and painful. The pain is referred to the medial side of the knee. There is limitation of abduction and rotation of the hip. X-ray reveals flattening of the head, followed by fragmentation. The femoral neck becomes thickened. Treatment is orthopaedic. The condition should be distinguished from tuberculosis of the hip in which the pain *precedes* the limp. Osteoarthritis may develop ten or more years after apparent healing.

Other sites of osteochondrosis include the tibial tuberosity (*Osgood-Schlatter's disease*), the tarsal navicular (*Kohler's disease*) and the vertebral bodies (*Scheuermann's disease*).

Albright's disease

Polyostotic fibrous dysplasia is a rare disorder which may occur with or without endocrine disturbances. It is characterised by unilateral fibrous replacement of bones with multiple radiotranslucent areas (cysts) which have sclerotic margins. In addition there are large *café-au-lait* spots (areas of light brown pigmentation) of the skin on the ipsilateral side. Endocrine disturbances include precocious puberty, hyperthyroidism and hyperadrenalism.

Treatment
There is no treatment. Pathological fractures should be treated by curettage and, if the defect is large, by bone grafting. Once adulthood is reached, the lesions do not enlarge further. The disease does not shorten life.

INFECTIONS OF BONE AND JOINTS

Osteomyelitis and pyoarthrosis may complicate sepsis of the newborn or septicaemia at any age, particularly if there is depression of the immune mechanisms. Sickle-cell anaemia and trauma are known to predispose to osteomyelitis.

Osteomyelitis

Osteomyelitis is almost always due to *Staphylococcus aureus* but *Haemophilus influenzae*, streptococci and other organisms may also cause it. It usually begins in the vascular part of the bone, the metaphysis. Intense pain, fever and toxaemia develop rapidly while local tenderness, swelling and heat are present over the affected area. X-ray of the affected bone usually shows nothing abnormal in the bone in the first ten days, but soft-tissue swelling may be present. There is always a marked polymorphonuclear leucocytosis.

Differential diagnosis

Acute rheumatic fever often seems to begin with pain in one limb, but other features of the disease are usually present. Osteogenic sarcoma may cause confusion. In babies it may be difficult to locate whether the lesion is in the bone or joint (it may be in both!).

Treatment

It may be possible in many cases to control the infection with antibiotic therapy (cloxacillin, fusidic acid or erythromycin are effective for staphylococci), but it may be at the cost of extensive bone destruction. In our opinion the bone should be opened to relieve tension and to allow the pus to drain. At the same time the pus should be cultured and sensitivity tests done. Immobilisation of the limb is recommended but bed exercise, under guidance of a physiotherapist, is advised until full recovery.

Acute suppurative arthritis

This disease may be due to a number of organisms including staphylococci, pneumococci, gonococci, *S. typhi* and *E. coli*. In the newborn *E. coli* and staphylococci are the common infecting organisms. Any joint may be infected but usually the knee, ankle, hip and shoulder are likely to be affected. There is local pain, swelling and toxaemia, while limitation of movement with extreme pain on attempts to move the joint are to be expected.

Diagnosis

Diagnosis is confirmed by aspiration of the pus *via* a fairly thick needle. It should be sent for culture and sensitivity.

Treatment

Treatment should begin as soon as the pus is sent for culture. An antistaphylococcal antibiotic combined with gentamicin may be given in large doses until the results of the sensitivity tests are available. The joint should be immobilised but bed exercises encouraged.

Tuberculosis of bone and joints

Infection is usually secondary to pulmonary or gastro-intestinal tuberculosis. Infection in the bone usually breaks through the epiphyses into the joint. The common sites are the spine, hip, knee, ankle, shoulder and elbow. Sometimes it affects several fingers (tuberculous dactylitis) causing spindle-shaped swellings. Caseous material forms and usually burrows through to the surface. The treatment is discussed on p. 327.

Transient synovitis of the hip (irritable hip syndrome)

Limp and pain referred to the knee in children aged 5–10 years may be due to transient synovitis of the hip. It is probably traumatic in origin. Needling of the joint reveals a sterile, clear or slightly turbid fluid. X-ray is normal. Differential diagnosis includes Perthes' disease, osteomyelitis, rheumatic fever and tuberculosis of the hip. Treatment is bed rest until symptoms have subsided.

Tumours of bone

An expanding *bone cyst* may be found as the result of a pathologic fracture or as an unexpected finding on an X-ray taken for other reasons. Most patients do not require therapy as the cyst stops growing when the patient does. Fracture is said to result in cure in some cases. In others the cyst should be curetted and filled with bone chips.

Multiple exostoses (diaphyseal aclasis)

This is an autosomal dominant disorder in which the exostoses grow from the diaphyses of the long bones. They sometimes cause pressure symptoms or they may retard the growth of the affected limb.

Osteoid osteoma

This is usually a solitary lesion which causes severe boring pain, especially at night. The lesion consists of a dense nidus of bone which is easily excised. Aspirin is said to be a specific pain reliever in this condition.

Malignant Tumours

1 Ewing's tumour

This is a rare malignant tumour of the shaft of a long bone, or the flat bones of the skull or pelvis, and usually occurs between five and ten years. It causes local pain and swelling and metastasizes to the lungs or to other bones. Any bone may be involved. On X-ray it is seen that the tumour extends through the shaft, sometimes raising the periosteum in layers ('onion skin'). New bone is laid down in the medullary cavity. The tumour may be arranged in radial lines ('sun ray'). It must be carefully differentiated from osteomyelitis and neuroblastoma. Treatment consists of high dose radiotherapy and chemotherapy using agents such as vincristine, cyclophosphamide and doxorubicin. The condition is almost unknown in blacks.

2 Osteogenic sarcoma

Osteogenic sarcoma is commonest between 10 and 20 years and tends to arise at the ends of long bones. It tends to produce islands of new bones which may extend into the soft tissues, as well as causing destruction of existing bone. Treatment consists of extensive surgery and radiotherapy, but cures are infrequent. Recently chemotherapeutic regimens using high dose methotrexate with citrovorum factor rescue, doxorubicin and cyclophosphamide have been tried.

3 Secondary neoplasms

Leukaemia, neuroblastoma, Wilms' tumour and osteogenic sarcomas can metastasise to bones causing pain, swelling and pathological fractures.

Neurofibromata of nerve roots are non-malignant tumours which cause pressure symptoms. Scoliosis is common.

CHAPTER 22

CHILD HEALTH AND COMMUNITY PAEDIATRICS

Previous chapters in this book have concentrated mainly on how to examine, diagnose and treat sick children. This is in keeping with the definition of paediatrics as 'the study of disease in children'.

The report 'Fit for the Future' of the Committee of Child Health Services (1976) noted:

'We believe that children have a right to basic health care which comprehends not only treatment at times of illnesses or injury, but also continuing surveillance to promote health and detect disability or handicap'.

We should thus see paediatrics as 'the branch of medicine dealing with children'.

CHILD HEALTH

Comprehensive Paediatrics

Health ——————— | ——————— **Care**

Mental   Preventive
Physical   Promotive
Emotional   Curative
Social   Rehabilitative

The Child

Home   School

Family

Community

Environment

Child health

Child health encompasses the comprehensive care of the individual child—preventive, promotive, curative and, if necessary, rehabilitative. It interprets health in its broadest sense, aiming to enable all children to reach their full potential—physically, mentally, socially and emotionally. The child is also considered in relation to his family, his community and his environment. These latter factors are major determinants of health especially for children who, being immature and dependent, are particularly vulnerable to external circumstances.

Community paediatrics

Community paediatrics is concerned with the health and well-being of all the children in a community. The community may consist of a national population, or simply a group of children within a school or family practice.

The techniques of epidemiology are used to study the determinants and distribution of health and disease in such populations of children. Priorities can then be determined, suitable solutions considered, implemented and evaluated (see Bryant's Problem Solving Cycle as described in D. C. Morley's *Paediatric Priorities in the Developing World*', Butterworths, 1973). It is valuable for all doctors to have this broader prospective. They should know about other available health services or community resources for children in their care and, as necessary, any legislation pertaining to them.

Infant and childhood morbidity and mortality patterns and rates allow awareness of specific problem areas such as low birth-weight babies, congenital malformations, malignancy, accidents and problems related to nutrition and infection.

Children at risk may be identified and special provision made for those with handicapping conditions. This often calls for multidisciplinary team work.

The management of diseases or disorders in individuals has little impact on the general health and well-being of communities. These latter are largely determined by socio-economic, environmental, political and cultural factors. In some Third World situations child mortality is stated to be 50 times as great as in Europe. The priority needs to correct this are adequate nutrition, a safe water supply and sanitation, as well as the control of specific infections and the provision of health care.

In the United Kingdom, the infant mortality rate in social cass V (unskilled) is twice the mortality rate in social class I (professional occupations). Morbidity and development are similarly adversely influenced with a multifactorial background of disadvantage in class V families.

In all situations, 'if one wants to help children, help families!' (see D. P. Hymovich and R. W. Chamberlain's *Child and Family Development: Implications for Primary Health Care*, McGraw-Hill). The clinician therefore also requires an understanding of child rearing practices and family dynamics.

The scope of child health and community paediatrics is vast and attention can only be drawn to a few important aspects.

Preventive paediatrics

Preventive paediatric care involves not only doctors but many others with whom they should learn to communicate and work.

Primary prevention
Action aimed to prevent a problem occurring:

1 Immunisation.
2 Chemoprophylaxis for malaria.
3 Administration of INH to the newborn babies of tuberculotic mothers.
4 Health and nutrition education.
5 Enhancing maternal-infant bonding and encouraging breast feeding by ensuring early close and continuing contact of mothers with their newborn babies. This together with any necessary support or advice may have implications in nutrition, allergy and child abuse.
6 Environmental control, e.g. water and sanitation.

Secondary prevention
Measures to minimise the ill-effects of an abnormality or deviation from normal:

1 Early detection of congenital dislocation of the hips or cerebral palsy where effective intervention is available to improve the future outlook.
2 Prolonged penicillin prophylaxis after rheumatic fever to prevent recurrence, possible cardiac crippling and the consequent need for surgery.
3 Crisis intervention—counselling for the family and, when appropriate, the child in stress situations such as hospitalisation, chronic or serious illness or death, thus reducing avoidable psychosocial disturbances.

Tertiary prevention
Action to contain or minimise an established abnormal condition:

1 Rehabilitation.
2 Use of available community resources.
3 Reshaping the physical environment, e.g. special facilities for the handicapped.

In preventive clinical care usually the initiative must be taken by the doctor, as opposed to curative help being directly sought by the patient or family. It therefore calls for expertise to identify when and how to intervene and to evaluate the results. In fact, if preventive care is successful one has to measure 'non-events', for instance the number of

children who did *not* get measles following an immunisation pro-
gramme. This lacks the drama of the child with post-measles pneumonia
recovering after weeks in an intensive care unit, but the overall benefits
are obvious.

Preventive practice assumes importance both on humanitarian and
financial grounds. The term 'Paediatrics in the community' has been used
in contradistinction to paediatrics practiced in hospitals. As such it has
little virtue, but it is important to realise that many health problems of
children will not normally be encountered in a ward or hospital setting.
These include various behavioural problems, minor illnesses and feeding
difficulties. Students would be well advised to gain experience with
general practitioners who have the art, skills and attitudes needed to deal
with frequently ill-defined clinical problems, where sound judgement
and the use of time as a diagnostic tool replace expensive laboratory and
radiological investigation. Much of this cannot be gleaned from lectures
or books. As R. S. Illingworth (*The Practitioner*, **22**, 701–2, May 1979)
has pointed out, the likelihood of one case of cystic fibrosis or congenital
dislocation of the hip presenting in an average general practice is about
once in every 37 years.

Attention is drawn to two serious paediatric problems:

1 Child abuse (non-accidental injury, battered baby syndrome)

The abuse of infants and children may be physical, mental or sexual.
Neglect, deprivation or rejection are other variants.

The true incidence of child abuse is difficult to assess but has been
considered to be about 6–10 cases per 1000 live births with resultant
suffering, disability and death.

Child abuse is more likely to occur when the parents are youthful and
immature, if they are of low intelligence, if they themselves have been
deprived, or if there is a history of psychiatric disorder. The single
unsupported mother is also more likely to abuse her child, particularly if
he was born early and separated from her in the neonatal period.
However, the problem exists in all social classes. Suspicion should lead to
appropriate action when history, findings and the backgrounds of the
families suggest this dangerous pathological state.

If the child has been physically abused the parents may delay seeking
medical advice. Multiple fractures of varying age, burns, bruises and
other injuries may be found. Bruises about the face and injuries to the
eye, mouth and genitalia should arouse suspicion. The child may seem
watchful and subdued. Infants may be deprived of food or drink, or
suffer whiplash cerebral trauma from violent shaking. The parents'
explanations of how the injuries occurred are unconvincing and often
inconsistent. The social services department may know, and already be
involved with the family. The police or National Society for the

Prevention of Cruelty to Children may have received complaints about the care of the children. If necessary, these agencies should be contacted for more information.

Whenever child abuse is suspected admission to hospital is advised, preferably to a unit experienced in handling the problem. If the parents should refuse to allow admission to hospital then, in the United Kingdom, one can insist by asking the social services department (or police) to arrange for a 'Place of Safety Order' which enables one to retain the child for 7–28 days pending a court hearing.

The child's injuries may need emergency treatment. A full radiological skeletal survey should be done to look for old or new fractures. If there has been bruising or bleeding then a haemorrhagic disorder should be excluded by appropriate investigation.

After the facts of the case have been collected together a case conference should be held with all interested parties (parents excepted) to discuss the diagnosis and to work out a plan of action. Unhelpful condemnation should be avoided for the parents need sympathetic understanding, long-term social support and perhaps psychiatric help. It is the *paediatrician's* duty to act in the best interests of the *child*. In serious cases an application to the court for a Care Order will have to be made to allow free access to the child, or to remove him from his parents. A review case conference is held some months later to discuss progress.

2 Sudden infant death syndrome

This accounts in Britain for approximately half the post-neonatal deaths occurring at home, the peak incidence being between 12 and 16 weeks.

At autopsy one-third are found to have a previously unrecognised disease such as meningitis, laryngotracheobronchitis or gastroenteritis, one-third show evidence of minor illness, but in the other third no abnormality can be detected.

Many explanations have been offered including accidental suffocation (now considered unlikely), apnoeic spells, cow's milk anaphylaxis, cardiac arrhythmias and inhalation. Identification of risk factors and possible preventive measures are being studied.

Until the problem is solved, the immediate task is to assist and support the parents and siblings who suffer such a devastating tragedy.

Surveillance of growth

Finally mention will be made of the importance of monitoring growth in infancy and childhood. This is a valuable index of health and nutrition, the rate of growth being plotted on percentile weight charts (or similar records for height or skull circumference). See Chapter 6.

Such nutritional surveillance should allow necessary and appropriate intervention to avoid the hazards of excess, imbalance or deficiency.

It is well established that children whose weight for age falls below the

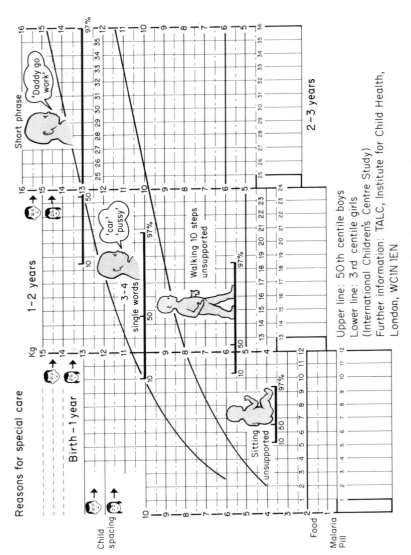

Fig. 22.1 'Road to Health' card. The age at which children sit up, walk ten steps unsupported and say three to four words and short sentences, with the percentile variations when these are achieved (courtesy of David Morley)

third percentile are at risk—in terms of morbidity, mortality and development. Conversely, those manifesting early obesity may be subject to cardiovascular or other disease in early adult life.

The Road to Health Card (Fig. 22.1) provides a comprehensive record of weight, developmental progress, immunisation and various risk factors. It can also be used as a health education tool.

Many important topics such as long-term care of handicapped children, risk registers and school medical services could not be included in this brief review; selected companion manuals of comprehensive and integrated child care are listed:

Suggested Reading

Fit for the Future: Review of the Committee on Child Health Services, Vol. 1 (1976) HMSO, London.

Mitchell, R. G. (Ed.) (1977) *Child Health in the Community*: A Handbook of Social and Community Paediatrics. Churchill Livingstone.

Hymovich, D. P. and Chamberlain, R. W. (1980) *Child and Family Development*: Implications for Primary Health Care. McGraw Hill Book Company.

Morley, D. C. (1973) *Paediatric Priorities in the Developing World.* Butterworths.

Illingworth, R. S. (1979) *The Incidence of Disease in General Practice.* Practitioner, **222**, 701–2.

Notes on the Promotion of Child Health in Southern Africa. Institute of Child Health, University of Cape Town.

Sheridan, M. D. (1981) *Children's Developmental Progress from Birth to Five Years.* NFER Publishing Company.

PAEDIATRIC DRUGS AND DOSES

The dose of drugs for the *newborn* have been worked out from pharmacokinetic data and should be given according to *body weight, gestation,* and *age*.

Outside the neonatal period children respond to medicine in a similar way to adults. Certain drugs, however, such as aspirin, morphine and aminophylline should be used with great caution as they are more likely to cause dangerous side-effects if the therapeutic doses are not carefully calculated. We are satisfied that for the majority of drugs used for children the dose can be scaled down from the adult dose using the *percentage method*. In order to use this method the prescriber refers to the table below to find the percentage of the adult dose suitable for children of different ages or weights. If the surface area dose is given, the surface area may be obtained from the same table.

Table A Surface area and percentage dose for children

Age	Weight kg	Surface area m^2	Percentage of adult dose
Adult	100	2.35	125
Adult	**65**	**1.76**	**100**
16 years	54	1.58	90
14 years	45	1.40	80
12 years	**40**	**1.32**	**75**
10 years	30	1.05	60
7 years	**23**	**0.87**	**50**
5 years	18	0.70	40
3 years	15	0.58	33
$1\frac{1}{2}$ years	11	0.53	30
1 year	10	0.49	28
8 months	**8.5**	**0.44**	**25**
4 months	6.5	0.36	20
2 months	4.5	0.28	15
Full term, (two weeks)	3.2	0.22	12.5

From: Catzel, P. and Olver, R. *The Paediatric Prescriber* (5th Edition) Blackwell Scientific Publications (1981)
NB For an 'in-between' age, weight or surface area, an 'in-between' percentage of the adult dose should be used.

Example

Estimate the dose of phenoxymethylpenicillin for a seven year old child with streptococcal sore throat. The adult dose is 500 mg four times daily for ten days.

According to the table the seven year old requires 50 % of the adult dose; i.e. 250 mg four times daily for ten days.

The practitioner should not use any drug that he is not familiar with, and is advised to consult the following books which should be part of his library:

1 Martindale *The Extra Pharmacopoeia* (The Pharmaceutical Press), which is an encyclopaedia of drugs, their uses, toxic effects and doses.
2 Goodman, L. and Gillman, A. *The Pharmacological Basis of Therapeutics*, (Macmillan), which is an excellent all-round large text. Being American, it is somewhat hamstrung by the Federal Drug Administration, which results in parts being ten years out of date.
3 Laurence, D. R. *Clinical Pharmacology* (Churchill Livingstone), which is an up-to-date and easy-to-read textbook with delightful stories and snippets of history presented with good humour—highly recommended.

    An alternative comprehensive and readable textbook is *A Textbook of Clinical Pharmacology* (Hodder and Stoughton) by H. J. Rogers, R. G. Spector and J. R. Trounce.
4 Catzel, P. and Olver, R. (5th Edition) *The Paediatric Prescriber* (Blackwell Scientific Publications), which is the only book devoted entirely to drugs used for infants and children. The author has conducted a campaign in successive editions to convince fellow paediatricians that estimation of doses should be standardised and that all workers in this field should state doses in mg/m^2 of body surface area, in preference to mg/kg body weight.

    The percentage method for estimating doses is based on this concept and to date seems to predict accurately doses in children in at least 90 % of cases—an essential work.

Many other useful textbooks are available and it is always advisable to buy the *latest edition*. In addition, the authors strongly recommend the *Drug and Therapeutics Bulletin* for well-balanced strictly non-commercial advice on drugs; the fact that it does not accept advertising and is not printed on expensive glossy paper is almost a guarantee of its lack of bias!

APPENDIX II

FURTHER READING

If the student wishes to acquire further information he should ascertain what paediatric text books and journals are available at the local medical library. It is useful to look up the latest edition of any large paediatric reference book. Nelson's *Textbook of Paediatrics* (Vaughan, McKay and Behrman; W. B. Saunders), Forfar and Arneil's *Textbook of Paediatrics* (Churchill Livingstone) and Schaffer and Avery's *Diseases of the Newborn* (W. B. Saunders) will often supply the information that is sought. Texts on child development, community paediatrics and therapeutics have been referred to elsewhere in this book. Most large textbooks give references to original papers and monographs which in turn will supply more references. A *recent relevant reference* should be chosen first in order to avoid getting bogged down with too much detail.

Other sources of information which may also be helpful are the paediatric specialist journals, for example *Archives of Disease in Childhood, Paediatrics, Journal of Paediatrics, Australian Journal of Paediatrics*, and others. The subject under investigation may conveniently be looked up in the annual index of the journal. Sometimes one may find useful editorials, paediatric articles or annotations in general journals such as the *British Medical Journal, The Lancet* and *The New England Journal of Medicine*. Abstracts from leading papers published in previous years are to be found in the *Year Book of Paediatrics* (Year Book Medical Publications) while useful monographs appear in *Advances in Paediatrics* by the same publishers. Lists of *titles* of papers published week by week are to be found in the weekly edition of *Current Contents* (The Institute for Scientific Information).

Occasionally one has to resort to the *Index Medicus* or the Medical libraries computer for a suitable list of papers. In all cases of difficulty we have always found the medical librarian a mine of useful information.

APPENDIX III

SI UNITS

The Système International d'Unités (SI) was formulated in 1960 by the International Committee of Weights and Measures to provide an international language of measurements. Its base units include:

Physical quantity	Name of SI unit	Symbol
length	metre	m
mass	kilogramme	kg
time	second	s
amount of substance	mole	mol
electric current	ampere	A
energy	joule	J

Decimal multiples and submultiples of the units are formed by prefixes. Note that the symbols are printed without a full stop and do not alter in the plural:

Multiple	Prefix	Symbol	Submultiple	Prefix	Symbol
10^{12}	tera	T	10^{-1}	deci	d
10^{9}	giga	G	10^{-2}	centi	c
10^{6}	mega	M	10^{-3}	milli	m
10^{3}	kilo	k	10^{-6}	micro	μ
10^{2}	hecto	h	10^{-9}	nano	n
10^{1}	deca	d	10^{-12}	pico	p
			10^{-15}	femto	f
			10^{-18}	atto	a

The decimal point is a full stop or comma on the line. Thus 1·5 is now written 1.5 or 1,5. The comma is preferred on the Continent. The raised point is a multiplication sign. Thus 1×5 is now written 1·5.

In writing large numbers, groups of three figures are separated by a space and not by a comma. Thus one million five hundred thousand should read:

$$1\,500\,000 \text{ or } 1,5 \times 10^6$$
$$\text{or } 1.5 \times 10^6$$

When there is a combination of units the divider or 'per' may be expressed as a single oblique (/) or by the use of negative powers.

Thus: grammes per metre squared is g/m^2 or $g \cdot m^{-2}$ and grammes per metre squared per second is $g/m^2/s$ or $g \cdot m^{-2} \cdot s^{-1}$

The familiar litre (l) continues to be used because the derived base unit for volume is the metre cubed (m^3) which is too large a volume for medical purposes. The litre is a decimetre cubed (dm^3) and is more easily handled.

The Celcius scale for temperatures is used in clinical medicine, the term being used in preference to 'centigrade'.

Some countries have not converted to SI units.

CONVERSION OF SI UNITS TO TRADITIONAL NORMAL VALUES

Chemical pathology	SI units	Traditional normal values	
glucose	3–5 mmol/l	54–90	mg/100 ml
urea	2.4–6.5 ,,	15–39	,,
creatinine	30–60 μmol/l	0.33–0.67	,,
urate (uric acid)	0.1–0.4 mmol/l	1.6–6.8	,,
calcium	2.1–2.6 ,,	8.4–10.4	,,
phosphorous	0.8–1.4 ,,	2.5–4.4	,,
bilirubin	5–17 μmol/l	0.3–1.0	,,
cholesterol	3.6–7.8 mmol/l	140–300	,,
triglycerides	0.4–2.52 ,,	25–150	,,
proteins (total)	62–82 g/l	6.2–8.2	g/100 ml
albumin	36–52 ,,	3.6–5.2	,,
thyroxine	70–180 mmol/l	5.4–14	μg/100 ml
cortisol	275–700 nmol/l	10–25	,,
serum iron	13–32 μmol/l	70–180	,,
iron binding capacity	45–70 ,,	250–390	,,
P_{CO_2}	4.53–6.4 kPa	34–48 mmHg	
P_{O_2}	12–15 kPa	90–112 mmHg	

Values vary with age and method of analysis so the 'normal range' should always be checked with the laboratory.

Height in cm = height in inches × 2.54   2.5 cm = 1 inch
                                          30 cm = 1 foot
Mass in kg = mass in pounds × .4536   10 kg = 22 lb
                                          23 kg = 50 lb
                                          36 kg = 80 lb
                                          65 kg = 143 lb
Energy in kJ = energy ın kcal (medical calorie; Calorie) ÷ 4.2 (approx)
                                          4.2 kJ = 1 kcal

INDEX